International Perspectives on Aging

Volume 28

Series Editors
Jason L. Powell, Department of Social and Political Science,
University of Chester, Chester, UK
Sheying Chen, Department of Public Administration, Pace University
New York, NY, USA

The study of aging is continuing to increase rapidly across multiple disciplines. This wide-ranging series on International Perspectives on Aging provides readers with much-needed comprehensive texts and critical perspectives on the latest research, policy, and practical developments. Both aging and globalization have become a reality of our times, yet a systematic effort of a global magnitude to address aging is yet to be seen. The series bridges the gaps in the literature and provides cutting-edge debate on new and traditional areas of comparative aging, all from an international perspective. More specifically, this book series on International Perspectives on Aging puts the spotlight on international and comparative studies of aging.

More information about this series at http://www.springer.com/series/8818

Kieran Walsh • Thomas Scharf
Sofie Van Regenmortel • Anna Wanka
Editors

Social Exclusion in Later Life

Interdisciplinary and Policy Perspectives

EUROPEAN COOPERATION IN SCIENCE & TECHNOLOGY

Funded by the Horizon 2020 Framework Programme of the European Union

Springer

Editors
Kieran Walsh
Irish Centre for Social Gerontology,
Institute for Lifecourse and Society
National University of Ireland Galway
Galway, Ireland

Sofie Van Regenmortel
Department of Adult Educational Sciences
Vrije Universiteit Brussel
Brussels, Belgium

Thomas Scharf
Population Health Sciences Institute
Newcastle University
Newcastle upon Tyne, UK

Anna Wanka
Research Training Group 'Doing Transitions'
Goethe University Frankfurt am Main
Frankfurt am Main, Germany

ISSN 2197-5841 ISSN 2197-585X (electronic)
International Perspectives on Aging
ISBN 978-3-030-51405-1 ISBN 978-3-030-51406-8 (eBook)
https://doi.org/10.1007/978-3-030-51406-8

This Springer imprint is published by the registered company Springer Nature Switzerland AG
The registered company address is: Gewerbestrasse 11, 6330 Cham, Switzerland

Acknowledgements

Social exclusion in later life involves the marginalisation of older individuals and groups from mainstream society. It represents a complex set of research questions, a critical public and social policy challenge, and a profound societal concern for older people, families and communities in ageing societies. This has only been reinforced, across Europe and internationally, by the outbreak of the coronavirus disease 2019 (COVID-19) pandemic. The ways in which social exclusion can have a multifaceted impact on the daily lived experiences of older adults, and reflect the engrained position of older people and ageing within our structures and institutions, render it a particularly difficult issue to disentangle and tackle. With significant and welcomed advances in life expectancy, the task of answering these questions, overcoming these policy challenges and addressing these societal concerns has become critical – and even more so in the wake of the continuing developments related to COVID-19 and the implications for ageing societies. As co-editors of this book, we believe it is only by drawing together interdisciplinary and policy perspectives that we can provide the necessary scientific evidence to inform how best to undertake this task and advance this field of scholarship.

This book is a result of a collaboration between members of the COST Action CA15122 *Reducing Old-Age Social Exclusion* – ROSEnet (www.rosenetcost.com), supported by COST (European Cooperation in Science and Technology). COST is a funding agency for research and innovation networks (www.cost.eu). The book stems directly from the research and analyses that were engaged in across the period of ROSEnet's work programme, from 2016 to 2020. Although not all members are represented within this book, the debates and discussions that occurred as a part of ROSEnet seminars and conferences have contributed to the development of its themes and perspectives. It is on this basis we want to thank the PhD students; the early-stage, mid-career and senior researchers and academics; the policy stakeholders – particularly Patricia Conboy of HelpAge International and Maciej Kucharczyk of AGE Platform Europe for their expertise and guidance; and the Older Adult Reference Group who participated as members of ROSEnet. We would like to thank COST for giving us the opportunity to collaborate with these excellent colleagues from across the world, and we wish to acknowledge their financial support in facilitating the open access license for this book.

We would like to especially thank all of the contributors to this volume for embracing its aim, approach and collaborative nature with commitment and scientific excellence. We would like to thank the ROSEnet working group co-leaders and the section introduction authors for their dedication to this project and for providing a critical framing of the different aspects of exclusion. As co-editors of this volume we are indebted to Niamh Hennelly for her editorial assistance, to Christine De Largy for her support throughout the development of the text, and Celia Sheridan for her assistance in the final proofing stages. Without the contributions of all of these individuals, this book would not have been possible.

Galway, Ireland
Newcastle, UK
Brussels, Belgium
Frankfurt, Germany
August, 2020

Kieran Walsh
Thomas Scharf
Sofie Van Regenmortel
Anna Wanka

Contents

Editors and Contributors

About the Editors

Kieran Walsh is Professor of Ageing & Public Policy and Director of the Irish Centre for Social Gerontology at the National University of Ireland Galway, Ireland. Kieran's research interests include: social exclusion in later life, the relative nature of disadvantage in cross-national contexts, place and life-course transitions, and informal and formal infrastructures of care. Kieran is Chair of the European COST Action CA15122 on 'Reducing Old-Age Social Exclusion' (ROSEnet).

Thomas Scharf (PhD) is Professor of Social Gerontology in the Population Health Sciences Institute at Newcastle University, United Kingdom. His research explores issues relating to multidimensional forms of inclusion and exclusion in later life, particularly in relation to the places in which people age.

Sofie Van Regenmortel is an affiliated postdoctoral researcher in Vrije Universiteit Brussel, Brussels, Belgium. She is a member of the Belgian Ageing Studies (BAS) research group and completed her PhD research on social exclusion in later life in September 2017. She was part of the European project 'WeDO2! For the wellbeing and dignity of older people' (2013-2015). In 2016, she joined the ROSEnet COST action on 'Reducing Old-Age Social Exclusion: Collaborations in Research and Policy'.

Anna Wanka studied sociology and law at the University of Vienna, Austria. From 2009 to 2016 she was a researcher at the Research Group 'Family / Generations / Life Course / Health and Ageing' in the Department of Sociology. She completed her PhD in environmental gerontology in 2016 and since 2017 has worked as a postdoctoral researcher at Goethe University Frankfurt am Main, Germany. Her main research areas are environmental and social exclusion in later life, life-course transitions, technology and ageing, and lifelong learning.

About the Contributors

Marja Aartsen is Research Professor at Oslo Metropolitan University, Norway. Her research is on longitudinal developments in older adults' social networks, social participation and loneliness in relation to cognitive, physical and mental health. She is involved in the European research collaboration on social exclusion in older adults (GENPATH) and co-leader of the working group on exclusion from social relations of the COST Action ROSEnet.

Monika Alisch is Professor in the Department of Social Work and Director of the Centre of Research for Society and Sustainability – CeSSt, Fulda University of Applied Sciences, Germany. Monika is a sociologist working on social space research, sociology and social planning. At the CeSSt – Centre of Research for Society and Sustainability, Fulda University of Applied Sciences – she leads research projects (regional, national and international) on participation, older migrants, civic engagement in later life and democratic processes in rural areas.

John Andersen holds a PhD in sociology and is Professor of Planning, Sociology and Action Research in the Department of People and Technology (IMT), Roskilde University, Denmark. He was a member of the Copenhagen City Council from 2013 to 2017. He is inspired by the action research tradition: knowledge as a tool to people's empowerment, social justice and sustainability. His research areas include urban planning, age-friendly neighbourhoods, community empowerment and affordable housing.

Francesco Barbabella (PhD) is Research Fellow at the Centre for Socio-Economic Research on Ageing at the National Institute of Health and Science on Ageing (INRCA), Italy. He is a social scientist whose research intersects social gerontology, gerontechnology and social policy. His main research interests concern the investigation of experience, expectations and patterns of use of traditional care services and digital health solutions by older people.

Hande Barlin is an Assistant Professor in the Economics Department of Gebze Technical University, Turkey. Previously she designed and implemented socio-economic development, empowerment and social inclusion projects and carried out research on regional development and European economics. Currently, her academic work concentrates on disadvantaged groups and social inclusion.

Ahmet Melik Bas is an MA student of cultural anthropology in the Graduate School of Humanities and Studies on Public Affairs, Chiba University, Japan. He graduated from the gerontology undergraduate programme, Akdeniz University, in 2018. He has participated in the European Volunteer Program in Italy and helped people who have learning difficulties and has participated in exchange programmes in Germany and Japan. His research interests are cultural aspects of ageing and quantitative and qualitative methods in ageing research.

Annette Bilfeldt (PhD) is an Associate Professor of Social Science at the University of Greenland and an external Lecturer at Roskilde University, Denmark. Her research focuses on participatory action research with residents, relatives and care workers at nursing homes in relation to residents' rights, empowerment and quality in eldercare.

Vanessa Burholt BSc, PhD, FAcSS, is Professor of Gerontology in the School of Nursing/School of Population Health at the University of Auckland, New Zealand, and in the Centre for Innovative Ageing at Swansea University, Wales, UK. She is the Co-leader of the ROSEnet Working Group on Social Relations. She is a Fellow of the Academy of Social Sciences (UK). Her research focuses on older people's attachment to people and places, and she has published on rurality, loneliness, intergenerational relationships, ethnicity and migration.

Maria Cheshire-Allen is a doctoral candidate at Swansea University, Wales, UK. Her disciplinary background lies in philosophy and sociology. She has held policy and public affairs roles within NGOs and the public sector before pursuing an academic career in critical social gerontology. Her PhD study is a conceptual exploration of 'well-being' in the context of family care for older people focusing on its application within social care policy in the UK.

Florent Cholat is a PhD student of geography and urban sociology at Grenoble Alpes University, France and at the University of Milan Bicocca, Italy. He is Co-founder of the Young University Company '45.5 Sustainable Engineering' focused on the optimisation of reversed mobilities. Florent is a member of the COST ROSEnet PhD forum and coordinator of the ERASMUS+ TERAPI programme which addresses links between territories and learning.

Patricia Conboy is the Head of Global Ageing, Advocacy and Campaigns with HelpAge International. She has extensive work experience in the policy arena, ranging from partnership working at community level through to policy influencing at national, European and global levels. Her specialist area is analysis of policy design and implementation on ageing and older people. Prior to joining HelpAge in 2016, Patricia was Director of Older & Bolder, a national alliance of NGOs campaigning with older people to advance their rights in Ireland.

Luca Daconto PhD in Urban and Local European Studies (URBEUR), is a Postdoctoral Researcher in the Department of Sociology and Social Research at the University of Milan Bicocca, Italy. He carries out teaching and research activities with particular attention to the topics of accessibility, mobility, food, social vulnerability, ageing and GIS techniques applied to socio-territorial analysis.

Lena Dahlberg is Associate Professor of Social Work at Dalarna University, Sweden, and Senior Researcher at the Aging Research Center, Karolinska Institutet and Stockholm University, Sweden. Her primary research interests include social exclusion and loneliness in older adults and inequalities in access to formal and informal care. Currently, she is leading a project on social exclusion among older adults in Sweden and a Nordic project on loneliness in old-age.

Liesbeth De Donder is Associate Professor of Adult Educational Sciences at the Vrije Universiteit Brussel (VUB) in Belgium. Her research focuses on social participation and inclusion, caring communities, safety and elder mistreatment, all with a particular interest in participatory methodologies.

Alexandra V. Dmitrieva is Co-founder and Researcher at the Support, Research and Development Center (SRDC) based in Kyiv, Ukraine. She specialises in qualitative research in the fields of drug use, drug policy and HIV/AIDS since 2009. She has authored more than 20 scientific publications on different aspects of educational ICT and ICT adoption by older people.

Veerle Draulans is Associate Professor in the Centre for Sociological Research at KU Leuven, Belgium. She is Chairperson of the 'Flemish Interuniversity Council Taskforce Gender' and of the Vlir UOS 'Gender, Diversity and Development' expert group, university collaboration with South partners. Veerle coordinates a gender-sensitive Joint Doctoral Summer School in Ethiopia. She is a member of the Board of Governors of Emmaus, a set of care and welfare facilities, including eldercare, in Flanders, Belgium.

Matthias Drilling studied Social Geography and Economics in Germany and Ghana and Spatial Planning at the ETH in Zürich, Switzerland. He is co-speaker of the Neighbourhood Research Network of the German Geographical Society (www.quartiersforschung.de) and Co-editor of the series Quartiersforschung/Neighbourhood Research at Springer Publishers. He is an expert/reviewer for the GRF, SNCF, and DAAD and consultant for several ministries and departments in Switzerland, Luxemburg and Germany on the topics of neighbourhood, neighbourliness, urban poverty and homelessness.

Marceline Filbig was a master's student in the Management and Coaching in Education and Social Sciences (MAMACO) programme at the University of Luxembourg, Luxembourg. She completed her master's thesis titled 'Unemployment in later life – A study on needs, attributions and coping strategies' (Arbeitslosigkeit in der späten Erwerbsphase. Eine Studie zu Bedürfnissen, Attributionen und Bewältigungsformen) in 2018.

Ada Lui Gallassi is a doctoral candidate in social work at Örebro University, Sweden. She has a multidisciplinary background in International Human Rights Law and Social Sciences and conducts her research from a human rights-based approach. Her PhD project lies within the fields of ageing and migration, with a focus on investigating the correlation between the working life trajectory of migrants and their socio-economic situation in later-life.

Vera Gallistl MA, studied sociology at the University of Vienna. She is currently a PhD student in the Department of Sociology at the University of Vienna, Austria, where she studies cultural participation in later life. Her main research interests lie in the field of social gerontology, where she specialised in Lifelong Learning, Gerontechnology and late-life social inequalities.

Elena Golubeva Dr (Gerontology and Geriatrics), is a Professor in the Department of Social Work and Social Security at the Northern (Arctic) Federal University, Russia. She is a member of the Gerontological Society of the Russian Academy of Sciences. Professor Golubeva has more than 146 research and methodological publications and 70 conference reports in Russia and abroad.

Irina A. Grigoryeva is a Professor of Sociology at the University of St. Petersburg, Russian Federation. After completing her second doctorate at the University of St. Petersburg in 2005, she received special education in Gerontology in 2008. She has written five monographs and more than 140 articles on social policy and the comparative theory of social work, and more recently social gerontology and 'the old people issue' in modern Russia.

Hannah Grove is a PhD student of Health Geography at Maynooth University, Ireland, and is funded by the Health Research Board (SPHeRE/2013/1). She studied Town Planning at the University of Brighton and Geography at the University of Sussex, and has previously worked as a Planning Policy Officer in the UK. Her research interests include promoting healthy and age-friendly environments and exploring the connections between people, place and health through qualitative and spatial methods.

Lars Harrysson holds a PhD in Social Work and is a Senior Lecturer at Lund University, School of Social Work, Sweden. He has researched pensions, cancer rehabilitation, and learning and collaboration in and between organisations. His latest publications are in journals and reports on these subjects.

Byron Ioannou (PhD) is an Associate Professor at Frederick University, Cyprus. He has taught urban planning and sustainable urbanism in a number of institutions of the Eastern Mediterranean Region. He studied architecture, spatial planning and planning law in Greece and the UK. Byron is an expert/ reviewer on sustainable built environment issues for European and local governmental bodies. His current research focuses on urban design and public space, inclusive urban development, density and sprawl. He currently coordinates the Urban Planning and Development Unit.

Norah Keating is a social gerontologist whose theoretical and empirical research has created evidence, challenged discourses and influenced policy in global, social and physical contexts of ageing. She has placed this work on the international stage through the Global Social Issues on Ageing, which fosters collaboration and critical thinking about ageing at the interfaces of regional issues and global trends. Professor Keating holds academic appointments in three world regions.

Nilufer Korkmaz-Yaylagul is Associate Professor in the Gerontology Department at Akdeniz University, Antalya, Turkey. She has trained as a landscape architect and has completed her MSc studies in the same field. Nilufer earned a PhD degree in Social Anthropology-Urban Anthropology and carried out postdoctoral research on 'Older Turkish immigrants and Health'. She has been involved in teaching sociology and anthropology of ageing in the Gerontology Department at the Akdeniz University since 2009. Nilufer has a particular interest in socio-cultural aspects of ageing and environmental gerontology.

Ioannis Kostakis (PhD) is an Economist at the University of Crete, Greece. He holds a Master's in Economics and Econometrics (University of Kent, UK) and a Doctorate in Applied Economics (Harokopio University, Greece). Dr Kostakis has experience both in private and public sectors, while in recent years, he has taught several economic modules at Harokopio University and Hellenic Open University. His current research fields include applied economic theory, quantitative methods in economics and econometrics.

Maciej Kucharczyk is Secretary General of AGE Platform Europe since July 2020 – a network of over 100 organisations "of" and "working for" people aged 50 and over – Maciej has overall responsibility for managing the network and implementing AGE's strategic objectives. Prior to taking over as Secretary General, Maciej had been working on social policy issues since 2006, such as the adequacy and sustainability of social protection, minimum income, the promotion of human rights, social justice and dignity. From 2014 to 2020, he was vice-president of the Social Platform, the largest European network of rights-based NGOs working in the social sector. Maciej has a degree in International Economic Relations from the University of Lodz, Poland, and holds post-graduate degrees in European Affairs from the College of Europe, Belgium, and in Public Administration from the ENA, France.

Susanne Kümpers Prof Dr, is Professor of Qualitative Health Research and Social Health Inequalities in the Department of Nursing and Health, Fulda University of Applied Sciences, Germany. Susanne is an educational and health scientist. Her research and teaching areas are ageing, social and health inequalities, poverty in old-age, and prevention and health promotion approaches in neighbourhood settings from a European perspective. Her methodologies include qualitative and participatory approaches.

Giovanni Lamura leads the Centre for Socio-Economic Research on Ageing at INRCA (Italy's National Institute of Health and Science on Ageing, Italy). He graduated in economics, achieved a PhD in 'Life course and social policy' (University of Bremen, Germany) and was visiting fellow at University of Hamburg-Eppendorf

(Germany) and the European Centre for Social Welfare Policy & Research (Austria). Research interests: international research on family and long-term care, migrant care work and interdisciplinary research on ageing.

Joe Larragy (PhD) is Lecturer in Social Policy at Maynooth University, Ireland. He has also worked as policy analyst in think tanks on age-related research and policymaking, and maintains an interest in pensions, care and social citizenship in old-age.

Lauri Leppik is a Senior Research Fellow in the Estonian Institute for Population Studies, School of Governance, Law and Society, Tallinn University, Estonia. His research interests relate to social policy, pension reform, social exclusion, social legislation, public policy analysis and the history of the population of Estonia. He is a member of the Estonian SHARE team and a former member of the European Committee of Social Rights.

Anu Leppiman is Professor of Marketing in the Department of Business Administration, Tallinn University of Technology, Estonia. She obtained her PhD in Social Work and Service Design from the University of Lapland in 2010 and is a Certified Experience expert and communication consultant. Anu is also Head of the Experience Marketing Research Group at Tallinn University of Technology. Her research interests include service design, family work, experience marketing and old-age social exclusion.

Ariela Lowenstein Gerontology Prof Emerita, Haifa University, Israel. Ariela established the Gerontology Graduate Department and the Center for Research & Study of Aging. She was also President of Yezreel Valley Academic College from 2012 to 2016. Reputed as a leading national and international expert in ageing, her past roles and achievements include: past Chair, *Eu Behavioral, Social Science & Research,* International Association of Gerontology; 5 years Chair, *Israeli Gerontological Society*, receiving the *life achievement* prize. Ariela is Co-chair of the ROSEnet Civic Exclusion working group and currently leads the Israeli group in the EU Horizon – Gendernet project, GENPATHS.

Marianne Mahler completed an MA in history at the University of Copenhagen in 1968. In 1981, she became a registered nurse, thereafter she received a doctorate of public health from the Nordic School of Public Health in Gothenburg. Marianne has worked in primary healthcare with practical and theoretical gerontology with the development of democracy in institutions and democracy in everyday life. Participatory research involving residents, relatives and staff is her recent research focus and she has written scientific articles and book chapters. She is a member of the Nordic Health Promotion Research Network.

Murat Anil Mercan is a Professor at Gebze Technical University, Turkey. His research interests include labour economics and demography and he has published several articles on these subjects. He is also a Management Committee Member of

Cost Action IS1409 Gender and Health Impacts of Policies Extending Working Life in Western Countries.

Maria Gabriella Melchiorre collaborated with the Department of Economic Sociology, at the University of Ancona in Italy, on several national and international research projects on migrants and care policies for the family from 1989 to 1997. Since 1997, she has been a researcher at the Centre for Socio-Economic Research on Ageing, INRCA-IRCCS, in Italy, working on social aspects of family caregiving, long-term care, elder abuse, migrant care workers, multi-morbidity, frailty and eHealth.

Sarmitė Mikulionienė is a Director of Lithuanian Social Research Centre, Vilnius, Lithuania. Her research interests are ageism, demography of ageing, generations, social exclusion and lifelong learning. She is a member of the EAST Network of Oxford Institute on Ageing, International Network for the Study of Intergenerational Issues. Currently, she is involved in the project 'Building older people's well-being: empowerment policies, monitoring indicators and the voice of older people'.

Aleksandra Milicevic-Kalasic MD, has an MSc in neuropsychology, a PhD in medical science on neuropsychiatric disorders in the elderly, and is a specialist in neuropsychiatry and an associated researcher in psychiatry. She is head of the mental health team since 1987 and is Associate Professor at the Department for Social Work FMK, at Singidunum University, Serbia since 2013. Aleksandra was the National Contact in the WHO Mental Health Programmes (2003–2011). She has also held a Fogarty Fellowship (2012–2015) from the University of California, Berkeley and served as Associate Editor of the IPA bulletin (1997–2012) and the International Journal of Psychology (2007–2013).

Deborah Morgan is a Senior Research Officer at the Centre for Innovative Ageing at Swansea University, Wales, United Kingdom. Her research is on loneliness and social isolation in later life, health/social inequalities, disability and chronic illness. She is the European Representative for the International Association for Gerontology Council of Student Organisations.

Thibauld Moulaert is Associate Professor at the PACTE Social Sciences Laboratory, Université Grenoble Alpes & CNRS, Sciences Po Grenoble, France. He studied sociology at the Université Catholique de Louvain (UCL), Belgium. His research critically focuses on active ageing and employment, international discourses on ageing, and on Age-friendly cities and communities in close collaboration with the University of Sherbrooke, Canada. Since arriving in Grenoble, his focus is on the relations between older people's citizenship and environments.

Elke Murdock is a Research Scientist at the Institute for Life Course Development, Family and Culture at the University of Luxembourg, Luxembourg. A cross-cultural psychologist by training, she has lived, studied and worked in Germany, Scotland, the USA, England and now Luxembourg. Her research interest focuses on identity construal processes and families in multicultural contexts. Her book 'Multiculturalism, Identity and Difference. Experiences of Culture Contact' was published in 2016.

Michal Myck is Director of the Centre for Economic Analysis, Szczecin, Poland. His research has focused on labour market and savings decisions and on the implications of exposure to shocks on long-term employment patterns and welfare. He has also worked on issues related to measurement of poverty, inequality and deprivation. He was the Polish Country Team Leader for the SHARE survey (2005-2017). He wishes to acknowledge the support of the Polish National Science Centre through project no. 2015/17/B/HS4/01018.

Rita Borges Neves is a Sociologist and Research Associate at the Centre for Decent Work, Management School, University of Sheffield, United Kingdom, where she formerly worked in the Public Health Department. Her PhD explored unemployment in late career and its effects on mental health under different welfare regimes in Europe. Her research interests broadly fall under topics related to social inequalities and mechanisms of exclusion in a context of changing labour market structures and population ageing.

Mia Niemi (M.Soc.Sc) is a PhD candidate at the University of Helsinki, Finland. Her previous work has been in the field of gerontological social work, focusing in particular on families in crisis and elder abuse interventions. Her PhD research focuses on vulnerability in the family life of older people. Most recently, she has worked in projects concerning older people's meaningful relationship at the end of life and home hospital services.

Jim Ogg is Head of the Ageing Research Unit at the National Pension Fund (Caisse nationale d'assurance vieillesse), Paris, France and Honorary Research Fellow at the College of Human and Health Sciences, Swansea University, Wales, United Kingdom. His research focuses on the sociology of the family in the context of ageing populations, the transition to retirement, social exclusion and housing environments. He is the Editor-in-Chief of the journal Retraite et société.

Frank Oswald PhD, is Professor for Interdisciplinary Ageing Research (IAW), Chair of the Frankfurt Forum for interdisciplinary Ageing Research (FFIA) at the Goethe University, Germany, and Director of the 'Center Aging' for Early Career Researchers at the Goethe Graduate Academy (GRADE). His research interests are contexts of adult development, issues of person-environment transaction and transitions in old-age, housing, ageing in place, relocation and the role of technologies in later life.

Oksana A. Parfenova is a research fellow at the Sociological Institute of FCTAS RAS, St. Petersburg, Russian Federation. In 2017, she defended her PhD Dissertation

'Care for older people in state social services in modern Russia'. She has publications on social policy for older people and ageing in modern Russia.

László Patyán is an associate professor at the University of Debrecen, Faculty of Health, Department of Gerontology, Nyíregyháza, Hungary. He is a also a social worker and a sociologist and has a PhD in sociology and social policy. His main research areas are social work, care policy, quality of life of older adults, and social exclusion in later life.

Jolanta Perek-Białas (Phd) is professor at Jagiellonian University, Institute of Sociology, and Director of the Center for Evaluation and Public Policy Analysis of the Jagiellonian University, Kraków, Poland. Jolanta's research interests are in gerontology, public policy analysis (including senior policy) and social science methodology. She is the principal investigator or co-investigator in many international projects on activating older people, ageism in the labour market and supporting the caregivers of older people. She collaborates with international, national, regional and local institutions on senior policy and labour market policies.

Anneli Pohjola is Professor Emerita at the University of Lapland, Rovaniemi, Finland. She has worked in various teaching and research positions in social work and as a researcher at the Academy of Finland. She has worked in the expert group on national social and health reform, and in various working groups and social organisations of the Ministry of Social Affairs and Health. Her research interests focus on the development of well-being services and the role of clients in the service system, disability and mental health, and old-age exclusion.

Arianna Poli (M.Psy.) is a doctoral student in ageing and later life at the Division Ageing and Social Change (ASC), Linköping University, Sweden. Previously she was a Research Assistant at the Centre for Socio-Economic Research on Ageing at the Italian National Institute of Health and Science on Ageing (INRCA). She conducts research in the field of social gerontology, particularly at the intersection of ageing, inequality, and new technologies. Her research focuses on digital technologies as contributing factors to rising old-age inequalities and increased risk of exclusion.

Allan Puur is a Professor of Demography at the Estonian Institute for Population Studies, School of Governance, Law and Society, Tallinn University, Estonia. His research interests are related to the development of the population of Estonia from a comparative perspective. In recent years he has published articles on fertility and family demography, the demographic behaviour of immigrants and their descendants, and topics related to historical demography. He is also actively involved in developing the infrastructure for register-based demographic research in Estonia.

Gražina Rapolienė is a research fellow at the Lithuanian Social Research Centre, Lithuania. She is a member of the working group on civic exclusion in the COST Action on Reducing Old-Age Social Exclusion (ROSEnet) and was a Management

Committee member in the COST Action on ageism. Examples of her publications include 'Ageing Identity: Do Theories Match Experiences?' and 'Old Age Stigmatization'. Her research interests include: social exclusion, ageism, ageing identity, representations in media, and consumption.

Iivi Riivits-Arkonsuo is Associate Professor of Marketing in the Department of Business Administration, Tallinn University of Technology, Estonia. She defended her PhD in 2015. Her research focuses mainly on the digital divide, digital exclusion in older-age and consumer engagement. She has been a Research Manager in one of the leading market research companies in Estonia, Turu-uuringute AS, for more than 20 years.

Luule Sakkeus is Head of the Estonian Institute for Population Studies and a Senior Research Fellow in the School of Governance, Law and Society, Tallinn University, Estonia. Her research is focussed on the demographic and health-related behaviours of the immigrant-origin population as compared with the native population. In recent years, she has published articles on various aspects of demographic ageing, and she is the Estonian Research Coordinator for SHARE. She also has long-term research interests in migration studies and reproductive health.

Marjaana Seppänen is Professor of Social Work at the University of Helsinki, Finland. Her background is in social sciences (especially social work), and she has extensively studied and published on questions connected to ageing, well-being, gerontological social work and the living conditions of older adults. Prof Seppänen is part of several international research networks in gerontology and social work, having several leading positions in their organisation and implementation.

Rodrigo Serrat (PhD) is a Serra Húnter tenure-track lecturer in the Department of Cognition, Development, and Educational Psychology at the University of Barcelona, Spain. His research focuses on civic participation in later life, with a particular focus on issues of inclusion and diversity.

Lone Sigbrand is an architect at MMA, and senior consultant in the Department of the Built Environment, at Aalborg University, Denmark. Her field of work focuses on users, especially users with disabilities, and inclusion in the built environment, and in relation to the process and the outcomes of development, and the subsequent operation of the built environment through education and counselling activities aimed at the construction industry. Since 2015, her main field has been optimising the physical framework of people with dementia in order to create well-being and quality of life.

Anu Siren PhD in psychology, is a senior researcher at the Danish Center for Social Science Research in Copenhagen, Denmark. Her previous affiliations include Technical University of Denmark and University of Helsinki in Finland. Her areas of interest are related to the institutional and cultural contexts of ageing, age-related policies, and family arrangements in late-life. She has authored over 90 publications.

Merle Sumil-Laanemaa is an Advisor to the Estonian Social Insurance Board and a PhD student of social work at Tallinn University, Estonia. She has worked as a practitioner in the field of social protection for more than 20 years. In 2016, she began her doctoral studies at Tallinn University. Her main areas of research are the social and material well-being of older persons. Her latest research is focussed on the recipients of minimum pensions in Estonia.

Zsuzsa Széman is Professor of Sociology in the Doctoral Programme at the Institute of Mental Health, Semmelweis University, Budapest, Hungary. She has given numerous lectures and is the author and editor of many books and articles, elaborated model programmes and intervention programmes. The most important research projects that she has been involved in include: PIE, EUROFAMCARE, MOBILATE, ENABLE-AGE, Employment Initiatives for an Ageing Workforce, Elder-friendly House, CARICT, HELPS, FUTURAGE, MOPACT, Skype-Care and ROSEnet.

Angelika Thelin is an Associate Professor of Social Work at Linnaeus University, Växjö, Sweden. She wrote a dissertation in Swedish about relative income poverty among older people in Sweden. After that she has continued with cross-national studies on the matter. She is also a member of the Norma Elder Law Research Environment, Faculty of Law, Lund University, through research on self-neglect and social services among older people with dementia.

Sandra Torres is Professor of Sociology and Chair of Social Gerontology at Uppsala University, Sweden. Most of her scholarly contributions aim to expand the gerontological imagination on ethnicity/race and migration. Her latest books include: *Ethnicity & Old Age: Expanding our Imagination* (Policy Press, 2019) and the first *Handbook on Migration & Aging* (Edward Edgar Publishing, 2022) for which she is lead editor.

Isabelle Tournier studied psychology and holds a Master of Arts degree in Clinical Psychology (oriented on psychogerontology) as well as a PhD in Psychology from the University of Bordeaux (France). After completing postdoctoral positions at the LPC (Mobility and Behavior Psychology Laboratory; IFSTTAR, French Institute of Science and Technology for Transport, Development and Networks, Versailles), in the domain of elderly road users' safety, and at INSIDE (Integrative Research Unit on Social and Individual Development, University of Luxembourg, Luxembourg) for various projects related to ageing or dementia. She is now project manager and coordinator at the Info-Zenter Demenz (Luxembourg). This independent service aims to raise awareness, inform and orient citizens regarding dementia diagnosis and care in Luxembourg.

Anna Urbaniak is a postdoctoral researcher on the GENPATH project – a life course perspective on the GENdered PATHways of exclusion from social relations – in the Department of Sociology in Vienna, Austria. She is a sociologist by training and worked as a researcher at the Irish Centre for Social Gerontology at the National University of Ireland, Galway, Ireland and in the Department of Sociology in Kraków, Poland. Her research interests comprise spatial aspects of ageing, life-course transitions, the re/production of social inequalities across the life course, ageing migrants and people living with dementia.

Lucie Vidovićová (Phd) is Assistant Professor in the Office for Population Study at the Faculty of Social Studies, Masaryk University, Brno, Czechia. Lucie is a sociologist. Her long-term research interests include the sociology of ageing, topics of age discrimination, social exclusion, environmental gerontology, penology, social robotics and active ageing. She is also involved in research projects in the field of family and social policy. Lucie conducts research for national as well as European bodies and works as a consultant on a number of implementation projects, including senior advocacy.

Feliciano Villar (PhD) is an associate professor in the Department of Cognition, Development, and Educational Psychology at the University of Barcelona, Spain. His research focuses on two fields: generativity and older people's contributions in later life, and nursing home policies and practices regarding participation and residents' rights.

Katarina Vojvodic MD, is a specialist in Social Medicine and Master of Health Care Management. She is also a PhD candidate in Public Health, Serbia. Katarina is working at the Institute of Public Health in Belgrade as Head of the Unit for Health Care Quality Improvement with experience of working in all levels of healthcare, data analysis, policymaking and education.

Charles Waldegrave coordinates the Family Centre Social Policy Research Unit, Lower Hutt, Wellington, New Zealand. He has been a joint leader of the New Zealand Poverty Measurement Project and the New Zealand Longitudinal Study of Ageing. Currently he is jointly leading three National Science Challenge projects: Loneliness and Social Isolation; Revitalising the Production of Affordable Homes; and Māori and Ageing. He is an international member of the COST Action ROSEnet.

Bethan Winter is an honorary research associate in the Centre for Innovative Ageing, College of Human and Health Sciences, Swansea University, Wales, UK. She completed her PhD research in 2017 titled 'Disadvantage and advantage among older people in rural communities: A multilevel and life-course perspective'. In 2019, Bethan was elected as a Member of Parliament for the Labour Party in the UK.

List of Figures

List of Tables

Section I
Introduction

Chapter 1
The Intersection of Ageing and Social Exclusion

Kieran Walsh, Thomas Scharf, Sofie Van Regenmortel, and Anna Wanka

1.1 Introduction

This book examines social exclusion in later life, its key attributes and manifestations, and its construction and amelioration through policy structures and systems. The significance of demographic ageing, inequalities amongst older populations, and rising economic, social and political uncertainty, is clear for many advanced industrial societies. So too is the potential for these trends and processes to intersect and reinforce each other (Nazroo 2017; Hargittai et al. 2019; Dahlberg et al. 2020). Despite these circumstances suggesting the need for a strong focus on the exclusion of older people, research and policy debates on this topic have stagnated in recent years. This has contributed to the absence of a coherent research agenda on old-age social exclusion, and a lack of conceptual and theoretical development (Van Regenmortel et al. 2016; Walsh et al. 2017). It has also meant that innovative policy responses, that are effective in reducing exclusion for older people, are in relatively short supply (ROSEnet 2020).

K. Walsh (✉)
Irish Centre for Social Gerontology, Institute for Lifecourse and Society,
National University of Ireland Galway, Galway, Ireland
e-mail: kieran.walsh@nuigalway.ie

T. Scharf
Population Health Sciences Institute, Newcastle University, Newcastle upon Tyne, UK

S. Van Regenmortel
Department of Adult Educational Sciences, Vrije Universiteit Brussel, Brussels, Belgium

A. Wanka
Research Training Group 'Doing Transitions', Goethe University Frankfurt am Main,
Frankfurt am Main, Germany

K. Walsh et al. (eds.), *Social Exclusion in Later Life*, International Perspectives
on Aging 28, https://doi.org/10.1007/978-3-030-51406-8_1

As a societal issue in a globalised world, it can be argued that social exclusion in later life has become more complex in its construction, and potentially more pervasive in its implications for individual lives and for societies. There is now a growing evidence base that points to how it can implicate interconnected economic, social, service, civic (civic participation and socio-cultural), and community and spatial domains of daily life (Dahlberg et al. 2020; Prattley et al. 2020). Understanding social exclusion of older people is, however, not just about a focus on older-age and the way that age-related changes, and a society's response to those changes, can give rise to exclusionary mechanisms. It is also about providing insight into processes of risk accumulation across the life course, identifying crucial points for early intervention, and highlighting the degree of impact when earlier forms of exclusion go unaddressed (Grenier et al. 2020).

Against this background, there is a pressing need to address stagnated debates on social exclusion in later life, and the deficits in research and policy that they sustain. These circumstances have become more urgent in the wake of the outbreak of the coronavirus disease 2019 (COVID-19) pandemic. This edited volume responds to this need.

1.2 Rationale – Stagnated Policy and Research

The lack of advances in research and policy may, in part, be due to a number of political factors that betray a research-policy misalignment.

First, is the traditional absence of ageing from social equality agendas (Warburton et al. 2013). In many jurisdictions, ageing remains entrenched within a health framing and, although social protection portfolios pursue goals around pension adequacy and sustainability, it appears largely to be considered the domain of health policy. Second, demographic ageing is more likely to be seen as a threat to the sustainability and effectiveness of social inclusion orientated structures (*i.e.* institutions; policies), than a focus of those structures (Phillipson 2020). This is both at the level of national states and within European political forums, where there can be a problematisation of demographic ageing in relation to maintaining social protection systems. Third, more entrenched, and sometimes subtle, ageist discourses negatively locate older people within our societies. As such, there can be a systemic political complacency towards the concerns of ageing populations, or even a more active discriminatory marginalisation of their needs and position (Ayalon and Tesch-Römer 2017). It can certainly be argued that the COVID-19 pandemic has only served to intensify each of these three factors.

Fourth, and perhaps most significant of all, there are questions around whether or not social exclusion of older people is a critical public policy issue, with debates around the extent to which older adults are experiencing exclusion. Within Europe, the European Commission's 'At-Risk of Poverty and Social Exclusion' (AROPE) measure suggests a need to focus on children (of whom 26.9% are identified as being at risk of poverty and social exclusion), single parents (50%) and particularly the unemployed (66.6%). People aged 65 years and over appear to be less at risk (18.1%) (Eurostat 2019), with policymakers unlikely to be as motivated to drive innovation to address social exclusion in later life. However, the AROPE measure focuses on economic forms of disadvantage concentrating on those at-risk of poverty, or those experiencing severe material deprivation, or those households with low work intensity. This is in contrast to the significant body of empirical research that illustrates the need to broaden our thinking about exclusion in older-age, and how older people may simultaneously be susceptible to multiple and interconnected forms of disadvantage (Kendig and Nazroo 2016; Dahlberg and McKee 2018; Macleod et al. 2019). The AROPE measure, therefore, is likely to fall short in capturing complex, multidimensional exclusion.

Stagnated debates are also likely to be due to conceptual factors, and the awkwardness of the social exclusion concept. Although the comprehensiveness of the construct is credited with providing valuable insights into multidimensional disadvantage for older people, there is a difficulty in empirically and conceptually representing that comprehensiveness (Van Regenmortel et al. 2016). Common critiques focus on the concept's failure to foster an analytical frame that supports theoretical elaboration and the development of actionable policies (Bradshaw 2004). This fundamentally undermines the establishment of large-scale research programmes, and meaningful policy and practice implementation plans. As a result, much of our knowledge continues to reside in single domain fields, such as services or social relations, with a failure to adequately account for the interrelationships across domains (Walsh et al. 2017). Additionally, even though there is recognition that exclusion in later life involves both individual and societal/policy levels, most existing work continues to neglect multilevel analyses – again, functioning to impede effective progress in research and policy. Therefore, from a research perspective, how to account for disadvantages in different domains of life, while exploring their interrelated and multilevel construction, is a fundamental challenge.

Like other complex social phenomena, social exclusion in later life is relative. Just as with multidimensionality (Atkinson 1998), this represents both a valuable conceptual attribute and a challenge that impedes the development of frameworks for researching and reducing exclusion in different jurisdictions. For ageing societies, there are four parameters that can influence the construction and meaning of exclusion in later life (Scharf and Keating 2012; Macleod et al. 2019). First, there are different patterns of demographic ageing, with heterogeneity (related to ethnicity, sexual orientation, class and expectations around rights) across and within older populations. Second, there are different degrees of age-related institutional infrastructure, underpinned by diverse value systems. Third, there are distinct sets of cohort experiences linked to context-specific cultural, socio-economic and geopolitical forces (*e.g.* conflict; recession; immigration). And fourth, there are country/region specific scientific paradigms that influence views on disadvantage in older-age and that remain outside the English-language literature (Walsh et al. 2017). Addressing and harnessing the relative nature of older adult exclusion is essential if we want to pursue meaningful cross-national comparisons. It is also essential if we want to design policy responses that are appropriate both within and across nations.

Aside from political and conceptual factors, it is also necessary to consider our capacity to advance the agenda on social exclusion of older people. International research has a long-standing engagement with the construction of inequalities for older adults, driven by a commitment to critical perspectives in gerontology. While this scholarship has expanded our understanding of disadvantage in later life, it has in relative terms not been as influential in progressing debates on older adult exclusion as might have been expected. Instead, a more applied approach has dominated, which has typically been more descriptive. Secondly, research capacity on this topic has been underdeveloped and undermines our ability to critically analyse the topic of old-age social exclusion into the future. As a result, questions persist about how we engage a new audience of early-stage researchers and policy analysts in these debates. There is a need to create collaborative initiatives that will foster engagement opportunities for some and illustrate the value of such opportunities for others.

1.3 Aim and Objectives

Drawing on interdisciplinary, cross-national perspectives, this book aims to advance research and policy debates on social exclusion of older people by presenting state-of-the-art knowledge in relation to scholarship and policy challenges. In doing so, it seeks to develop a forward-looking research agenda on the multilevel, multidimensional and relative construction of social exclusion in later life.

The book has four key objectives:

1. To produce a comprehensive analysis of social exclusion of older people, deconstructing its multidimensionality across different life domains, the interrelationship between these domains, and the involvement of individual and societal/policy levels.
2. To present cross-national and interdisciplinary perspectives on social exclusion of older adults so as to account for the relative nature of exclusion and establish shared understandings of its meaning and construction.
3. To institute a dialogue between conceptual and empirical perspectives, in order to strengthen the critical potential of empirical studies, and the empirical application of critical concepts.
4. To nurture research capacity in the field of social exclusion and ageing, establishing meaningful collaborations between early-stage researchers and senior scholars across countries.

This book has emerged from a cross-national, and collaborative networking platform that focuses on *Reducing Old-Age Social Exclusion – ROSEnet* (COST Action CA15122). Involving established and early-career researchers, policy stakeholders and older people, ROSEnet comprises 180 members from 41 countries. ROSEnet aims to overcome fragmentation and critical gaps in conceptual innovation on old-age exclusion across the life course, in order to address the research-policy disconnect and tackle social exclusion amongst older people. ROSEnet is dedicated to developing shared understandings of old-age exclusion that are underpinned by state-of-the-art research and innovation, and that help to direct meaningful policy and practice development. The network involves five working groups that address different domains of exclusion (economic; social; service; civic; and community and spatial) and a programme of activities around domain interrelationships, and policy. ROSEnet, therefore, provides a strong foundation for addressing challenges around the comprehensive and relative nature of exclusion of older people.

In the remainder of this chapter, we will set out the central tenets of old-age exclusion and how they inform the book's approach and structure. We begin by drawing on the findings of two recent reviews of the international literature (Van Regenmortel et al. 2016; Walsh et al. 2017) to conceptualise and define social exclusion in later life. We then consider the political evolution of social exclusion as a policy concept and the ways in which exclusion can be mediated by policy discourses. We conclude by outlining the book's structure and approach.

1.4 Conceptualising and Defining Social Exclusion of Older People

There have been relatively few attempts to define social exclusion in later life, or indeed to conceptualise its construction (Van Regenmortel et al. 2016). While this reflects the paucity of scientific research on the topic, it also reflects the longstanding ambiguities concerning the general concept itself (Levitas et al. 2007).

Definitions of social exclusion have though typically engaged with what Atkinson (1998) identifies as a set of common characteristics of the construct. These features enhance the concept's power to explain multifaceted and complex forms of disadvantage, but they also pose inherent challenges for the identification and assessment of the phenomenon. They include the conceptual attributes of multidimensionality (where older people can be excluded across multiple domains of life, or can be excluded in one domain and not in others) and that of its relative nature (where exclusion is relative to specific populations, institutions, values and a normative level of integration within a particular society) – which are the prime consideration of this volume. But they also include two other aspects of the construct. Social exclusion is dynamic, where older people can drift in and out of exclusion, and experience different forms of exclusion at different points of the life course. Social exclusion also involves agency or the act of exclusion, where older people, for instance, can be excluded against their will, may lack the capacity and resources for self-integration, and, whether consciously or sub-consciously, may choose to exclude themselves in certain situations.

While there is renewed interest in conceptualising exclusion of older people, there has been a noticeable lack of innovation in theorising the intersection between ageing and exclusion. Adapted from Walsh et al. (2017), Table 1.1 reveals a small number of frameworks that attempt to explain old-age exclusion. Although these

Table 1.1 Old-age exclusion conceptual frameworks

Guberman and Lavoie (2004)	Scharf et al. (2005)/Scharf and Bartlam (2008)	Jehoel-Gijsbers and Vrooman (2008)	Barnes et al. (2006)/Kneale (2012)	Feng (2012)	Hagan Hennessy et al. 2014	Van Regenmortel et al. 2016	Walsh et al. (2012)/(2019)	Macleod et al. (2019)
1. Economic exclusion	1. Exclusion from material resources	1. Socio-economic exclusion: material deprivation	1. Exclusion from material resources/ common consumer goods 2. Exclusion from financial products	1. Economic situation	1. Poverty and social welfare	1. Financial resources 2. Material resources 3. Employment labour market	1. Income and financial resources	1. Economic factors
2. Institutional exclusion *(e.g. decreased services)*	2. Exclusion from basic services	2. Socio-economic exclusion: social rights *(e.g. exclusion from government provisions)*	3. Exclusion from basic services 4. Local amenities	2. Social rights	2. Spatial and transport connectivity 3. Virtual connectivity	4. Access to health services 5. Exclusion from basic services or information 6. Transport 7. Housing	2. Access to services 3. Transport and mobility	2. Service provision and access
3. Exclusion from meaningful relations	3. Exclusion from social relations	3. Socio-cultural exclusion: social integration *(e.g. lack of social relations)*	5. Exclusion from social relationships	3. Social participation 4. Perceptions of loneliness 5. Social support 6. Social integration	4. Social participation 5. Intergenerational relationships	8. Social relations/ social isolation	4. Social connections and social resources	3. Social relations and resources

4. Socio-political exclusion	4. Exclusion from civic activities		6. Exclusion from civic activities and access to information		6. Civic engagement	9. Participation in civic activities		4. Civic participation
5. Territorial exclusion	5. Neighbourhood exclusion		7. Neighbourhood exclusion		7. Landscape connectivity	10. Neighbourhood exclusion	5. Safety, security and crime	5. Environment and neighbourhood
6. Symbolic exclusion 7. Identity exclusion		4. Socio-cultural exclusion: normative integration	8. Exclusion from cultural activities		8. Group identity 9. Imaginative connectivity	11. Ageism 12. Ostracism 13. Self-reported exclusion		
						14. Health 15. Psychological Well-being 16. Self-dependence		6. Health and well-being

Adapted from Walsh et al. (2017)

frameworks vary in their conceptual depth, common to all is the capacity of social exclusion to detract from a full model of participation (Van Regenmortel et al. 2016). In this regard, each conceptualisation attempts to unpack the multidimensionality of the exclusion construct in older-age across a set of domains. There is also a recognition that interrelationships are likely to exist between different forms of exclusion where outcomes in one domain may contribute to broader processes that result in outcomes in other domains [see Dahlberg, and section VII in this volume for a full exploration of these interrelationships]. While the relative nature of exclusion is not explicitly articulated, it is implied. Some frameworks are grounded in specific settings (*e.g.* rural Ireland/Northern Ireland – Walsh et al. 2012/2019), while others note the capacity of macro contexts (institutions, norms, values) in shaping exclusionary experiences (*e.g.* Jehoel-Gijsbers and Vrooman 2008).

For the most part, an in-depth theoretical elaboration of how ageing and exclusionary processes intersect is largely neglected in these frameworks, with less of a focus on identifying the drivers of multidimensional exclusion. There are, however, a number of exceptions to this. Jehoel-Gijsbers and Vrooman (2008) highlight the influence of macro risks surrounding social processes (*e.g.* population ageing; individualisation) and government policy/provision (*e.g.* inadequate policy), meso risks relating to official bodies, business and citizens (*e.g.* discrimination; inadequate implementation), and micro risks at the individual/household level (*e.g.* health). Walsh et al. (2012/2019) describe the influence of individual capacities, life-course trajectories, place characteristics, and macro-economic forces in mediating multilevel rural age-related exclusion. Finally, Macleod et al. (2019) identify economic factors, environment and neighbourhood, and health and well-being as key determinants of social exclusion in later life.

It is also worth noting that while not presenting formal conceptualisations, important edited volumes on social exclusion of older people (*e.g.* Scharf and Keating 2012; Börsch-Supan et al. 2015), seminal works on related concepts (such as cumulative advantage/disadvantage – Dannefer (2003); precarity – Grenier et al. (2020)), and recent empirical/measurement papers (Dahlberg and McKee 2018; Feng et al. 2018; Van Regenmortel et al. 2018; Prattley et al. 2020; Keogh et al. 2021) have significantly expanded our conceptual understanding of multifaceted forms of disadvantage in later life.

With reference to Fig. 1.1, Walsh et al. (2017) broadly summarise the conceptual structures of the different frameworks into six key domains of exclusion, and identify a series of domain sub dimensions (which represent processes and outcomes) from a review of 425 publications. Together with Scharf and Keating (2012), they also highlight three elements of old-age exclusion arising from this review. First, exclusion can be accumulated over the course of older people's lives, contributing to an increased prevalence into older-age (*e.g.* Kneale 2012). Second, older people may have fewer opportunities and pathways to lift themselves out of exclusion (*e.g.* Scharf 2015). Third, older people may be more susceptible to exclusionary processes in their lives. This reflects the altered positioning of older adults with time, and specifically the potential to encounter ageism and age-based discrimination;

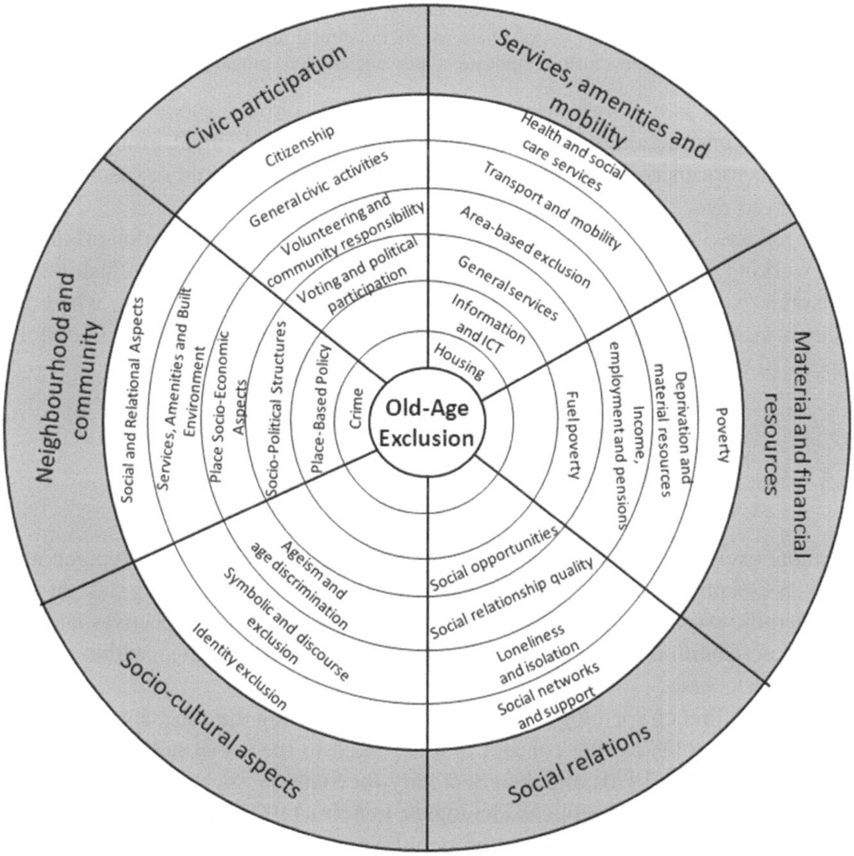

Fig. 1.1 Old-age exclusion framework depicting interconnected domains and sub dimensions

Source: Walsh et al. 2017

age-related health declines; contracting social and support networks; and depleted income generation opportunities (Jehoel-Gijsbers and Vrooman 2008).

We can now turn to the task of defining social exclusion amongst older people. A number of contributions within this volume present slightly different views of what exclusion in later life is. This is necessary to illustrate the variety of different perspectives, and to allow for more domain-specific mechanisms to be described. However, in order to set out the broad parameters of our focus – the same parameters that provided a conceptual scope for the ROSEnet COST Action – we adopt the following definition:

> 'Old-age exclusion involves interchanges between multilevel risk factors, processes and outcomes. Varying in form and degree across the older adult life course, its complexity, impact and prevalence are amplified by old-age vulnerabilities, accumulated disadvantage for some groups, and constrained opportunities to ameliorate exclusion. Old-age exclusion leads to inequities in choice and control, resources and relationships, and power and rights

in key domains of neighbourhood and community; services, amenities and mobility; material and financial resources; social relations; socio-cultural aspects of society; and civic participation. Old-age exclusion implicates states, societies, communities and individuals'.

Therefore, and as highlighted within this definition, old-age social exclusion is a life-course construction that is influenced and shaped by individual, group and institutional factors encountered across the life course, and not just those specific to the stage of old-age.

As reflected in the work of the ROSEnet Action, and its organisation around its five working groups, in this volume we condense the domains of exclusion into: economic; social relations; services; community and spatial; and civic, where the latter is an amalgamation of exclusion from civic participation and socio-cultural aspects of exclusion.

1.5 Social Exclusion, Policy and COVID-19

Defining exclusion in this manner, and acknowledging its various conceptual attributes, is essential for a volume committed to presenting and advancing state-of-the-art scientific research. However, focusing solely on scholarly perspectives neglects how these traditions are intertwined with the construct's lineage within policy/political discourse.

Although French sociology is credited with elaborating the core semantic meaning of social exclusion, the concept first appeared in the social policy analysis of Rene Lenoir in the 1970s, the then Secretary for State on Social Action in France. Building upon French republican ideologies, Lenoir's (1974) book *Les Exclus* identified a two-tier society where certain population groups were disconnected from, and unprotected by, core societal institutions. Although originally concentrating on manifestations of structural unemployment, social exclusion began to evolve as a broader descriptor of social disadvantage that was associated with new forms of urban poverty during the 1970s and 1980s. Social exclusion became 'institutionalised' in French public policy in the early 1990s when it was defined as a rupture in the social fabric, and a deficiency in solidarity (Mathieson et al. 2008; Silver 2019).

The concept was also adopted and developed as a core focus of social policy within other contexts around the same period – sometimes drawing on the evolving French political discourse, and sometimes harnessing other policy traditions (Mathieson et al. 2008). As described by Silver (2019), social exclusion and poverty became tied as core policy concerns within Europe's social agenda when a commitment to combating social exclusion was made in 1989. By 2001, European member states had agreed to report on progress on a set of social indicators within National Action Plans for Social Inclusion (later termed National Social Reports), and the commitment to tackle social exclusion remains evident within contemporary European policy frameworks. In the UK, the 1997 New Labour Government embraced the multidimensionality of exclusion to underpin a joined-up approach for tackling complex multifaceted social problems (Mathieson et al. 2008). This built upon longstanding critical social policy interests in the study of structural inequalities and power imbalances that construct a 'moral underclass' (Townsend, 1979). But social exclusion is also evident within the social policy agendas of international settings such as in North America, Australasia, and Asia (Warburton et al. 2013).

While the concept has altered in meaning over the years, and has at times been used interchangeably with social inclusion, it has once again come to espouse a focus on economic disadvantage within many jurisdictions. Labour market participation thus represents the main mechanism to combat exclusion, and a lack of attachment to the labour market its ultimate example (European Commission 2011). This gives rise to an uncomfortable tension with respect to how to reduce exclusion in later life, and the relevance of such measures.

Consequently, the fates of research and policy discourse need to be considered intertwined if advancement in the field is truly sought. It is for this reason that ROSEnet has attempted to produce shared understandings of old-age exclusion across research and policy communities. This has been as much to benefit from the intersectoral knowledge of policy actors, as to foster research-informed policy development. However, it has also been to illuminate the role of policy in mediating late-life exclusionary experiences. Narrow formulations of ageing within public policy can reinforce notions of homogeneity, propagate ageism and strip back complex identities of older populations to single age-related dimensions and associations (Biggs and Kimberley 2013; North and Fiske 2013). Even when policy is more comprehensive in its approach, a lack of implementation and resource allocation has often plagued the ageing sector. But clearly, policy can also have a substantial role to play in promoting fairness and inclusivity for older adults, protecting against exclusion. There are now a number of policy frameworks and initiatives that have considerable potential to enrich the lives of older people. This includes the EU Pillar for Social Rights, the United Nation's (UN) Sustainable Development Goals [both of which are considered within this volume], and the World Health Organization's (WHO) Age-Friendly Environments programme and the Decade of Healthy Ageing (2020–2030).

Ultimately, the dynamic nature of public policy environments, and older peoples' lives, demands that the impact of policies are continuously evaluated. The COVID-19 pandemic marks a recent and a significant global example of the need to attend to the multilevel interplay between policy and exclusionary experiences in older-age. We are writing this chapter in the midst of the global pandemic, with an ever growing number of cases and deaths announced each day across Europe and internationally. It is apparent that the impact of this traumatic crisis will live long in our global collective memory. It is also apparent that it is likely to be etched across many core aspects of our societies, including our public health policies, economies and, very possibly, demographic age structures with a disproportionate, and an alarming, number of deaths in older-age groups. Notwithstanding the significant risk to the health of older individuals (particularly those resident in nursing homes), and the immediate consequences of the virus for well-being, there has been a clear emergence of exclusionary mechanisms for older people associated with policy responses during the pandemic.

First, there are those mechanisms that stem directly from the strategies employed to control the spread of COVID-19, which produce exclusions in older people's daily lives (Le Couteur et al. 2020). These include: profound forms of digital exclusion, where some older adults may struggle to access critical online health information; barriers to attending essential medical appointments for the fear of contracting the virus or stigmatisation related to health service use during the pandemic; and the, well-publicised, increased risk of loneliness, and lack of support, due to self-isolation and "cocooning" (Brooke and Jackson 2020). Many of these exclusions are only intensified for older people living in nursing homes, where access to external social connections, services and other formal and informal supports is likely to be greatly diminished.

Second, there are direct exclusionary processes and outcomes that may arise from decision-making practices, informal or otherwise, that are integral to COVID-19 treatment pathways. Evidence suggested, that in some jurisdictions, the shortage of intensive care unit beds and ventilators led to the prioritisation of younger, healthier patients with a higher chance of recovery in treatment centres. While these circumstances place considerable moral strain and ethical responsibility on front-line health professionals, they also side-line need as a basis for resource allocation and exacerbate the risk of poorer outcomes for older individuals.

Third, public and policy discourses on ageing and older people have the potential to act as powerful exclusionary and discriminatory processes. This has emerged across two dimensions. While not many would argue with what appears to be a strong sentiment of concern, the paternalistic nature of protectionist endeavours, such as cocooning, have functioned to homogenise older people as highly vulnerable, passive agents in the pandemic (AGE Platform 2020). This has superseded the massive diversity of needs across older populations, and undermined the informal practices engaged in by older people that are emerging in response to the outbreak. More critically, however, there has been evidence of a problematisation of ageing in the context of the pandemic, where older people have been framed in some sections of the public sphere as en masse consumers of valuable and limited resources, blocking the access of younger, healthier individuals to treatment services. This has given rise to questions about the need to re-evaluate the social contract in favour of people who are deemed to be more "productive", and more tangibly contributing to the development, sustainability and economic welfare of societies (United Nations 2020). Aside from serving as a destabilising threat to solidarity across the generations, such discourses function to devalue not only the status of older people as equal citizens, but the value that we place on their contributions, and their lives, in our society. If such discourses are operational at a policy and practice level, then "cocooning" could be viewed in a very different light, where it is less about protecting people in older-age and more about protecting the health system and its resources for younger cohorts. This is, of course, played out at the level of our formal care settings, our communities, and to a degree within our own homes, and may have very real consequences for resource allocation and health outcomes.

The treatment of nursing homes and nursing home residents in many western nations during the pandemic has epitomised the most severe form of this problematisation. Indeed, it may have exposed a more systemic collective ease at the segregation of these facilities, and the health vulnerabilities of their older populations, away from mainstream society. The fact that many countries failed to count COVID-related deaths in nursing homes can be argued to be the ultimate exclusion, stripping individual identities and devaluing individual lives.

While the chapters in this book will not engage directly with this topic, having been written primarily before the onset of the pandemic, they have a strong relevance to the COVID-19 crisis and a capacity to illustrate why exclusion is occurring as a result of the outbreak. On a more general level, these dynamics draw attention to how significant shocks, be they from public health, environmental, or economic sources (*e.g.* Adams et al. 2011), can quickly alter the social, economic and symbolic circumstances of older people with short-, medium- and long-term consequences for ageing societies.

1.6 Approach and Structure of This Book

Current conceptualisations of social exclusion in later life, in terms of its multidimensional and relative nature, and its relevance and relationship to policy, has directly informed the approach and structure of this book. This edited volume involves 77 contributors working across 28 nations, and comprises 34 chapters. Twenty-four chapters are co-authored by cross-national interdisciplinary writing teams, fostering sensitivity to relative differences in jurisdictional circumstances, and integrating diverse understandings, literatures and empirical data from national settings that are not typically featured in English-language volumes. Twenty-four chapters also represent writing partnerships between early-career researchers and established international experts at the forefront of academic scholarship, with approximately 40 early-career researchers contributing to the volume.

Across this volume, contributors have been encouraged to adopt a life-course and critical gerontological understanding of social exclusion in later life. While direct engagement with these perspectives is certainly evident in some chapters more than others, authors generally are cognizant within their analysis of earlier life events, changes over time, turning points and transitions, the influence of structural and institutional factors, and the positionality of ageing and older people within cultural and normative value systems. A number of contributions also directly address the intersectionality of key social locations, ageing and exclusion, and/or the position of marginalised sections of the older population. This includes gender, ethic and migration background, socio-economic status and class, dementia, and homelessness.

The book is divided into eight sections, with the main body organised in accordance with the multidimensional structure of social exclusion in later life, and policy related challenges.

Sections II–VI will consider the five domains of old-age social exclusion: economic; social relations; services; community and spatial; and civic exclusion. Each section comprises four chapters. A short introductory chapter, written by co-leaders of the relevant ROSEnet working groups, will introduce the exclusion domain. It will also frame the subsequent three chapters, with each of these exploring a different sub dimension of the exclusion domain.

Section II focuses on economic exclusion. Jim Ogg and Michal Myck introduce economic aspects of exclusion in later life in Chap. 2. The authors emphasise the need to consider its many dimensions from a life-course perspective. As such, they highlight the importance of exploring multidimensional economic outcomes in older-age as a product of the combination of all life stages. In Chap. 3, Sumil-Laanemaa et al. assess the variation in material deprivation of the population aged 50+ across four geographic clusters of welfare regimes in Europe. Murdock et al., in Chap. 4, explore job loss in older-age, as a form of acute economic exclusion, and its implications for mental health in later life. Barlin et al., in Chap. 5, chart the economic exclusion and coping mechanisms of widowed, and divorced and separated older women in Turkey and Serbia.

Section III focuses on exclusion from social relations. In Chap. 6, Vanessa Burholt and Marja Aartsen introduce exclusion from social relations in later life. In addition to highlighting risk factors and the dynamic nature of exclusion from social relations, Burholt and Aartsen emphasise the impact of psychological resources, socio-economic processes and immediate neighbourhood environments on the exclusion process. In Chap. 7, Van Regenmortel et al. analyse the manifestations and drivers of exclusion from social relations, in Belgium and rural Britain, and consider links with other forms of disadvantage. In Chap. 8, Morgan et al. examine the impact of micro- and macro-level drivers of loneliness and changes in the experiences of loneliness in eleven European countries. In Chap. 9, Waldegrave et al. explore the complex nature of the conflicted, abusive and discriminative relations of older people and their differential impacts across countries.

Section IV focuses on exclusion from services. Veerle Draulans and Giovanni Lamura introduce exclusion from services in Chap. 10. The authors highlight the need to consider particular macro- and micro-level factors in the construction of exclusion from services, with the focus on the former relating to the increasing individualisation of risk, and the latter on the intersection of age and other social locations. In Chap. 11, Cholat and Daconto explore how reverse mobilities, where services travel to service users, may promote older people's inclusion in mountain areas. Széman et al. in Chap. 12, investigate patterns and construction of exclusion from home care services in Central and Eastern European countries, focusing on Hungary and Russia. Finally, in Chap. 13, Poli et al. examine the provision of care and support through digital health technologies, and present a conceptual framework for old-age digital health exclusion.

Section V focuses on community and spatial aspects of exclusion. In Chap. 14, Isabelle Tournier and Lucie Vidovićová introduce this form of exclusion and explore the notion of a "good place". Drawing on a model of life space, they emphasise the intersection of multilevel spatial environments and the needs of older adults with respect to engagement and inclusion. In Chap. 15, Drilling et al. present a theoretical model that integrates the dimensions of age, space and exclusion in one perspective, and explores its potential to explain older people's exclusion. Urbaniak et al., in Chap. 16, investigate how relationships with place and old-age social exclusion intersect during the life-course transitions of bereavement and retirement. In Chap. 17, Vidovićová et al. explore how exclusion from care provision in rural areas can be understood as a form of place-based disadvantage in three central European countries.

Section VI focuses on civic exclusion. Sandra Torres introduces civic exclusion in later life in Chap. 18. Torres provides an overview of existing understandings of both exclusion from civic participation and socio-cultural aspects of exclusion and outlines the importance of considering the heterogeneity of older populations and their life-course experiences within this topic. In Chap. 19, Serrat et al. present an analysis of older people's exclusion from civic engagement, and emphasise the importance of considering its multidimensionality, and its cultural embeddedness. Gallistl, in Chap. 20, examines patterns of cultural participation for older people, drawing out the relationship of changes in these patterns with socio-economic status. Finally, in Chap. 21, Gallassi and Harrysson situate ageing and migration within the setting of international human rights law and how the principles of equality and non-discrimination can help combat exclusions for ageing migrants.

Section VII specifically explores the interrelationships between the exclusion domains. Illuminating ways in which different processes of exclusion can intersect, this section is pivotal in developing an understanding of old-age exclusion that goes beyond a collection of single domains. In the first of five chapters, Lena Dahlberg, in Chap. 22, introduces the study of interrelationships as developed in the international literature. Dahlberg charts the interconnections that have been identified across the domains before highlighting key knowledge gaps and outlining each of the remaining contributions. In Chap. 23, Villar et al. examines the circumstances of older people in long-term care institutions and the potential for exclusion from social relationships, civic participation and socio-cultural life. In Chap. 24, Myck et al. assess the relationship between material conditions and the level and dynamics of loneliness in later life. Siren, in Chap. 25, employs the concept of "structural lag" to analyse the links between transport mobility, well-being and wider constructions of multidimensional exclusion. In the final contribution, Korkmaz-Yaylagul and Bas in Chap. 26 explore the multidimensional aspects of old-age exclusion in the homelessness literature, and how homelessness can be a significant determinant of interrelated sets of disadvantages.

Section VIII is specifically dedicated to policy challenges in relation to social exclusion in later life. Comprising of an introduction and six chapters, the majority of authors are drawn from policy stakeholder organisations. In Chap. 27, Norah Keating and Maria Cheshire-Allen introduce social exclusion as a policy framework for population ageing and older persons. They highlight how values, political agendas and competition among multiple social goals require as much attention as scientific evidence in assessing current policy debates. Conboy, in Chap. 28, explores the potential of the 2030 Agenda for Sustainable Development to serve as a global framework for addressing multidimensional old-age exclusion. In Chap. 29, Ogg examines the role of pension policies in preventing exclusion of older people and analyses the main mechanisms of pension system reform that may help facilitate this. In Chap. 30, Grigoryeva et al. consider the case of the post-Soviet space, and the ways in which differential reforms may impact the capacity of social policies to protect older people from risks of exclusion. Andersen et al., in Chap. 31, explore the potential for innovative micro-level policy and practice to prevent social exclusion of nursing home residents from local life. In Chap. 32, Leppiman et al. focus on digital service policy in Finland and Estonia as a mediator of broader sets of exclusions and inclusions in older-age. Finally in Chap. 33, Kucharczyk analyses the potential of the European Pillar of Social Rights to address social exclusion of older people in Europe, and the measures necessary to ensure this comes about.

Section IX presents the book's conclusion chapter. The chapter seeks to draw together various threads from the preceding sections, and their contributions, and chart future directions for research and policy development on social exclusion in later life.

1.7 Concluding Remarks

This book aims to advance research and policy debates on social exclusion of older people. In both established and emerging ageing societies, the exclusion of older adults is harmful to individuals and the effectiveness and solidarity of communities and nations. Regardless of the future patterns of the COVID-19 outbreak, it appears that the pandemic, as with many other major crises, has exposed longstanding mechanisms of exclusion and entrenched, multiple forms of disadvantage for heterogenous older populations. It has also exposed the importance of factors like institutional structures, and their underlying values, in how they constitute policy responses to age-related risk and ultimately influence the relative nature of exclusion and real and perceived differences across contexts. The COVID-19 pandemic has as such only served to enhance the relevance and timeliness of this volume. In pursuing its four objectives, this book targets contributions that together will provide a critical analysis of current state-of-the-art knowledge, and the basis for the development of a forward-looking research agenda. It is hoped that through these contributions that this book will inspire a commitment to scholarship and evidence-informed action on social exclusion in later life.

References

Adams, V., Kaufman, S. R., Van Hattum, T., & Moody, S. (2011). Aging disaster: Mortality, vulnerability, and long-term recovery among Katrina survivors. *Medical Anthropology, 30*, 247–270.

AGE Platform Europe. (2020). *COVID-19 and human rights concerns for older persons*. https://www.age-platform.eu/sites/default/files/COVID-19_%26_human_rights_concerns_for_older_persons-April20.pdf

Atkinson, A. B. (1998). *Social exclusion, poverty and unemployment* (CASE paper).

Ayalon, L., & Tesch-Römer, C. (2017). Taking a closer look at ageism: Self- and other-directed ageist attitudes and discrimination. *European Journal of Ageing, 14*, 1–4. https://doi.org/10.1007/s10433-016-0409-9.

Barnes, M., Blom, A., Cox, K., & Lessof, C. (2006). *The social exclusion of older people: Evidence from the first wave of the English Longitudinal Study of Ageing (ELSA): Final report*. London: Office for the Deputy of Prime Minister.

Biggs, S., & Kimberley, H. (2013). Adult ageing and social policy: New risks to identity. *Social Policy and Society, 12*(2), 287–297. https://doi.org/10.1017/S1474746412000656.

Börsch-Supan, A., Kneip, T., Litwin, H., Myck, M., & Weber, G. (eds.) (2015). Ageing in Europe: Supporting policies for an inclusive society. Berlin: De Gruyter. ISBN 978-3-11-043704-1. https://doi.org/10.1515/9783110444414

Bradshaw, J. (2004). How has the notion of social exclusion developed in the European discourse? *Economic and Labour Relations Review, 14*(2), 168–186.

Brooke, J., & Jackson, D. (2020). Older people and COVID-19: Isolation, risk and ageism. *Journal of Clinical Nursing*. https://doi.org/10.1111/jocn.15274.

Dahlberg, L., McKee, K. J., Fritzell, J., Heap, J., & Lennartsson, C. (2020). Trends and gender associations in social exclusion in older adults in Sweden over two decades. *Archives of Gerontology and Geriatrics, 89*, 104032.

Dahlberg, L., & McKee, K. J. (2018). Social exclusion and well-being among older adults in rural and urban areas. *Archives of Gerontology and Geriatrics, 79*, 176–184.

Dannefer, D. (2003). Cumulative advantage/disadvantage and the life course: Cross-fertilizing age and social science theory. *The Journals of Gerontology. Series B, Psychological Sciences and Social Sciences, 58*, 327–337.

European Commission. (2011). *The European platform against poverty and social exclusion: A European framework for social and territorial cohesion*. Luxembourg: Publications Office of the European Union. Available online at: http://ec.europa.eu/social/main.jsp?catId=738&langId=en&pubId=6028&type=2&furtherPubs=yes.

Eurostat. (2019). *Archive: People at risk of poverty or social exclusion*. Eurostat Statistics Explained.

Feng, W. (2012). Social exclusion of the elderly in China: One potential challenge resulting from the rapid population ageing. In C. Martinez-Fernandez, N. Kubo, A. Noya, & T. Weyman (Eds.), *Demographic change and local development: Shrinkage, regeneration and social dynamics*. Paris: OECD.

Feng, Z., Phillips, D. R., & Jones, K. (2018). A geographical multivariable multilevel analysis of social exclusion among older people in China: Evidence from the China Longitudinal Aging Social Survey ageing study. *Geographical Journal, 184*, 413–428.

Grenier, A., Hatzifilalithis, S., Laliberte-Rudman, D., Kobayashi, K., Marier, P., & Phillipson, C. (2020). Precarity and aging: A scoping review. *The Gerontologist*, gnz135. https://doi.org/10.1093/geront/gnz135.

Guberman, N., & Lavoie, J. P. (2004). Equipe vies: Framework on social exclusion. In *Centre de recherche et d'expertise de gérontologie sociale*. Montréal: CAU/CSSS Cavendish.

Hagan Hennessy, C., Means, R., & Burholt, V. (2014). Countryside connections in later life: Setting the scene. In C. Hagan Hennessy, R. Means, & V. Burholt (Eds.), *Countryside connections: Older people, community and place in rural Britain* (pp. 95–124). Bristol: Policy Press.

Hargittai, E., Piper, A. M., & Morris, M. R. (2019). From internet access to internet skills: Digital inequality among older adults. *Universal Access in the Information Society, 18*, 881–890. https://doi.org/10.1007/s10209-018-0617-5.

Jehoel-Gijsbers, G., & Vrooman, C. (2008). *Social exclusion of the elderly: A comparative study of EU member states*. Brussels: CEPS.

Kendig, H., & Nazroo, J. (2016). Life course influences on inequalities in later life: Comparative perspectives. *Journal of Population Ageing, 9*, 1–7.

Keogh, S., O'Neill, S., & Walsh, K. (2021). Composite measures for assessing multidimensional social exclusion in later life: Conceptual and methodological challenges. *Social Indicators Research*. https://doi.org/10.1007/s11205-021-02617-7

Kneale, D. (2012). *Is social exclusion still important for older people?* The International Longevity Centre-UK (ILC-UK). Available at: https://ilcuk.org.uk/wp-content/uploads/2018/11/Social-exclusion-Report.pdf.

Le Couteur, D., Anderson, R., & Newman, A. (2020). COVID-19 through the lens of gerontology. *The Journals of Gerontology: Series A*, glaa077. https://doi.org/10.1093/gerona/glaa077.

Lenoir, R. (1974). *Les exclus: Un français sur dix* [The excluded: One French Person out of Ten]. Paris: Seuil.

Levitas, R., Pantazis, C., Fahmy, E., et al. (2007). *The multi-dimensional analysis of social exclusion*. London: Cabinet Office.

Macleod, C., Ross, A., Sacker, A., Netuveli, G., & Windle, G. (2019). Re-thinking social exclusion in later life: A case for a new framework for measurement. *Ageing and Society, 39*(1), 74–111. https://doi.org/10.1017/S0144686X17000794.

Mathieson, J., Popay, J., Enoch, E., Escorel, S., Hernandez, M., Johnston, H., & Rispel, L. (2008). *Social exclusion meaning, measurement and experience and links to health inequalities. A review of literature*. WHO Social Exclusion Knowledge Network Background Paper 1. https://www.who.int/social_determinants/media/sekn_meaning_measurement_experience_2008.pdf.pdf.

Nazroo, J. (2017). Class and health inequality in later life: Patterns, mechanisms and implications for policy. *International Journal of Environmental Research and Public Health, 14*, 1533. https://doi.org/10.3390/ijerph14121533.

North, M. S., & Fiske, S. T. (2013). Subtyping ageism: Policy issues in succession and consumption. *Social Issues and Policy Review, 7*, 36–57. https://doi.org/10.1111/j.1751-2409.2012.01042.x.

Phillipson, C. (2020). Austerity and precarity: Individual and collective agency in later life. In A. Grenier, C. Phillipson, & R. Settersten (Eds.), *Precarity and ageing: Understanding insecurity and risk in later life* (Ageing in a global context) (pp. 215–235). Chicago: Policy Press.

Prattley, J., Buffel, T., Marshall, A., & Nazroo, J. (2020). Area effects on the level and development of social exclusion in later life. *Social Science & Medicine, 246*, 112722.

ROSEnet. (2020). Multidimensional Social Exclusion in Later life: Briefing Paper and a Roadmap for Future Collaborations in Research and Policy. In: K. Walsh and T. Scharf (series Eds.), *ROSEnet Briefing Paper Series: No. 6. CA 15122 Reducing Old-Age Exclusion: Collaborations in Research and Policy*. ISBN: 978-1-908358-76-9.

Scharf, T. (2015). Between inclusion and exclusion in later life. In K. Walsh, G. Carney, & A. Ní Léime (Eds.), *Ageing through austerity: Critical perspectives from Ireland* (pp. 113–130). Bristol: Policy Press.

Scharf, T., & Bartlam, B. (2008). Ageing and social exclusion in rural communities. In N. Keating (Ed.), *Rural ageing: A good place to grow old?* (pp. 97–108). Bristol: The Policy Press.

Scharf, T., Phillipson, C., & Smith, A. E. (2005). Social exclusion of older people in deprived urban communities of England. *European Journal of Ageing, 2*, 76–87.

Scharf, T., & Keating, N. (2012). Social exclusion in later life: A global challenge. In T. Scharf & N. Keating (Eds.), *From exclusion to inclusion in old age: A global challenge* (pp. 1–16). Bristol: The Policy Press.

Silver, H. (2019). Social exclusion. In A. Orum (Ed.), *The Wiley Blackwell encyclopedia of urban and regional studies* (pp. 1–6). Wiley. https://doi.org/10.1002/9781118568446.eurs0486.

Townsend, P. (1979). *Poverty in the United Kingdom: A survey of household resources and standards of living*. Aylesbury: Hazel Watson & Viney Ltd, Great Britain.

United Nations. (2020). A defining moment for informed, Inclusive and targeted response. *Issue brief: Older persons and COVID-19*. Available at: https://www.un.org/development/desa/ageing/wp-content/uploads/sites/24/2020/04/POLICY-BRIEF-ON-COVID19-AND-OLDER-PERSONS.pdf

Van Regenmortel, S., De Donder, L., Dury, S., Smetcoren, A. S., de Witte, N., & Verté, D. (2016). Social exclusion in later life: A systematic review of the literature. *Journal of Population Aging, 9*, 315–344. https://doi.org/10.1007/s10262-016-9145-3.

Van Regenmortel, S., De Donder, L., Smetcoren, A., et al. (2018). Accumulation of disadvantages: Prevalence and categories of old-age social exclusion in Belgium. *Social Indicators Research, 140*, 1173–1194. https://doi.org/10.1007/s11205-017-1817-8.

Walsh, K., O'Shea, E., & Scharf, T. (2012). *Social exclusion and ageing in diverse rural communities: Findings of a cross border study in Ireland and Northern Ireland*. Galway: Irish Centre for Social Gerontology.

Walsh, K., O'Shea, E., & Scharf, T. (2019). Rural old-age social exclusion: A conceptual framework on mediators of exclusion across the life course. *Ageing & Society*, 1–27. https://doi.org/10.1017/S0144686X19000606.

Walsh, K., Scharf, T., & Keating, N. (2017). Social exclusion of older persons: A scoping review and conceptual framework. *European Journal of Ageing, 14*, 81–98. https://doi.org/10.1007/s10433-016-0398-8.

Warburton, J., Ng, S. H., & Shardlow, S. M. (2013). Social inclusion in an ageing world: Introduction to the special issue. *Ageing & Society, 33*, 1–15.

Section II
Economic Exclusion

Chapter 2
Introduction: Framing Economic Exclusion

Jim Ogg and Michal Myck

2.1 Introduction

Economic exclusion is a multidimensional concept that has particular relevance in the context of ageing populations and globalised economies. Sustaining adequate incomes in old-age and protecting older citizens from poverty are major challenges for governments and policy makers and they have been amplified in the face of the economic consequences of the COVID-19 pandemic. Over the past few decades most countries have made adjustments to their pension systems and other welfare related policies that concern older citizens, and these reforms have already had and will continue to have a differential impact on economic exclusion. For some, extending the working life and pushing back the legal age of retirement can be a safeguard against inadequate incomes in old-age, while for others who are excluded from the labour market, or who are working in low paid jobs, economic exclusion remains a reality. The labour market implications of the pandemic are likely to exacerbate this risk for those whose situation was already fragile before the crisis.

However, as the current situation around the world makes clear, economic exclusion in later life and old-age is not confined to pension reforms alone. Economic exclusion should be perceived from a life-course perspective and understood as a process with many dimensions, with all life stages and all dimensions combining to determine outcomes in later life and old-age. This perspective sheds light on the importance of the economic consequences of the COVID-19 pandemic both for the current older generations as well as those for whom retirement is still a distant prospect. The purpose of this chapter is to first briefly introduce the topic of economic

J. Ogg (✉)
Ageing Research Unit, National Pension Fund (Caisse nationale d'assurance vieillesse), Paris, France

College of Human and Health Sciences, Swansea University, Swansea, UK
e-mail: jim.ogg@cnav.fr

M. Myck
Centre for Economic Analysis, Szczecin, Poland

K. Walsh et al. (eds.), *Social Exclusion in Later Life*, International Perspectives on Aging 28, https://doi.org/10.1007/978-3-030-51406-8_2

exclusion, with a particular focus on the life-course dimensions of economic forms of hardship. The second purpose is to introduce the three chapters within this section as exploring different facets of economic exclusion.

2.2 Economic Exclusion and the Life Course

Social class, education, and migration play an important part in individual chances to secure adequate resources over the life course. Labour market opportunities and the balance between family life and paid work are also important in determining access to resources in later life. These dimensions are manifest in different social policy regimes as well as in organisational policies and practices within the workplace before retirement. However, they encompass new and existing social risks in general and life-course risks in particular, as well as life-course events and experiences, all of which shape life time trajectories of health, social relations and material conditions. Moreover, these dimensions relate not only to the macro-level of economics, but also to climates of political and social change as well as economic crises.

In order to understand how events in the life course affect economic exclusion outcomes in later life, Myck et al. (2017) identify key factors that influence material well-being over the life course and the capacity of individuals to respond to expected and unexpected changes in the level of their material conditions. In the worst-case scenario, permanently low levels of material resources in relation to the needs of individuals endure over long spans of the life course. Long-term unemployment, precarious working conditions, and low-paid jobs combine to prevent the build-up of pension rights and assets that are needed to safeguard against economic exclusion in later life. Poor health and disability over the life course can also be an important factor that limits the capacity to build up wealth and secure regular sources of income for old-age. Accumulated over time, a low level of material resources leads to insufficient buffers of assets to ensure sufficient resources in old-age and individuals are subsequently ‘trapped’ in poverty. From this perspective various elements of welfare systems are crucial to ensure that not only such individuals can meet their basic needs, but that they also can participate fully in civic society.

A second trajectory that influences economic exclusion in later life is the arrival of unexpected shocks to the level of resources in relation to individual needs. Certain events in the life course, such as divorce, widowhood, illness, and redundancy, are often accompanied by a sharp drop in income and a depletion of savings. The consequence of such shocks is that it may not only be difficult to maintain the prior levels of material well-being, but the altered circumstances may lead to significant worsening of material conditions due to inability to earn income and the need to run down accumulated assets. Significant negative shocks may thus lead to a fall in current income and a permanent reduction in material well-being due to inability to further accumulate assets for future use.

Finally, despite the absence of prolonged periods of unpaid work or life-course shocks, individuals may fail to direct their economic resources towards future needs in old-age. Old age can be accompanied by significant costs related to home care and residential accommodation fees. In the current climate of budgetary constraints to welfare systems, which are likely to be exacerbated by the economic slowdown induced by the COVID-19 pandemic, this feature of economic exclusion has particular importance. The nature of the risks involved and the potentially very high costs of providing the necessary level of care imply that provision of insurance against the need of extensive long-term care cannot be provided by private insurers. In recent decades, however, many governments have been either reducing the degree of collective societal obligations to provide age-related welfare support or essentially ignoring the implementation of systemic solutions of provision of care for future generations. The consequence of both approaches is a shift of responsibility for the financing of old-age care on to the individual.

Income and the process of asset accumulation on the one hand, and the development of risks and the related material needs on the other are therefore essential components in understanding how economic exclusion can arise in later life and old-age. However, unlike traditional approaches to material well-being that tend to focus on the dimension of poverty and income, the concept of economic exclusion extends beyond financial aspects of material conditions to a broader perspective (non-financial) that includes different aspects of individual lives. Given the growing evidence for the weaknesses and failures of the traditional approaches with respect to identification of disadvantaged groups of the society through the lens of current income, there has been growing interest in the development of more adequate and more internationally comparable measures of material well-being. An alternative approach to income-base measures has been the analysis of material well-being using measures of material deprivation, defined as 'the inability to possess the goods and services and/or engage in activities that are ordinary in the society or that are socially perceived as "necessities"' (Fusco et al. 2010, p. 7).

Increasingly, research in this area is adopting a variety of measures to capture those elements of economic exclusion that go beyond monetary aspects and it seems that such a broader approach will be essential to understand the consequences of the combination of the health and economic crises brought about by the COVID-19 pandemic. Central to this approach is the place of subjectivity and how individuals perceive their financial situation and material conditions. Subjective measures are strongly correlated with other aspects of quality of life in old-age (Adena and Myck 2013). As such, they underpin the notion of unmet needs and provide a very broad indicator of material conditions and thus material exclusion. At the same time, they suffer both from a high degree of cultural bias, and from adjustments by individuals to the assessment of their material situations over prolonged periods of time spent in a given material situation. There are theoretical arguments and empirical results that older people who experience economic hardships adjust their preferences to scarce economic resources over time (Berthoud and Bryan 2011). For this reason they become satisfied with their living standards and everyday lives despite facing economic hardship in old-age. Another way of explaining this counter intuitive finding is that current coping among older people – such as focusing on positive aspects of everyday life and adjusting one's preferences according to what is possible to achieve—results in satisfaction with everyday life despite the negative consequences of economic hardship.

Taking into consideration the complex and multi-layered domain of economic exclusion, it is not surprising that estimates of the extent of the phenomenon are difficult to undertake. However, broadly speaking, research on economic hardship in Europe reveals that a significant proportion of older people face problems in meeting their material needs and that substantial differences in material conditions exist in Europe both between and within countries. These poor material conditions include low levels of income and assets, difficulties in financing basic expenditures on food, housing, transport, health and social care. Older people facing economic hardship also can be excluded from participation in leisure and other civic activities. As the above review demonstrates, though, only a broad and comprehensive approach to the problem of poor material conditions among older people is likely to succeed in significant reductions of the number of individuals facing economic hardship. Moreover, only complex measures of material conditions will be able to capture the influence of both, the resources individuals have at their disposal on the one hand, and the public services they receive such as health or long-term care on the other. At all stages of life, but in particular in old-age, it is the combination of these two factors that determine individual material well-being, a fact that has been so strongly evident in the light of the COVID-19 pandemic. Any policy measures aimed at protecting and improving the welfare of senior citizens should take this into account.

2.3 Outline of This Section

The three chapters in this section present original research that focuses on specific dimensions related to economic exclusion reviewed above, notably the subjective experience of economic exclusion in later life and the measurement of material deprivation. All chapters have been written in the pre-pandemic reality, but they provide arguments and evidence which are extremely relevant in the current situation and which can support policy response to the crisis.

In Chap. 3, Merle Sumil-Laanemaa and colleagues examine the differences in the role of factors which influence the level of material deprivation in four categories of countries participating in the Survey of Health, Ageing and Retirement in Europe (SHARE) divided with regard to their broad welfare regimes into: Continental, Nordic, Southern and Eastern European. They analyse the differences in the degree of association of socio-demographic characteristics with a material deprivation index and report results which are of high relevance for the discussion of the role of the welfare state in ensuring sufficient material resources in old-age. Results confirm a significant role of the welfare regime with respect to the degree of material deprivation in later life.

Unemployment is strongly associated with economic exclusion. Elke Murdock and colleagues in Chap. 4 examine the under-researched aspect of the economic and psychosocial consequences of unemployment in later life. Using data from a study of sixty-seven older unemployed persons in Luxembourg, the authors show that the length of time in unemployment is associated with lower life satisfaction. Notwithstanding this finding, the research points to a diversity of the profiles of unemployed older persons, suggesting that measures to reduce social exclusion should take into account different needs and different profiles of personal and social competence.

In Chap. 5, Hande Barlin and colleagues examine the coping strategies that older divorced and separated, and widowed women in Turkey and Serbia employ to compensate for low incomes. This qualitative study that compares the experiences in the two countries is firmly rooted in a life-course perspective, demonstrating the strong influence of early divorce on incomes in later life and the importance of survivor pensions and other welfare pensions that compensate for the absence of acquired pension rights. The authors show the continued importance of family support whilst at the same time emphasising the relevance that older divorced and widowed women attach to their independence.

References

Adena, M., & Myck, M. (2013). Poverty and transitions in key areas of quality of life. In A. Börsch-Supan, M. Brandt, H. Litwin, & G. Weber (Eds.), *Active ageing and solidarity between generations in Europe: First results from SHARE after the economic crisis* (pp. 55–73). Berlin: De Gruyter.

Berthoud, R., & Bryan, M. (2011). Income, deprivation and poverty: A longitudinal analysis. *Journal of Social Policy, 40*(1), 135–156.

Fusco, A., Guio, A.-C., & Marlier, E. (2010). *Income poverty and material deprivation in European countries* (Theme: Population and social conditions, collection: Methodologies and Working Papers, 2010, Cat. No. KS-RA-10-030-EN-N). Luxembourg: European Union.

Myck, M., Ogg, J., Aigner-Walder, B., Kareholt, I., Kostakis, I., Motel-Klingebiel, A., Marban-Flores, R., Murdock, E., Perek- Bialas, J., & Thelin, A. No 1 (2017). *Economic aspects of old age exclusion: A scoping report*. Knowledge synthesis series. Rosenet Cost Action (CA15122) Reducing Old-Age Social Exclusion: Collaborations in Research & Policy.

Chapter 3
Socio-demographic Risk Factors Related to Material Deprivation Among Older Persons in Europe: A Comparative Analysis Based on SHARE Data

Merle Sumil-Laanemaa, Luule Sakkeus, Allan Puur, and Lauri Leppik

3.1 Introduction

The concept of social exclusion encompasses the processes and interplay of factors that hinder personal well-being and, consequently, full and equal participation in society. The ageing of the population warrants research on social exclusion in older age, examining the processes and risk factors of exclusion that can predominate in later life (Walsh et al. 2017). Scharf et al. (2005) conceptualise social exclusion in old-age as a phenomenon with five dimensions: material resources, social relations, civic activities, basic services, and neighbourhoods. Myck et al. (2017) point out that economic exclusion in later life – a process that relates to the focus of this chapter – is rooted in the development of material well-being over the life course and entails an incapacity to address expected and unexpected changes in the level of material conditions and needs. In addition to current income, economic exclusion involves low assets, a shortage of durable goods accumulated over the life course, limited access to services, and other types of non-monetary material wealth. The concept of material deprivation also includes non-monetary aspects of economic exclusion (Boarini and Mira d'Ercole 2006).

Only few studies to date have explored the individual risk factors of material deprivation (such as sex, age, education, household size and socio-economic status) among older persons from a broad cross-national comparative perspective (*e.g.* Jehoel-Gijsbers and Vrooman 2008). Lacking an understanding of how the influence of these factors might vary across different jurisdictions and different types of welfare regimes not only impacts negatively on scholarly knowledge but on our capacity for meaningful pan-European policy development. In this study, we aim to identify differences in material deprivation among older persons in Europe, analyse

M. Sumil-Laanemaa (✉) · L. Sakkeus · A. Puur · L. Leppik
Estonian Institute for Population Studies, School of Governance, Law and Society, Tallinn University, Tallinn, Estonia
e-mail: merle.sumil-laanemaa@tlu.ee

K. Walsh et al. (eds.), *Social Exclusion in Later Life*, International Perspectives on Aging 28, https://doi.org/10.1007/978-3-030-51406-8_3

the associations between socio-demographic risk factors and material deprivation, and the ways in which these associations differ across welfare regimes. The analysis provides further insights into the individual components of material deprivation and the complexity of the disadvantages experienced by older persons (Saunders 2008; Scharf 2015).

3.2 Material Deprivation: Operationalisation and Risk Factors

3.2.1 Concept and Operationalisation

Fusco et al. (2010) define material deprivation as an inability to possess the goods and services and/or engage in activities that are customary in society, or that are socially perceived as "necessities". The concept of material deprivation thus addresses aspects of economic exclusion that are not covered by current income, such as effective economic hardship and limited access to basic goods and services (Renahy et al. 2012). Myck et al. (2017) suggest that measures of material deprivation have several important advantages over traditional income-based and subjective measures of material well-being and exclusion. They refer directly to failures in effective capacity, while measuring material conditions more objectively than a subjective self-assessment of one's overall material situation, and are consequently more comparable across population groups and between countries. However, Myck et al. also note that measures of material deprivation are somewhat arbitrary in terms of their construction and composition, given that needs, expectations and preferences vary across subgroups of the population and may change over time.

The operational definitions of material deprivation vary according to the items that are included in the "basket" of basic goods and services considered ordinary or necessary, and the weights assigned to them (Guio 2009). These choices thus have a normative element.

The EU portfolio of social inclusion indicators defines the material deprivation rate (MDR) and severe material deprivation rate (SMDR) as the proportion of the population living in households that are unable to afford at least three (for the MDR) or four (for the SMDR) of the following nine items: (1) to pay rent or utility bills; (2) to keep their home adequately warm; (3) to meet unexpected expenses; (4) to eat meat, fish or a protein equivalent every second day; (5) to take a week's holiday away from home; or could not afford if they wanted to have: (6) a car; (7) a washing machine; (8) a colour television; or (9) a telephone. Although the total household is taken into account, the unit of analysis for the EU indicators is the individual within his/her household (Fusco et al. 2010). The MDR and SMDR are calculated based on EU-SILC (EU Statistics on Income and Living Conditions) data (Eurostat 2019). Fusco et al. (2013) comment that such indicators aggregate information on some key aspects of material living conditions, but do not cover all dimensions of economic exclusion. The selection of items in the aggregate indicator is based on a lack of affordability rather than on personal choice or lifestyle preferences.

An alternative measure – the Material Deprivation Index (MDI) – has been developed within the framework of the Survey of Health, Ageing and Retirement in Europe (SHARE). The composition have this assessment of material deprivation bears some similarities to the Eurostat indicators, but there are also differences. The MDI is based on a set of 11 material deprivation indicators that refer to a household's financial difficulties and inability to meet basic needs (Adena et al. 2015).

Basic needs include the ability to: (1) have meat, fish or chicken; and (2) fruits or vegetables, in the household diet at least three times a week; (3) purchase necessary groceries and household supplies; (4) pay for adequate heating; (5) replace worn-out shoes; and (6) clothes; (7) purchase new glasses when needed; and (8) see a doctor; and (9) dentist. Indicators of financial difficulties include the inability to afford: (10) a week-long holiday; and (11) to pay unexpected expenses without borrowing. Compared with the EU-SILC-based material deprivation indicators, SHARE's MDI does not include possession of or ability to afford durable goods such as a car, washing machine, or colour television. Instead, the MDI focusses more on immediate basic needs, such as the affordability of fruits and vegetables, shoes and clothes, and seeing a doctor or dentist. It is argued that this approach makes the MDI more suitable for measuring material deprivation among older persons (Adena et al. 2015).

3.2.2 Risk Factors Related to Material Deprivation

A considerable number of earlier studies have analysed the links between material deprivation and socio-demographic risk factors such as sex, age, education, household size and socio-economic status. Several studies have found higher rates of material deprivation among women, although the material deprivation gender gap remains largely unexplained (Bárcena-Martín et al. 2014). Numerous studies have examined the connection between material deprivation and age, with somewhat contradictory results. Jehoel-Gijsbers and Vrooman (2008) and Dewilde (2008) observed that in almost all European countries material deprivation decreases with age. This is explained by the large proportion of older persons who own their home, which allows them to manage on a smaller income (Dewilde 2008); furthermore, the author posits that older people have better budgeting skills or grew up in an era when people had fewer material desires. In contrast, Hrast et al. (2013) showed that older people in Central and Eastern Europe experience significantly higher levels of exclusion than the rest of the population, identifying material deprivation as one of the biggest problems, and pointing to the failure of post-socialist welfare states to promote social inclusion among older people.

Several studies have established that less well-educated persons face a greater risk of material deprivation, whereas higher levels of education reduce the risk (Bárcena-Martín et al. 2014; Saltkjel and Malmberg-Heimonen 2017). The link between socio-economic status and the risk of material deprivation has also been well established. Unemployed or inactive persons have a higher risk [see Murdock et al. this section for an analysis of the impact of unemployment in later life], while households with one or more employed workers exhibit lower deprivation scores (De Graaf-Zijl and Nolan 2011; Bárcena-Martín et al. 2014).

Regarding the relationship between material deprivation and the structure of the household, studies have revealed fairly similar results across European countries. Those living alone, single parents, and families with small children are especially vulnerable (Boarini and Mira d'Ercole 2006; Dewilde 2008). From a life-course perspective, those in later life are particularly susceptible to specific events that affect the composition of the household. Adult children leaving home, divorce, or the death of a spouse [see Barlin et al. this section for a discussion of the material circumstances of widowed, and separated and divorced older women] may increase the risk of material deprivation (Bárcena-Martín et al. 2014).

A number of other key risk factors have also been identified. Franzese (2015), for example, has shown that material deprivation is strongly correlated with both physical and mental health. According to Hunkler et al. (2015), migrants experience greater material deprivation in older-age than non-migrants [see Gallassi and Harrysson this volume for a discussion of the economic and social situation of older migrants]. Levasseur et al. (2015) observed that despite higher residential density and social deprivation in urban areas with larger populations, material deprivation was greater among older adults in rural areas.

Several studies have attempted to ascertain the capacity of welfare states to modulate the risk of material deprivation (Muffels and Fouarge 2004; Jehoel-Gijsbers and Vrooman 2008; Nelson 2012; Saltkjel and Malmberg-Heimonen 2017). Muffels and Fouarge (2004) analysed 11 European countries and observed a higher prevalence of material deprivation in Southern and Liberal welfare regimes compared with Corporatist and Social-democratic regimes, concluding that the practices of welfare regimes concerning the distribution of resources and opportunities do have an effect on differences in material deprivation across countries. Jehoel-Gijsbers and Vrooman (2008) examined material deprivation among older people (aged 55 and over) in 26 European countries and observed the highest rates of material deprivation in Eastern Europe, followed by the Mediterranean welfare cluster. Nelson (2012) found the rate of material deprivation to be lower in countries with higher levels of social benefits. Similarly, Saltkjel and Malmberg-Heimonen (2017) demonstrated that the generous benefits of welfare states moderated the risk of material deprivation. However, it should be noted that, while Jehoel-Gijsbers and Vrooman (2008) focused on the 55+ age group, all of these other studies concentrate on those aged between 18–64 years. Consequently, how these risk factors vary across welfare regimes in later life remains poorly understood.

In summary, despite the sizeable number of studies investigating the links between material deprivation and socio-demographic risk factors and their variation across European countries, most existing studies do not focus specifically on older persons, are based on the EU material deprivation rate, and sometimes include only a limited set of individual risk factors. These gaps in existing research provided the motivation for our study.

3.2.3 Research Questions

In this study we pose two research questions:

(i) How does material deprivation among older persons vary according to socio-demographic risk factors?
(ii) How do the relationships between material deprivation and socio-demographic risk factors vary between groups of countries with different welfare regimes?

We base our analysis on cross-sectional SHARE data, which means that the target population of our study is comprised of individuals aged 50 years and over. By using the SHARE-based MDI as opposed to the EU-SILC-based MDR, we anticipate some differences in the results compared with the studies that utilised the latter measure. In contrast to the earlier SHARE-based analyses of associations between material deprivation and socio-demographic risk factors (*e.g.* Adena et al. 2015; Bertoni et al. 2015; Franzese 2015), we address a wider set of risk factors and investigate the variation in their effects across welfare clusters.

3.3 Data and Analytical Approach

The data used in this study come from SHARE, which is a pan-European survey. It produces cross-sectional and longitudinal data on a wide range of issues related to ageing and how it affects individuals in different societal contexts, with a central focus on socio-economic circumstances, physical and mental health, living arrangements, kinship and social networks. The main advantages of SHARE are comparability across a large number of countries, representative data on older persons without imposing an upper age limit, and the relatively large sample size (Börsch-Supan et al. 2013).

Our analysis is based on the fifth wave of the SHARE carried out in 2013 in 15 countries—Austria, Belgium, the Czech Republic, Denmark, Estonia, France, Germany, Israel, Italy, Luxembourg, Sweden, the Netherlands, Spain, Slovenia, and Switzerland (Börsch-Supan 2018). The fifth wave included a series of questions related to material deprivation (Adena et al. 2015).

As discussed above, the SHARE-based MDI includes 11 material deprivation items that refer to the inability of households to afford basic needs and to their financial difficulties (Adena et al. 2015). The MDI was computed as the weighted sum of these failures with respect to the items described above. The MDI used in this study is based on so-called hedonic weighting, which employs the correlation between the set of deprivation items and with self-assessed satisfaction with life. The resulting

MDI yields a score between 0 and 1 (for additional information on alternative weighting schemes and the Index, see Bertoni et al. 2015). In this study, we focus on whether individuals are materially deprived. A binary dependent variable is therefore constructed on the basis of the MDI, which is set at one if the respondent scored higher than zero on material deprivation, and zero otherwise. Our independent variables are: gender, age, living arrangements, number of children, educational attainment, labour market status, the presence of chronic diseases and activity limitations, area of residence, and migrant origin, which, based on the literature, can be expected to modulate the risk of material deprivation.

In this study our main interest relates to the variation in the relationship between material deprivation and socio-demographic risk factors across larger groups of countries, categorised as Anglo-Saxon, Continental, Nordic, Southern and Eastern European welfare regimes (*e.g.* Aiginger and Leoni 2009). As neither the UK nor Ireland is covered by SHARE, we omit the Anglo-Saxon welfare regime and group 15 SHARE countries into four clusters. Denmark, Sweden and the Netherlands comprise the Northern cluster. The inclusion of the Netherlands in the Northern cluster is supported by analyses of the Dutch welfare state (Sapir 2006; Eleveld and van Vliet 2013). Austria, Belgium, France, Germany, Luxembourg and Switzerland are included in the Western cluster. The Southern cluster is made up of Italy, Spain and Israel. While Israel bears some resemblance to a liberal welfare regime, the emphasis on family and religion allows the country to be included in the "extended family" of Mediterranean welfare regimes (Tarshis 2017). The Eastern cluster is comprised of the Czech Republic, Estonia, and Slovenia. Figure 3.1 presents the mean MDI values for the four clusters, which reveals marked contrasts in the levels of deprivation.

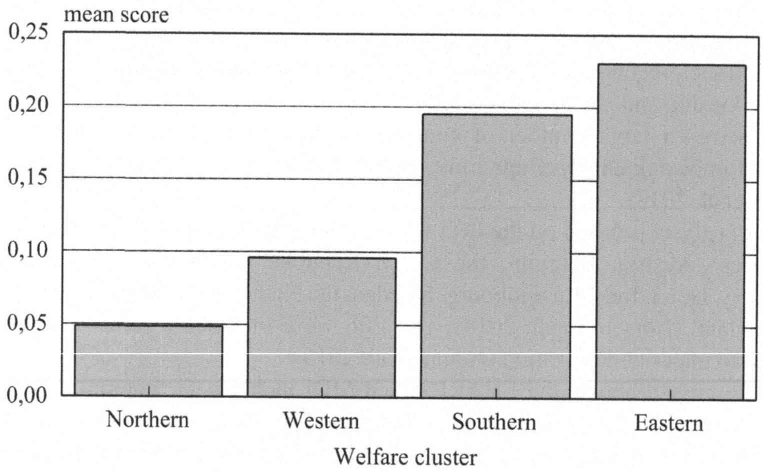

Fig. 3.1 Mean MDI score by welfare cluster, 2013

Source: SHARE database, authors' calculations

We employ logistic regression (SPSS Version 20) to analyse the relationship between material deprivation and the risk factors. Our modelling strategy is straightforward. For each cluster of countries, we estimate a series of hierarchical models. At the exploratory stage of analysis, we also estimated models with interactions between the risk factors and the clusters of countries. As the patterns were similar, we opted for separate models. In order to produce non-adjusted estimates, we insert one independent variable at a time into the models.

The adjusted models include the full complement of independent variables. Our working sample consists of 28,578 male and 36,270 female respondents, for a total of 64,848 respondents. Table 3.1 provides information on the number of persons at different levels of the independent variables and the related percentage distributions for the clusters of countries.

3.4 Results

Tables 3.2, 3.3, 3.4 and 3.5 present the odds ratios from the logistic regression models. The modelling results for the different clusters for each independent variable are discussed below.

Gender In accord with previous research, the non-adjusted odds ratios reveal a moderately elevated risk of material deprivation for women in all clusters. After adjusting for the effects of the other covariates, the statistically significant female disadvantage (1.12 times) persists only in the Eastern cluster. In the Northern and Western clusters, gender makes no significant difference to the odds of material deprivation. By contrast, the Southern cluster features an inversion of the gender gradient: according to the adjusted model, women are less deprived.

Age Our results indicate considerable diversity in the age pattern of material deprivation across clusters. With regard to the non-adjusted estimates, the Northern and Western clusters exhibit no cross-cutting change in material deprivation in relation to age. The observed pattern is curvilinear with an increase in the odds ratio from 50–64 year-olds to 65–79 year-olds followed by a decrease among the 80+ age group. As a result of these opposing shifts, the non-adjusted deprivation risks among the youngest and oldest age groups are similar. By contrast, the Southern and Eastern clusters feature a systematic age-related increase in material deprivation to markedly high levels. Similar to the findings for gender, adjustment for the effects of other covariates produces a substantial transformation of the pattern. In the Northern and Western clusters, adjustment leads to the emergence of an inverse relationship between age and deprivation. Among the 80+ age group, the odds of material deprivation are 0.59 and 0.64 times lower compared with 50–64 year-olds, respectively. However, the Eastern and Southern clusters show no statistically significant association in the adjusted model between advanced age and the odds of

Table 3.1 Descriptive statistics of socio-demographic variables used in the models, SHARE countries, 2013

	Northern cluster		Western cluster		Southern cluster		Eastern cluster	
Variable	Count	%	Count	%	Count	%	Count	%
Gender								
Male	5836	46	10,934	45	6029	45	5779	41
Female	6928	54	13,607	55	7348	55	8387	59
Age group								
50–64	5507	44	11,497	48	5488	42	5830	42
65–79	5589	44	9527	40	5578	42	6328	45
80+	1504	12	3083	13	2095	16	1830	13
Living arrangements								
Living alone	2788	22	5686	23	1935	14	3285	23
Couple	8223	64	13,291	54	6227	47	7160	51
Couple with others	1462	11	4393	18	4159	31	2602	18
Single with others	291	2	1171	5	1056	8	1119	8
Number of children								
Childless	1064	8	2928	12	1233	9	901	6
1 child	1577	12	4685	19	2283	17	2717	19
2 children	5370	42	9015	37	4965	38	6756	48
3–4 children	4033	32	6651	27	3729	28	3279	23
5+ children	693	5	1212	5	925	7	485	3
Education								
Low	4251	34	7147	29	8952	68	4850	34
Medium	4139	33	10,895	45	2405	18	6840	48
High	4201	33	6262	26	1849	14	2422	17
Labour market status								
Retired	5841	46	12,116	50	5853	44	8467	60
Employed	5557	44	9025	37	4254	32	4695	34
Homemaker	515	4	2023	8	2377	18	243	2
Other	663	5	987	4	749	6	606	4
Chronic diseases								
0–1	7115	56	12,960	53	6813	51	6820	48
2+	5625	44	11,425	47	6526	49	7300	52
Activity limitations								
No	7409	58	13,554	55	8026	60	6467	46
Yes	5333	42	10,917	45	5314	40	7660	54
Area of residence								
Rural	2676	22	10,164	42	2057	16	4934	36
Smaller town	2795	23	5886	24	4177	33	3498	26
Larger town	3065	25	2391	10	2614	21	2297	17
Suburb	2538	21	2637	11	1198	10	817	6
City	1264	10	2927	12	2494	20	2089	15
Origin								
Native	11,711	92	20,758	85	11,116	83	12,097	85
Immigrant	1053	8	3783	15	2261	17	2069	15

Source: SHARE database, authors' calculations

Table 3.2 Odds ratios for material deprivation by gender and age (logistic regression models), SHARE countries, 2013

	Northern cluster		Western cluster		Southern cluster		Eastern cluster	
Variable	Non-adjusted	Adjusted	Non-adjusted	Adjusted	Non-adjusted	Adjusted	Non-adjusted	Adjusted
Gender								
Male	1	1	1	1	1	1	1	1
Female	1.25***	1.07	1.21***	1.01	1.13**	0.81***	1.23***	1.12*
Age group								
50–64	1	1	1	1	1	1	1	1
65–79	0.89**	0.79***	0.88***	0.80***	1.07	0.81***	1.17***	0.99
80+	1.03	0.59***	1.03	0.64***	1.54***	0.86	1.72***	1.07

*p < 0.05; **p < 0.01; ***p < 0.001

Model: The dependent variable is the binary index of material deprivation. In the non-adjusted models, the independent variables were added to the model one at a time. The adjusted model includes controls for gender, age group, living arrangements, number of children, educational attainment, labour market status, chronic diseases, activity limitations, area of residence, and origin

Table 3.3 Odds ratios for material deprivation by living arrangements and number of children (logistic regression models), SHARE countries, 2013

	Northern cluster		Western cluster		Southern cluster		Eastern cluster	
Variable	Non-adjusted	Adjusted	Non-adjusted	Adjusted	Non-adjusted	Adjusted	Non-adjusted	Adjusted
Living arrangements								
Living alone	1	1	1	1	1	1	1	1
Couple	0.43***	0.45***	0.56***	0.55***	0.65***	0.64***	0.60***	0.67***
Couple with others	0.57***	0.63***	0.67***	0.61***	1.00	0.98	0.61***	0.72***
Single with others	1.19	1.24	1.33***	1.17*	1.36***	1.23*	1.15	1.12
Number of children								
Childless	1.48***	1.10	1.15**	0.95	0.90	0.82*	1.63***	1.39***
1 child	1.34***	1.12	1.21**	1.12**	0.93	0.90	1.44***	1.31***
2 children	1	1	1	1	1	1	1	1
3–4 children	1.22***	1.21***	1.27***	1.27***	1.39***	1.26***	1.41***	1.38***
5+ children	1.63***	1.45***	2.48***	2.21***	2.80***	1.98***	2.35***	1.95***

* p < 0.05; ** p < 0.01; ***p < 0.001

Model: The dependent variable is the binary index of material deprivation. In the non-adjusted models, the independent variables were added to the model one at a time. The adjusted model includes controls for gender, age group, living arrangements, number of children, educational attainment, labour market status, chronic diseases, activity limitations, area of residence, and origin

Table 3.4 Odds ratios for material deprivation by education and labour market status (logistic regression models), SHARE countries, 2013

Variable	Northern cluster		Western cluster		Southern cluster		Eastern cluster	
	Non-adjusted	Adjusted	Non-adjusted	Adjusted	Non-adjusted	Adjusted	Non-adjusted	Adjusted
Education								
Low	1.81***	1.68***	2.40***	2.20***	3.25***	3.08***	3.04***	2.44***
Medium	1.29***	1.23***	1.46***	1.51***	1.55***	1.63***	1.80***	1.76***
High	1	1	1	1	1	1	1	1
Labour market status								
Retired	1	1	1	1	1	1	1	1
Employed	0.85***	0.84*	0.96	1.02	0.83***	1.10	0.65***	0.91
Homemaker	1.03	0.76*	1.04	0.89*	1.88***	1.75***	1.85***	1.64*
Other	2.80***	1.76***	3.02***	2.01***	2.42***	1.57***	2.38***	1.92***

*p < 0.05; **p < 0.01; ***p < 0.001

Model: The dependent variable is the binary index of material deprivation. In the non-adjusted models, the independent variables were added to the model one at a time. The adjusted model includes controls for gender, age group, living arrangements, number of children, educational attainment, labour market status, chronic diseases, activity limitations, area of residence, and origin

Table 3.5 Odds ratios for material deprivation by health-related characteristics, area of residence and origin (logistic regression models), SHARE countries, 2013

Variable	Northern cluster		Western cluster		Southern cluster		Eastern cluster	
	Non-adjusted	Adjusted	Non-adjusted	Adjusted	Non-adjusted	Adjusted	Non-adjusted	Adjusted
Chronic diseases								
0–1	1	1	1	1	1	1	1	1
2+	1.39***	1.12***	1.43***	1.18***	1.88***	1.40***	1.59***	1.07
Activity limitations								
No	1	1	1	1	1	1	1	1
Yes	1.70***	1.49***	1.84***	1.62***	2.53***	2.08***	2.33***	1.92***
Area of residence								
Rural	1	1	1	1	1	1	1	1
City	0.94	0.91	0.99	0.98	0.63***	0.73***	0.77***	0.82*
Suburb	1.10	1.06	0.93	0.91	0.96	1.12	0.53***	0.57***
Larger town	0.96	0.92	1.11*	1.04	0.93	1.07	0.92	0.86*
Smaller town	1.01	0.99	1.00	1.00	0.84	0.90	0.90	0.94
Origin								
Native	1	1	1	1	1	1	1	1
Immigrant	1.80***	1.62***	1.66***	1.62***	0.94	1.38***	2.31***	2.44***

*p < 0.05; **p < 0.01; ***p < 0.001

Model: The dependent variable is the binary index of material deprivation. In the non-adjusted models, the independent variables were added to the model one at a time. The adjusted model includes controls for gender, age group, living arrangements, number of children, educational attainment, labour market status, chronic diseases, activity limitations, area of residence, and origin deprivation. Among the 65–79 age group, differences across welfare clusters are smaller.

Living Arrangements The association between household context and material deprivation is strong and relatively uniform. In all clusters, living as a couple markedly reduces the odds of deprivation relative to living alone. In the adjusted model, the reduction appears largest in the Northern cluster (0.45 times) and smallest in the Eastern cluster (0.67 times). Interestingly, the contrast between living as a couple and living alone peaks in the Northern cluster. Considering that the welfare systems in the Nordic countries are the least familistic, one might have expected a different result.

In most clusters, couples living with others are also better protected against material deprivation than older individuals living alone. The only exception is the Southern cluster in which the presence of other family members in the household is associated with the same risk of material deprivation as experienced by those living in one-person households. Finally, the highest odds of material deprivation are found among single persons living with others. In the Western and Southern clusters, their risk of deprivation significantly exceeds that of the reference group. The similarity of the adjusted and non-adjusted estimates suggests that the relationship between living arrangements and material deprivation is relatively independent of the other factors considered in the analysis.

Number of Children In most clusters, childlessness and having one child are associated with elevated risks of material deprivation relative to the reference group (individuals with two children) in the non-adjusted models. However, after adjustment, moderate excess risks persist only in the Eastern cluster, and to a limited extent in the Western cluster (only for those with one child). In the Southern cluster, childlessness is associated with lower odds of deprivation. However, having a large family distinctly increases the risks of material deprivation in all clusters. In the Western, Southern and Eastern clusters having five or more children is associated with a 1.95 to 2.21 increase in the adjusted odds of deprivation. Only in the Northern cluster does the excess risk appear somewhat smaller, plausibly reflecting the capability of Nordic welfare systems to bolster economic inequalities arising from family circumstances.

Education In all clusters, individuals with a medium or low education exhibit substantially higher risks of deprivation compared with those with high education. In the adjusted models, the odds ratio of deprivation ranges from 1.23 to 1.76 for medium-educated older persons, and from 1.68 to 3.04 for those with low education. Plausibly supported by generous welfare systems and lower economic inequality, differences in material deprivation according to the level of education appear smallest in the Northern cluster. By contrast, the largest differences are found in the Southern and Eastern clusters.

Labour Market Status The non-adjusted estimates show that being employed reduces the risk of material deprivation: with the exception of the Western cluster, the difference from the reference group (retirees) is statistically significant. However, after adjustment for the effects of the other covariates, the protective effect associated with employment loses significance in most clusters. This suggests that retirement in itself does not involve a significant increase in the risks of material deprivation. The opposite may hold true in the Northern cluster, although only to a limited extent.

The association between homemaking and material deprivation exhibits more variation. In the Northern and Western clusters, homemakers do not show any excess risk of deprivation. According to the adjusted estimates, the odds of being deprived are as much as 0.76 times lower for homemakers relative to the reference group. In the Eastern and Southern clusters, however, homemaking is related to a significant excess in risk of deprivation, ranging from 1.64 to 1.75. Individuals in the residual category feature substantially elevated risks of material deprivation, but, unlike for homemakers, the pattern is similar across clusters.

Chronic Diseases and Activity Limitations Having multiple chronic diseases and activity limitations adds substantially to the risk of deprivation. In all clusters but one (the Eastern), a significant association between deprivation and chronic diseases persists after the inclusion of the other covariates in the model. The effects of activity limitations are significant in all clusters. The effect appears more pronounced in Southern and Eastern clusters and more moderate in Northern and Western clusters. This suggests that welfare systems in the Northern and Western clusters are more supportive of the economic needs of older persons in poor health.

Area of Residence Area of residence makes only a limited difference in the risks of material deprivation. In the Northern and Western clusters, differences in the odds of deprivation associated with area of residence are not significant. In the Southern cluster, living in a city entails a reduction of 0.73 times in the odds of deprivation relative to rural residence. In the Eastern cluster, the largest advantage relates to living in suburbs. This finding is not surprising, as many countries of Eastern Europe experienced a tide of suburbanisation among the more affluent strata of the population after the fall of state socialism. Overall, in both the Southern and Eastern clusters, the results indicate a disadvantage for rural residents that is not counterbalanced by the welfare system [see Vidovićová et al. this volume for the consequences of such a disadvantage for care provision].

Origin Although arrival in the host country usually occurs relatively early in the life course, the disadvantage associated with immigrant origin does not disappear but persists well into old-age. Our results show that higher risks of deprivation among immigrants can be found in all clusters. However, there is a considerable variation in the odds ratios of deprivation for immigrants, ranging from 1.38 in the Southern cluster to 2.44 in the Eastern cluster in the adjusted model. We think that the observed differences stem not only from contrasts between host societies but also from the diverse origins and characteristics of immigrants across clusters.

3.5 Conclusion

In this chapter, we used SHARE data to investigate the risk of material deprivation of older persons as a dimension of economic exclusion associated with socio-demographic factors in 14 countries across Europe and Israel. In the context of research on material deprivation, the contribution of our study is derived from several elements. First of all, the SHARE material deprivation index employed in this study is specifically designed to consider the material needs of older persons (Adena et al. 2015). Furthermore, only a few comparative analyses of material deprivation have been conducted on the basis of SHARE data (Bertoni et al. 2015; Franzese 2015; Hunkler et al. 2015). However, to the best of our knowledge, none of the SHARE-based analyses have systematically investigated the variation in the role of socio-demographic risk factors across country clusters with different welfare regimes in contemporary Europe. An extended range of risk factors pertaining to individuals rather than the head of household also enhances its contribution to the literature. Finally, the strict harmonisation of the SHARE data circumvents the lack of comparability that plagues the findings from single-country studies.

The study found statistically significant effects for all the risk factors considered. In accordance with most previous research (Boarini and Mira d'Ercole 2006; Bárcena-Martin et al. 2014), lower education, living alone, having health-related activity limitations, and being of immigrant origin markedly elevated the risk of material deprivation among older persons, sometimes doubling the odds. For gender, age, and area of residence, the effects were less pronounced. Corroborating earlier comparative studies of the older population (Jehoel-Gijsbergs and Vrooman 2008; Bertoni et al. 2015), our findings suggest that older persons in the countries of Northern and Western Europe are generally less materially deprived than their counterparts in Southern and Eastern Europe. This indicates that the welfare regimes may play a protective role buffering against material deprivation in later life.

Separate models for clusters of countries revealed some interesting and seldom reported variations in the effects associated with the risk factors. Although most earlier studies have found that women are more deprived than men (Muffles and Fouarge 2004; Bertoni et al. 2015), in this study this was found to be true, and only to a limited extent, in the Eastern cluster. For other groups of countries women exhibited similar (Northern and Western) or even lower (the Southern cluster) risks of deprivation than men. A commonly reported pattern whereby deprivation risks decrease with age (Jehoel-Gijsbergs and Vrooman 2008) was observed only in the Northern and Western clusters; in other clusters the risks did not diminish or did so for only part of the older population. While previous research has focussed on the relationship between the number of children currently living in the household (Boarini and Mira d'Ercole 2006), our study provides insight into the effects associated with the number of offspring irrespective of co-residence with their parents. The results suggest that the disadvantage related to having a large family persists well into old-age in all clusters. Finally, there are also differences between clusters associated with the effects of homemaking, area of residence, and migrant status that have not been reported in previous studies. This suggests that material deprivation does not always affect vulnerable groups to the same degree in all countries.

Across clusters of countries, the smallest differences in deprivation risks associated with socio-demographic factors are characteristic of the Northern cluster. The results for the Western cluster appear quite similar. By contrast, the Southern and Eastern clusters exhibit much larger differences in the risks of material deprivation. A closer examination of the results suggests that the Eastern cluster more frequently ranks higher than the Southern cluster [see Grigoryeva et al. this volume for a discussion of welfare reform in Eastern and post-Soviet contexts]. These findings lend support to the notion that more generous welfare systems and greater equality provide better support to population groups at risk of material deprivation. With regard to policy implications that are relevant for economic exclusion, this study identifies subgroups of the older population that encounter disproportionately high risks of material deprivation, in some or all clusters, that will need consideration into the future as ageing populations grow and become increasingly diverse.

Editors' Postscript

Please note, like other contributions to this book, this chapter was written before the COVID-19 pandemic of 2020. The book's introductory chapter (Chap. 1) and conclusion (Chap. 34) consider some of the key ways in which the pandemic relates to issues concerning social exclusion and ageing.

Acknowledgements This study was supported by a grant from the Estonian Research Council (PRG71). The study uses data from SHARE wave 5 (DOI:https://doi.org/10.6103/SHARE.w5.700).

References

Adena, M., Myck, M., & Oczkowska, M. (2015). Material deprivation items in SHARE wave 5 data: A contribution to a better understanding of differences in material conditions in later life. In A. Börsch-Supan, T. Kneip, H. Litwin, M. Myck, & G. Weber (Eds.), *Ageing in Europe – Supporting policies for an inclusive society* (pp. 25–37). Berlin: De Gruyter.

Aiginger, K., & Leoni, T. (2009). *Typologies of social models in Europe*. Vienna: Austrian Institute of Economic Research WIFO.

Bárcena-Martín, E., Lacomba, B., Moro-Egido, A. I., & Pérez-Moreno, S. (2014). Country differences in material deprivation in Europe. *Review of Income and Wealth, 60*(4), 802–820.

Bertoni, M., Cavapozzi, D., Celidoni, M., & Trevisan, E. (2015). Assessing the material deprivation of older Europeans. In A. Börsch-Supan, T. Kneip, H. Litwin, et al. (Eds.), *Ageing in Europe – Supporting policies for an inclusive society* (pp. 49–56). Berlin: De Gruyter.

Boarini, R., & Mira d'Ercole, M. (2006). *Measures of material deprivation in OECD countries* (OECD Social, Employment And Migration Working Papers No. 37). Paris: OECD.

Börsch-Supan, A. (2018). *Survey of health, ageing and retirement in Europe (SHARE) Wave 5*. Release version: 6.1.0. SHARE-ERIC. Data set.

Börsch-Supan, A., Brandt, M., Hunkler, C., Kneip, T., Korbmacher, J., Malter, F., et al. (2013). Data resource profile: The survey of health, ageing and retirement in Europe (SHARE). *International Journal of Epidemiology, 42*(4), 992–1001.

De Graaf-Zijl, M., & Nolan, B. (2011). Household joblessness and its impact on poverty and deprivation in Europe. *Journal of European Social Policy, 21*(5), 413–431.

Dewilde, C. (2008). Individual and institutional determinants of multidimensional poverty: A European comparison. *Social Indicators Research, 68*(2), 233–256.

Eleveld, A., & van Vliet, O. (2013). The Dutch welfare state: Recent reforms in social security and labour law. *Diritto Pubblico Comparato Ed Europeo, 4*, 1371–1399.

Eurostat. (2019). *EU statistics on income and living conditions (EU-SILC) methodology*. https://ec.europa.eu/eurostat/statistics-explained/index.php/EU_statistics_on_income_and_living_conditions_(EU-SILC)_methodology. Accessed 3 Dec 2019.

Franzese, F. (2015). Slipping into poverty: Effects on mental and physical health. In A. Börsch-Supan, T. Kneip, H. Litwin, M. Myck, & G. Weber (Eds.), *Ageing in Europe – Supporting policies for an inclusive society* (pp. 139–147). Berlin: De Gruyter.

Fusco, A., Guio, A.-C., & Marlier, E. (2010). Characterising the income poor and the materially deprived in European countries. In A. B. Atkinson & E. Marlier (Eds.), *Income and living conditions in Europe* (Eurostat statistical books). Luxembourg: Publications Office of the European Union.

Fusco, A., Guio, A.-C., & Marlier, E. (2013). Building a material deprivation index in a multinational context: Lessons from the EU experience. In V. Bérenger & F. Bresson (Eds.), *Poverty and social exclusion around the Mediterranean Sea* (Economic studies in inequality, social exclusion and well-being 9) (pp. 43–71). New York: Springer.

Guio, A.-C. (2009). *What can be learned from deprivation indicators in Europe?* (Eurostat Methodologies and Working Paper). Eurostat: Luxembourg.

Hrast, M. F., Mrak, A. K., & Rakar, T. (2013). Social exclusion of elderly in Central and Eastern Europe. *International Journal of Social Economics, 40*(11), 971–989.

Hunkler, C., Kneip, T., Sand, G., & Schuth, M. (2015). Growing old abroad: Social and material deprivation among first-and second generation migrants in Europe. In A. Börsch-Supan, T. Kneip, H. Litwin, M. Myck, & G. Weber (Eds.), *Ageing in Europe-supporting policies for an inclusive society* (pp. 199–208). Berlin: De Gruyter.

Jehoel-Gijsbers, G., & Vrooman, C. (2008). *Social exclusion of the elderly: A comparative study of EU member states* (ENEPRI research report no. 57). Brussels: ENEPRI.

Levasseur, M., Cohen, A. A., Dubois, M. F., Généreux, M., Richard, L., Therrien, F. H., & Payette, H. (2015). Environmental factors associated with social participation of older adults living in metropolitan, urban, and rural areas: The NuAge study. *American Journal of Public Health, 105*(8), 1718–1725.

Muffels, R., & Fouarge, D. (2004). The role of European welfare states in explaining resources deprivation. *Social Indicators Research, 68*(3), 299–330.

Myck, M., Ogg, J., Aigner-Walder, B., Kåreholt, I., Kostakis, I., Motel-Klingebiel, A., et al. (2017). *Economic aspects of old age exclusion: A scoping report.* ROSEnet Economic Working Group, Knowledge synthesis series: No. 1. CA 15122 Reducing Old-Age Exclusion: Collaborations in Research and Policy.

Nelson, K. (2012). Counteracting material deprivation: The role of social assistance in Europe. *Journal of European Social Policy, 22*(2), 148–163.

Renahy, E., Alvarado-Llano, B., Koh, M., & Quesnel-Vallée, A. (2012). Income and economic exclusion: Do they measure the same concept? *International Journal for Equity in Health, 11*, 4. https://doi.org/10.1186/1475-9276-11-4.

Saltkjel, T., & Malmberg-Heimonen, I. (2017). Welfare generosity in Europe: A multi-level study of material deprivation and income poverty among disadvantaged groups. *Social Policy and Administration, 51*(7), 1287–1310.

Sapir, A. (2006). Globalization and the reform of European social models. *Journal of Common Market Studies, 44*(2), 369–390.

Saunders, P. (2008). Social exclusion: Challenges for research and implications for policy. *The Economic and Labour Relations Review, 19*(1), 73–92.

Scharf, T. (2015). Between inclusion and exclusion in later life. In K. Walsh, G. Carney, & Á. N. Léime (Eds.), *Ageing through austerity: Critical perspectives from Ireland* (pp. 113–130). Bristol: Policy Press.

Scharf, T., Phillipson, C., & Smith, A. E. (2005). Social exclusion of older people in deprived urban communities of England. *European Journal of Ageing, 2*(2), 76–87.

Tarshis, N. (2017). Israel as a welfare state: A visual essay. *Bulletin Articles*. http://taubcenter.org.il/israel-as-a-welfare-state/. Accessed 12 Sept 2019.

Walsh, K., Scharf, T., & Keating, N. (2017). Social exclusion of older persons: A scoping review and conceptual framework. *European Journal of Ageing, 14*(1), 81–98.

Chapter 4
Unemployment at 50+: Economic and Psychosocial Consequences

Elke Murdock, Marceline Filbig, and Rita Borges Neves

4.1 Introduction

In 2018, a record number of 71,338 people between the ages of 50 and 64 years old were unemployed in Europe (OECD 2018). The number of people aged 65 years or over in the world is forecast to increase by 46% between 2017 and 2030, outnumbering younger people in a huge social transformation (ILOSTAT 2019). Thus, the number of people aged 50 years and over in the labour force will increase significantly. Furthermore, the political shift towards extending working lives, by increasing statutory retirement age, makes early retirement financially less sustainable. This results in more older workers registering as unemployed when made redundant. The implications of these circumstances for experiences of economic exclusion have the potential to be severe. Despite this and the growing number of older people affected by unemployment, there is a marked lack of unemployment policies targeting late-career unemployed. There is also a general lack of research exploring how late career job loss may generate severe forms of economic exclusion in later life, with implications for material and other forms of economic outcomes. Although significant consequences for psychosocial well-being have been documented for other groups of unemployed people (McKee-Ryan et al. 2005; Paul and Moser 2009; Griep et al. 2015), there has been little consideration of these impacts for older workers.

E. Murdock (✉)
Institute for Life Course Development, Family and Culture, University of Luxembourg, Esch-sur -Alzette, Luxembourg
e-mail: elke.murdock@uni.lu

M. Filbig
Management and Coaching in Education and Social Sciences (MAMACO) Programme, University of Luxembourg, Esch-sur-Alzette, Luxembourg

R. Borges Neves
Centre for Decent Work, Management School, University of Sheffield, Sheffield, UK

K. Walsh et al. (eds.), *Social Exclusion in Later Life*, International Perspectives on Aging 28, https://doi.org/10.1007/978-3-030-51406-8_4

In this chapter, we draw attention to the latent functions of work and the psychosocial consequences of job loss in later life. Applying a life-course perspective, the aim of this chapter is to explore how job loss can be framed as a form of acute economic exclusion, and how this exclusion can have significant implications for poor mental health. We start by considering ageing and work and positioning the experience of work within the older adult life course. We provide a brief look at ageing in general, and the phase of middle adulthood in particular, before turning to the specifics of the older adult worker. We then look at the latent functions of work, which can be closely linked to the framework of old-age exclusion (Walsh et al. 2017; Walsh 2019). We then turn to the economic and psychosocial consequences of unemployment. As the German novelist Thomas Mann (2019) observed "Work is hard, is often a bleak and tedious prodding; but not working – that is hell". Focusing on the experiences of older unemployed persons in Luxembourg, we will present selected survey findings around the subjective experience of unemployment and coping processes, and their relationship with psychosocial well-being. We present this analysis in an effort to inform policy development for assisting older adults in dealing with the economic and psychosocial consequences of unemployment.

4.2 Ageing and Work

We are all ageing. To live is to grow older. As we move into adulthood, two aspects dominate – intimacy – forming close relationships, and generativity – being productive for and supporting future generations (Erikson 1963). Various terms have been suggested to describe these aspects including affiliation and achievement, attachment and productivity, commitment and competence. As observed by Freud (1935), adulthood is about love and work. A healthy adult is one who can love and work. For many adults, the answer to the question "Who are you?" depends on the answer to "What do you do?" Work can provide us with a sense of identity and opportunities for accomplishment (Myers 2006). Challenging and interesting positions enhance people's happiness. Research has shown that it is not the occupational role per se, but it is the quality of experience in the respective roles that mattered and affected well-being (Baruch and Barnett 1986). Happiness is about finding work that fits your interest and provides you with a sense of competence. Employment marks the transition into adulthood. Failure to make this transition into work and to establish an occupational identity can be accompanied by increased stress levels (Donovan and Oddy 1982; Tiggemann and Winefield 1984). The phase of middle adulthood is the phase of quiet transitions and has been characterised as an "in-between state." At 40 years plus, one is neither young nor old and the generational structure is changing (Perrig-Chiello and Höpflinger 2001; Höpflinger and Perrig-Chiello 2009). Children are in the process of leaving or having left home and individuals' parents are getting older and needing more care, requiring an intergenerational role reversal. In addition to this "in-between" positioning, this phase in life is accompanied by commitment and closure, as substantial decisions have been taken in the professional and private domain. Even though changes are still possible, these are increasingly effortful and complicated. It is a time of taking stock about goals accomplished – and a realisation that opportunities for professional change/mobility or future chances for professional re-orientation are reducing.

In that sense, ageing is the simultaneous accumulation of achievements and alternatives not taken (Perrig-Chiello and Höpflinger 2001). Paul and Moser (2009) noted that it is often assumed that this middle-aged group would be psychologically hardest hit by unemployment as this group often has family responsibilities, greater dependence on financial income and strong career commitment. However, in a meta-analysis these authors showed a curvilinear relationship between age, psychological stress and unemployment, with young unemployed and older unemployed nearing retirement showing the highest stress levels. The authors expressed surprise at this finding and commented that "studies with older unemployed workers are also rare, although most industrialised societies experience demographic changes that will lead to a higher proportion of elder persons in the labour market in the near future" (Paul and Moser 2009, p. 280).

Successful ageing means selective optimisation and compensation to maximise the use and mobilisation of available resources (Baltes et al. 1992). Yet, with increasing age, the range of options diminishes. Across the lifespan, the overall aim is thus to solidify gains and to minimise losses. As explained in the life-cycle theory of consumption (Modigliani and Brumberg 1954) people plan their lifetime economic activity. If unemployment hits in old-age – there may not be a chance to recover the losses. Older persons are not at greater risk to *become* unemployed – the age-specific risk is to *stay* unemployed (Brussig et al. 2006). As such, the risk of being long-term unemployed and never regaining access to the labour market increases with age.

4.2.1 The Meaning of Work

The increased stress levels among the older unemployed may be explained by considering the meaning of work. Marie Jahoda (1981, 1983, 1997) looked beyond the obvious economic consequences of (un-) employment and explored the psychological meaning of employment and unemployment. Jahoda developed the model of *manifest* and *latent* functions of employment. The manifest function of work is earning money – which maps to the domain of material and financial resources in the framework on old-age exclusion (Walsh et al. 2017). Yet work also fulfils latent functions and these include (a) providing a clear time structure, (b) an activity, (c) social status, (d) social contact beyond the nuclear family and (e) participation in a collective purpose, allowing meaningful societal engagement (Jahoda 1997). It can be argued that these latent functions mirror elements of other domains of social exclusion frameworks, namely social relations, socio-cultural factors, neighbourhood and community and civic participation. These latent functions of work satisfy important human needs with employment deprivation having psychosocial consequences.

If people are deprived access to these latent functions, their mental health will suffer. Jahoda's model has found empirical support (*e.g.* Paul and Batinic 2010; Selenko et al. 2011). However, Jahoda's model has also been criticised for placing not enough weight on the manifest factors (Fryer 1986). Paul and Moser (2006) suggest the incongruence hypothesis. They argue that a lack of fit between aspirations in terms of values and life goals and the current state of employment is the main source of stress. However, despite these differences, what these models have in common is that they link economic, social and psychological functions relating to the meaning of work.

4.2.2 Economic Consequences of Unemployment at 50+

In western capitalist societies, paid work is still the main source of income for most people and it allows access to vital material resources and to the "consumers' society'. Even in more generous welfare states that provide higher unemployment benefits, these are always a percentage of previous salaries and for a limited period. As noted by Brand (2015), job loss is an involuntary disruptive life event with far-reaching impact on workers' life trajectories. She clarifies the differences between job loss and unemployment. Whereas job loss is a discrete event, unemployment is a transitional state with a great deal of heterogeneity with respect to instigation and duration. Involuntary job loss may also indicate job separation as a result of health conditions – which becomes increasingly likely with advancing age. Job separation for health reasons may be worker initiated but can nevertheless be considered involuntary (Brand 2015). Ultimately, unemployment, and particularly long-term unemployment, represents financial deprivation and material ill-being [see Sumil-Laanemaa et al. this section]. Older unemployed adults can experience a longer duration before reemployment, with post-displacement jobs then tending to be of a shorter duration (Chan and Stevens 2001), to pay less than the lost job, and to be of lower quality (Samorodov 1999). Unemployment also diminishes income flows and represents a toll on retirement pensions. This heightens economic exclusion into older-ages (Chan and Stevens 1999; Arent and Nagl 2010; Myck et al. 2017). Commenting on the economic effects of job loss, Brand (2015) noted that the cumulative lifetime earning loss is estimated to be roughly 20%, with wage-scarring observed as long as 20 years post displacement. As noted above, older workers are at greater risk to stay unemployed and may therefore not have the opportunity to make up for losses. Thus, the economic consequences for older unemployed are potentially even more severe.

4.2.3 Psychosocial Consequences of Unemployment at 50+

A large body of research has focused on the relationship between unemployment and psychological well-being (*e.g.* McKee-Ryan et al. 2005; Paul and Moser 2009; Brand 2015). Paul and Moser (2009) compared mental health of employed and unemployed persons for the general population. Their study showed that 16% of the employed and 34% of the unemployed persons suffered from mental health problems. Thus, the unemployed have twice the risk of suffering from mental illness – unemployment having the potential to be a serious threat to public health. Paul and Moser's (2009) analyses also showed that the young and older unemployed are at particular risk in terms of mental health. Thus for the older-age group involuntary unemployment not only represents labour market exclusion or higher exposure to precariousness and economic deprivation, they are also more affected by psychosocial-related consequences as is confirmed by specific research on older unemployed workers (*e.g.* Chu et al. 2016). Later life unemployment may therefore threaten participation of older adults in the labour market as well as the realisation of ones' potential. Drawing on literature on the more general area of health and employment, unemployment is a risk factor for detriments in mental and physical health, physical disability and difficulties in performing basic activities of daily living (Gallo et al. 2009; Chu et al. 2016). This has the potential to widen the already steep health inequality at midlife and increase the risk of economic and social exclusion in later life. The onset of several illnesses has been attributed to experiences of job loss and older unemployed have a higher risk of physical disability (Gallo et al. 2009). Chu et al.'s (2016) study evaluated whether late-career unemployment is associated with increased all-cause mortality, functional disability, and depression among older adults in Taiwan. Their findings indicate that late-career unemployment increases the risks of future mortality and disability. Despite affecting a large number of people and its consequences being so severe, the literature that looks at the lived experience of unemployment in late career in relation to exclusion is not abundant.

One of the few in-depth studies focusing on psychosocial vulnerabilities of older adults following unemployment was conducted by Hansson et al. (1990). The aim of this study among 82 older unemployed adults was to gain a better understanding of the psychosocial consequences of unemployment – with a view to developing targeted unemployment counselling programmes for older adults. Their data suggested that support for older unemployed should attempt to differentiate between clients with different needs and different profiles of personal and social competence. Their findings point to the diversity of older unemployed. The authors observed that professional seniority does not offer protection for older workers in times of crisis. On the contrary – older workers in senior positions were found to have to compete with younger workers who were sometimes more mobile, whose education was more recent and possibly more extensive, and who often had more transferable skills. In addition, older workers were more likely to need training in interview skills and job-hunting strategies, given their time spent in stable employment. Again, older adults were found to be in danger of experiencing prolonged unemployment and often were found to have dropped out of the job market altogether. Prolonged unemployment also contributed to the decision to accept early retirement, even at reduced benefit.

Therefore, unemployment in late career may be the greatest threat to one's security and independence because of the risk of permanent exclusion from the labour market. The severity of health and psychological consequences were related to what a person lost when losing their job. Older workers, who had been loyal and productive for many years and committed more of their identity to work, were psychologically more affected by the unemployment. This is referred to as work-role centrality in McKee-Ryan and Kinicki's (2002) *life facet model* of coping with job loss. The authors explain the process of reacting to job loss in a coping – stress framework. Based on this model, McKee-Ryan et al. (2005) developed a taxonomy for their meta-analytic study on well-being during unemployment. Contributing elements to psychological and physical well-being following job loss include the aforementioned: (a) work-role centrality, that is the general importance of the work role to an individual's sense of self; (b) coping resources; (c) cognitive appraisal including attribution style; (d) coping strategies, *i.e.* the cognitive and behavioural efforts linked to managing the situation; and (e) human capital and demographics, *i.e.* education, ability and educational status.

To delve further into first-hand experiences of these impacts, in the next section we will consider a recent empirical study concerning coping strategies, well-being and job loss conducted in Luxembourg.

4.3 Coping Strategies and Well-being Among Older Unemployed in Luxembourg

In accordance with the life facet model of coping with job loss (McKee-Ryan and Kinicki's 2002), we investigated the role of cognitive appraisal, coping strategies and coping resources in subjective well-being of older unemployed. People differ in how they interpret job loss. How responsibility for job loss is assigned and interpreted, or cognitively appraised, is relevant to well-being in unemployment (McKee-Ryan et al. 2005). Coping strategies are also associated with increased psychological health during unemployment (Kanfer et al. 2001). Coping resources such as social support and personal traits (*i.e.* self-efficacy or emotional stability) also contribute to psychological well-being (McKee-Ryan and Kinicki 2002).

4.3.1 Methodology

4.3.1.1 Participants

Sixty-seven older unemployed individuals participated in this quantitative study in Luxembourg and completed a paper-based questionnaire. They were recruited at advisory and training centres for unemployed persons. Women were over-represented in this sample with n = 54 (80.6%). The average age was 52.65 (*SD* = 3.86, *range* = 46–61). The educational level was reasonably high with 34% of the sample holding a university degree and 21% holding the highest school leaving qualification (13 years of secondary education). Sixteen per cent held a professional qualification and 15% completed basic education (9 years of education) whilst 13% indicated other. Health restrictions were indicated by 28% of respondents. About 30% lived alone. A further 30% lived with their partner and their children: 20% lived with just their partner and 16% identified themselves as single mothers.

The (un-)employment history of respondents is summarised in Table 4.1 and illustrates a sample with a broad range of (un-)employment experiences. Participants with health restrictions are concentrated in the longer-term (>12 months) unemployment group.

Table 4.1 Participant's employment history

		Frequencies in %
Length of unemployment	<1 month	12
	1 – < 3 months	25
	3 – < 6 months	10
	6 – < 12 months	25
	12 – < 24 months	15
	>24 months	10
Length of former employment	<6 months	13
	6 – < 12 months	9
	12 – < 24 months	22
	2–10 years	30
	>10 years	18
Former contract	Fixed term	31
	Permanent	69
Unemployment history	Never before unemployed	34
	1 time before unemployed	34
	Several times unemployed	30

4.3.2 Measures

For cognitive appraisal processes, respondents had to rate to what extent a range of factors contributed to their job loss on a scale from one (not at all) to five (a lot). As shown in Table 4.2, some of these factors are external to the person, such as a crisis within the company or the economic climate. If a person associated their job loss with such an external event, we classified this as an external attribution (E). Other factors were associated directly with the person, which we classified as internal (I). While some of these internal factors could be potentially controlled by a person (*i.e.* engagement or skills) others, such as age or illness, were outside their control.

We also developed a series of items assessing coping strategies and resources. The items and domains are listed in Table 4.3. For proactive coping, the domains include persistence and flexibility of goal adjustment. Regarding coping resources, we included external and family support. In terms of personal resources, we included self-efficacy and hope. Since we focus on older unemployed persons, we also asked specifically about age as a barrier to regaining employment. Participants rated these items on a scale from one (does not apply at all) to four (totally applies).

Subjective well-being was assessed using the Satisfaction with Life Scale (SWLS, Diener et al. 1985, Diener 2006). The scale consists of five items, which are assessed on a seven-point Likert Scale. The Cronbach alpha coefficient for the SWLS scale was 0.80.

Table 4.2 Internal and external attribution of unemployment, ranked by mean scores

Categories:		Mean	SD	Frequency of mentions (%)
Crisis within the company	E	2.32	1.77	37.3
Age	I	2.28	1.42	**52.2**
Economic climate	E	2.11	1.42	43.3
Bad luck	E	1.98	1.45	37.3
Sickness/health problems	I	1.89	1.49	**28.4**
Fixed term contract	E	1.88	1.55	26.9
Disagreement with management	E	1.84	1.37	31.3
Mobbing	E	1.83	1.32	35.8
Lack of language skills	I	1.63	1.13	26.9
Problems with colleagues	E	1.56	1.11	23.9
Personal problems	I	1.51	0.98	25.4
Lack of specific skills	I	1.51	0.94	25.4
Family problems	I	1.47	1.08	19.4
Lack of personal engagement	I	1.31	0.79	17.9
Own misconduct	I	1.13	0.50	7.5

Table 4.3 Descriptive statistics: experience of unemployment and job seeking strategies

Item	*M*	*SD*	Domain	*M*	*SD*	*r*
I am confident to find a job in the near future.	2.85	0.88	Hope			
I believe that my professional profile fits the requirements of employers.	2.61	0.8	Self-efficacy	2.89	0.60	0.49**
I can present myself well in job interviews	3.17	0.6				
Even if I receive rejections, I continue searching for a job.	3.66	0.69	Persistence			
My age makes it difficult to find a job.	3.42	0.82	Age as perceived barrier	3.09	0.74	0.46**
My age is an important topic in job interviews.	2.76	0.92				
I am willing educate myself further to improve my chances on the job market.	3.58	0.7	Flexibility of goal adjustment	3.42	0.64	α = 0.69
I am willing to work in a completely different area/ sector.	3.44	0.78				
I am willing to accept a position I am actually overqualified for.	3.24	0.92				
I feel supported by my job agency.	2.71	0.99	Perceived external support	2.57	0.83	0.37**
I feel supported by other agencies.	2.44	1.01				
I am experiencing strong support from my family.	2.96	1.09	Family support			

Note: *p < .05, **p < .01

4.3.3 Results

Over half (55%) of the respondents attributed their unemployment, at least in part, to their age, but the extent of this designation was varied. While 45% indicated that age did not play a role in becoming unemployed, 9% indicated that age played a large role, 15% indicated it played a role, and a further 15% thought that age played a small role. For all other categories, the response pattern was different – with each factor either playing either an important role or none. Thus, when rating factors contributing to unemployment, gradations were hardly used, with the exception of age. With reference to Table 4.2, external attribution for job loss dominates, apart from age (2nd place) and illness. These latter factors are associated with the individual but are outside respondents' control.

Descriptive statistics for the items relating to the subjective experience of unemployment and coping strategies are presented in Table 4.3 and show *means* above the scale midpoint for all domains. There are no gender differences.

A comparison of groups according to length of unemployment (n = 24 < = 3 months; n = 14, 4–11 months; n = 29 > = 12 months) showed no significant differences for these items or domains with one exception: more recent unemployed had significantly lower mean scores for age as a barrier than the other two groups:

Table 4.4 Correlations between experiences of unemployment domains and SWLS

	1	2	3	4	5	6	7	8
Hope	1	0.23	0.17	−0.11	−0.02	0.09	0.26*	0.39**
Self-efficacy		1.00	0.21	−0.01	0.04	0.08	0.13	0.26*
Persistence			1.00	0.05	0.15	0.01	0.26*	0.20
Age as barrier				1.00	0.10	0.05	0.39**	−0.02
Flexibility					1.00	0.20	0.14	0.02
External support						1.00	0.13	0.21
Family support							1.00	0.39**
SWLS								1.00

Note: *p < .05, **p < .01

$F(2,64) = 3.2$ $p < 0.05$ ($M_{<=3\text{ m}} = 2.79$ $SD = 0.85$; $M_{4\text{-}11\text{m}} = 3.25$, $SD = 0.70$; $M_{>=12\text{m}} = 3.26$, $SD = 0.59$).

For the SWLS scale, the mean response at $M = 4.01$ $SD = 1.25$ was close to the scale midpoint of 4. Items with lower mean score were *The conditions of my life are excellent* ($M = 3.66$, $SD = 1.68$) and *If I could live my life over, I would change almost nothing* ($M = 3.74$, $SD = 1.9$).

The relationship between well-being and the various domains pertaining to coping with unemployment is presented in Table 4.4.

Family support and hope are significantly correlated with well-being. The length of unemployment, as a situational factor, is negatively correlated with SWLS $r = -0.42$**. To assess how well family support and length of unemployment predict well-being, a hierarchical multiple regression was performed, controlling for health restrictions. These were entered in Step 1 explaining 6% of the variance in SWLS scores. After entering length of unemployment and family support into the model, the total variance of the model was 26%, $F(3,61) = 8.33$, $p < 0.001$. These two variables explained 22% of the variance with an R squared change = 0.22, F change (2,61) = 9.33, $p < 0.001$. In the model both measures were statistically significant with length of unemployment recording a slightly higher beta value (beta = −2.87, $p < 0.01$) than family support (beta = 2.77, $p < 0.01$).

4.4 Discussion

This chapter set out to explore how job loss can be framed as a form of acute economic exclusion, and how this exclusion can have significant implications for poor mental health. As repeatedly noted, the age-specific risk of job loss, and a significant detractor of economic inclusion, is *prolonged* unemployment, or never gaining access to the labour market again, with potentially severe economic and psychosocial consequences. With increasing age, the range of income generation options diminishes, and the recovery of financial losses incurred through unemployment is increasingly difficult or even impossible. Not surprisingly, the meta-analytic study by Paul and Moser (2009) showed that young and older unemployed nearing retirement showed the highest stress levels. Older unemployed are at higher risk of *permanent* exclusion from the job market, being deprived of both, the manifest and latent functions of work. What is surprising is the relative scarcity of empirical studies on psychosocial consequences of job loss in later life – given the dramatic demographic change we face, with older people forecast to outnumber young people in a social transformation (ILOSTAT 2019). The empirical study conducted in Luxembourg is a first step to address this research gap.

In terms of cognitive appraisal of the job loss, it is important to point out that over half of the Luxembourg participants attributed their job loss, at least in part, to their age. Age was also seen as a barrier to regaining employment, with the effect being stronger for the longer-term unemployed workers. Our respondents feel discriminated against because of their age – and research evidence seems to confirm this assessment as studies have shown that prolonged or permanent unemployment *is* an age-specific risk (Brussig et al. 2006). The onset of illness is another risk factor whose relevance appears to increase with age and persons with health restrictions were indeed overrepresented in the long-term unemployed group in our sample. Furthermore, 28.4% of our respondents indicated that sickness or health related problems played a role in becoming unemployed.

The respondents in our study were, on average, very proactive in trying to get new employment – willing to retrain and even prepared to accept a job at lower wages. They were also optimistic in regaining employment – even though that optimism fades with increasing length of unemployment. This positive outlook in our sample may be a function of the flourishing Luxembourg job market, the high educational standing of the sample and a generous unemployment benefit system – factors that have been shown to buffer the negative effects of unemployment (Griep et al. 2015). The overall SWLS score at the midpoint of the scale is typical in economically developed nations (Diener 2006). The majority of people are generally satisfied, but have some areas where they would like improvements. Lower scores were obtained for the conditions of life item and participants would change things, if they could lead their lives over again. Not surprisingly, length of unemployment has a detrimental effect on subjective well-being. We also observed a buffering effect of family support.

Our sample of older unemployed is highly heterogeneous with different employment trajectories until the point of job loss. A glance at Table 4.1 depicting the employment history for our participants illustrates the very different (un-) employment trajectories that our participants have experienced. Consequently, assistance efforts to gain reemployment need to take this diversity and the different sets of coping resources and coping strategies into consideration. Even though we could not explore the dimension in depth, there were some precarious cases within our sample who would require a range of support measures – from building up relational capabilities to providing language training to specific skills training courses. Others may just need a refresher course in interview skills. Special support needs to be given to those with high work-role centrality as work as provider for meaning and fulfilment no longer exists – and this loss has been linked to lower psychological well-being (McKee-Ryan et al. 2005). Building on the beneficial role of family support, as indicated by our findings, assistance efforts might involve family members. Therefore, a "one-size-fits-all" approach is not appropriate for the 50 + unemployed group, who have less time remaining in their occupational career in which to recover from the consequences of the prolonged job loss, and are at heightened risk of economic exclusion.

4.5 Conclusion

There are limitations to this empirical research. First, the small sample size and the non-representative composition of the sample must be mentioned. The research is also correlational – so no conclusions about causality can be drawn. Some measures have been developed specifically for this study and need to be validated. We also only focused on subjective well-being and did not include specific measures to assess mental and physical health. However, there are surprisingly few studies focusing on the psychosocial consequences and lived experiences of older unemployed. The present study was a first attempt to address this imbalance. Ultimately, given the potentially severe consequences of late career unemployment (see Chu et al. 2016) and the rising number of older workers, dedicated research programmes that explore the diverse circumstances and experiences of this group are urgently needed.

Editors' Postscript

Please note, like other contributions to this book, this chapter was written before the COVID-19 pandemic of 2020. The book's introductory chapter (Chap. 1) and conclusion (Chap. 34) consider some of the key ways in which the pandemic relates to issues concerning social exclusion and ageing.

References

Arent, S., & Nagl, W. (2010). A fragile pillar: Statutory pensions and the risk of old-age poverty in Germany. *FinanzArchiv: Public Finance Analysis, 66*(4), 419–441.

Baltes, P. B., Smith, J., & Staudinger, U. M. (1992). Wisdom and successful aging. In T. B. Sonderegger (Ed.), *The Nebraska symposium on motivation: Vol. 39. The psychology of aging* (pp. 123–167). Lincoln: University of Nebraska Press.

Baruch, G. K., & Barnett, R. (1986). Role quality, multiple role involvement, and psychological well-being in midlife women. *Journal of Personality and Social Psychology, 51*, 578–585.

Brand, J. E. (2015). The far-reaching impact of job loss and unemployment. *Annual Review of Sociology, 41*, 359–375. https://doi.org/10.1146/annurev-soc-071913-043237.

Brussig, M., Knuth, M., & Schweer, O. (2006). *Arbeitsmarktpolitik für ältere Arbeitslose Erfahrungen mit „Entgeltsicherung" und „Beitragsbonus"*. IAT Report 02, Institut Arbeit und Technick, Wuppertal Institut für Klima, Umwelt, Energie.

Chan, S., & Stevens, A. H. (1999). Employment and retirement following a late-career job loss. *American Economic Review, 89*(2), 211–216.
Chan, S., & Stevens, A. H. (2001). Job loss and employment patterns of older workers. *Journal of Labor Economics, 19*(2), 484–521.
Chu, W. M., Liao, W. C., Li, C. R., Lee, S. H., Tang, Y. J., Ho, H. E., & Lee, M. C. (2016). Late-career unemployment and all-cause mortality, functional disability and depression among the older adults in Taiwan: A 12-year population-based cohort study. *Archives of Gerontology and Geriatrics, 65*, 192–198.
Diener, E. (2006). *Understanding scores on the satisfaction with life scale.* http://labs.psychology.illinois.edu. Accessed 10 Oct 2019.
Diener, E., Emmons, R. A., Larsen, R. J., & Griffin, S. (1985). The satisfaction with life scale. *Journal of Personality Assessment, 49*, 71–75.
Donovan, A., & Oddy, M. (1982). Psychological aspects of unemployment: An investigation into the emotional and social adjustment of school leavers. *Journal of Adolescence, 5*, 15–30.
Erikson, E. (1963). *Childhood and society*. New York: Norton.
Freud, S. (1935, reprinted 1960). *A general introduction to psychoanalysis*. New York: Washington Square Press.
Fryer, D. (1986). Employment deprivation and personal agency during unemployment: A critical discussion of Jahoda's explanation of the psychological effects of unemployment. *Social Behaviour, 1*, 3–23.
Gallo, W. T., Brand, J. E., Teng, H. M., Leo-Summers, L., & Byers, A. L. (2009). Differential impact of involuntary job loss on physical disability among older workers: Does predisposition matter? *Research on Aging, 31*(3), 345–360.
Griep, Y., Hyde, M., Vantilborgh, T., Bidee, J., De Witte, H., & Pepermans, R. (2015). Voluntary work and the relationship with unemployment, health, and well-being: A two-year follow-up study contrasting a materialistic and psychosocial pathway perspective. *Journal of Occupational Health Psychology, 20*(2), 190–204. https://doi.org/10.1037/a0038342.
Hansson, R. O., Briggs, S. R., & Rule, B. L. (1990). Old age and unemployment: Predictors of perceived control, depression, and loneliness. *Journal of Applied Gerontology, 9*(2), 230–240. https://doi.org/10.1177/073346489000900209.
Höpflinger, F. & Perrig-Chiello, P. (2009). *Hauptergebnisse eines empirischen Projekts zum Wandel des mittleren Erwachsenenalters – in Thesenform*. Retrieved from: http://www.hoepflinger.com/fhtop/fhmidage1.html. Accessed 9 Dec 2019.
ILOSTAT Labour Force Statistics. (2019). *Older workers are most discouraged in these countries*. https://ilostat.ilo.org/2019/10/01/older-workers-are-most-discouraged-in-these-countries/ Accessed 8 Dec 2019.
Jahoda, M. (1981). Work, employment, and unemployment: Values, theories, and approaches in social research. *American Psychologist, 36*(2), 184–191. https://doi.org/10.1037/0003-066X.36.2.184.
Jahoda, M. (1983). *Wieviel Arbeit braucht der Mensch? Arbeit und Arbeitslosigkeit im 20.* Weinheim: Jahrhundert.
Jahoda, M. (1997). Manifest and latent functions. In Nicholson, N. (Hrsg.), *The Blackwell encyclopedic dictionary of organizational psychology* (pp. 317–318). Oxford.
Kanfer, R., Wanberg, C. R., & Kantrowitz, T. M. (2001). Job search and employment: A personality-motivational analysis and meta-analytic review. *Journal of Applied Psychology, 86*, 837–855.
Mann, T. (2019). https://www.zitate.de/autor/Mann%2C+Thomas?page=2. Accessed 8 Dec 2019.
McKee-Ryan, F. M., & Kinicki, A. J. (2002). Coping with job loss: A life-facet model. *International Review of Industrial and Organizational Psychology, 17*, 1–29.
McKee-Ryan, F. M., Song, Z., Wanberg, C. R., & Kinicki, A. J. (2005). Psychological and physical well-being during unemployment: A meta-analytic study. *Journal of Applied Psychology, 90*(1), 53–76.
Modigliani, F., & Brumberg, R. (1954). Utility analysis and the consumption function: An interpretation of cross-section data. *Post-Keynesian Economics, 1*, 338–436.

Myers, D. (2006). *Psychology* (8th ed.). New York: Worth.
Myck, M., Ogg, J., Aigner-Walder, B., Kåreholt, I., Motel-Klingebiel, A., Marbán-Flores, R., & Thelin, A. (2017). *Economic Aspects of old age exclusion: a scoping report.* ROSEnet Economic Working Group Action, Knowledge Synthesis Series: No 1. CA 15122 Reducing Old-Age Exclusion: Collaborations in Research and Policy.
OECD. (2018). *Labour Force Statistics (LFS).* Retrieved from: https://stats.oecd.org/Index.aspx?DataSetCode=LFS_SEXAGE_I_R. Accessed 3 Dec 2019.
Paul, K. I., & Batinic, B. (2010): The need for work: Jahoda's latent functions of employment in a representative sample of the German population. *Journal of Organizational Behavior, 31*(1), 45–64.
Paul, K. I., & Moser, K. (2006). Incongruence as an explanation for the negative mental health effects of unemployment: Meta-analytic evidence. *Journal of Occupational and Organizational Psychology, 79*(4), 595–621.
Paul, K. I., & Moser, K. (2009). Unemployment impairs mental health: Meta-analyses. *Journal of Vocational Behavior, 74*(3), 264–282.
Perrig-Chiello, P., & Höpflinger, F. (2001). *Zwischen den Generationen. Frauen und Männer im mittleren Lebensalter*. Zürich: Seismo-Verlag.
Samorodov, A. (1999). *Ageing and labour markets for older workers*. Geneva: Employment and Training Department, International Labour Office.
Selenko, E., Batinic, B., & Paul, K. I. (2011). Does latent deprivation lead to psychological distress? Investigating Jahoda's model in a four-wave study. *Journal of Occupational and Organizational Psychology, 84*(4), 723–740.
Tiggemann, M., & Winefield, A. H. (1984). The effects of unemployment on the mood, self-esteem, locus of control, and depressive affect of school-leavers. *Journal of Occupational Psychology, 57*(1), 33–42.
Walsh, K. (2019). *Reducing old-age social exclusion in Europe*. Presentation at 5th ROSEnet European Policy Seminar on 11.01.2019 in Paris, France.
Walsh, K., Scharf, T., & Keating, N. (2017). Social exclusion of older persons: A scoping review and conceptual framework. *European Journal of Ageing, 14*(1), 81–98. https://doi.org/10.1007/s10433-016-0398-8.

Chapter 5
Coping Mechanisms of Divorced and Widowed Older Women to Mitigate Economic Exclusion: A Qualitative Study in Turkey and Serbia

Hande Barlin, Katarina Vojvodic, Murat Anil Mercan, and Aleksandra Milicevic-Kalasic

5.1 Introduction

Social exclusion goes beyond "depleted budgets" (Sen 2000) and involves broken social ties and marginalisation of specific groups in mainstream society (Sheppard 2012). It is both a dynamic process (Scharf 2015) and a multifaceted phenomenon (Levitas et al. 2007) manifesting in various aspects of social life (Walsh et al. 2017). Many adults are at risk of old-age social exclusion due to a higher probability of losing independence (Kneale 2012), reduced income, chronic disability and ageism (Phillipson and Scharf 2004). Amongst the older population some individuals are thus more prone to social exclusion, and its economic components (Barnes et al. 2006). While older women experience inequalities throughout their life (Sataric et al. 2013), disruptions such as divorce, separation and widowhood can exacerbate inequalities for previously married women, as it presents a reduction in income (Myck et al. 2017) and a drop in living standards (Calasanti 2010). It may affect housing decisions, downsizing and co-residing (Wagner and Mulder 2015).

Coupled with the challenges that old-age can bring (declining health; increased likelihood of bereavement, etc.), economic exclusion poses a threat to older people's capacity to pursue an independent and satisfactory quality of life (Whitley et al. 2018). Yet, some older people can adapt positively to adversely changing situations and can demonstrate a substantial capacity for resilience, as an "ability to

H. Barlin (✉) · M. A. Mercan
Gebze Technical University, Gebze, Turkey
e-mail: hbarlin@gtu.edu.tr

K. Vojvodic
Institute of Public Health of Belgrade, Belgrade, Serbia

A. Milicevic-Kalasic
Department for Social Work FMK, University Singidunum, Belgrade, Serbia

Institute for Gerontology and Palliative Care, Belgrade, Serbia

K. Walsh et al. (eds.), *Social Exclusion in Later Life*, International Perspectives on Aging 28, https://doi.org/10.1007/978-3-030-51406-8_5

incorporate both vulnerabilities and strengths across a range of areas and time frames" (Wiles et al. 2012, p. 243). This is also true for older adults with socio-economic disadvantages (Kok et al. 2018), and those faced with economic shocks (Fenge et al. 2012). While not all individuals can cope with such economic adversities (Bennett et al. 2016), understanding the coping mechanisms of older people who do adjust are important for devising policies and interventions for mitigating vulnerabilities and building more inclusive societies.

This chapter explores the economic exclusion experiences and coping mechanisms of materially deprived divorced, separated and widowed older women living in Serbia and Turkey – two countries whose ageing populations have received little study within the international literature. The two countries have many common cultural and social traits and family structure; such as extended families (Georgas 2006) and strong family ties (Ferra 2010). In both countries, older men fare better than women in many life domains, including employment and financial security (UNECE 2016). However, while Serbia is among the oldest populations in Europe (with 18.2% of people aged 65 years and over), Turkey is in comparison one of the youngest (with 8.7% of people aged 65 years and over) (United Nations 2019).

Previous research has examined resilience of older adults, especially with regards to health outcomes (Van Kessel 2013). More recently disadvantaged communities and groups (Thoma and McGee 2019) were also investigated. However, resilience and coping mechanisms of one of the most vulnerable older groups, materially deprived widowed and separated/divorced women, in the face of economic exclusion have never been studied in Turkey nor Serbia, with also little attention given to this topic in other jurisdictions. Drawing on a qualitative study, the chapter addresses four questions. Firstly, what are the economic exclusion experiences of materially deprived widowed and separated/divorced older women [also see Sumil-Laanemaa et al. this section]? Secondly, while these women are among the most vulnerable, do they demonstrate resilience *vis-à-vis* economic exclusion? Thirdly, if they do so, what coping mechanisms do they employ? Fourthly, how do similarities and differences in Serbian and Turkish contexts shape coping mechanisms of these women? We begin by outlining the qualitative study that underpins our analysis. This is followed by a description of the findings of the research, focusing on early life experiences, life during marriage, and life after disruption to marriage (*e.g.* bereavement; separation; divorce). Finally, a discussion and conclusion are presented.

5.2 Methodology

Data was collected through 11 semi-structured in-depth interviews conducted in Serbia and 16 conducted in Turkey during August and September 2019. The interview guide consisted of questions regarding: (1) socio-economic background; (2) current daily and social life; (3) economic and financial circumstances throughout the life course; (4) life with husband and family; and (5) changes experienced after disruption of marital ties, as well as fulfilled or unfulfilled aspirations and experiences of loneliness and exclusion. The questions were broad so as to allow participants to elaborate and express their experiences and perceptions freely.

The interviews were conducted in two cities in Serbia (Belgrade and Kraljevo) and two villages (Ćuvdin and Žiča) and three provinces in Turkey (Edirne, Mersin and Istanbul). A responsive interviewing approach was used, where researchers were flexible and adjusted to the personalities of the participants (Rubin and Rubin 2012). The interviews were audio recorded and lasted one hour approximately.

5.2.1 Recruitment and Participants

Participants were recruited through purposive sampling based on five criteria: (1) being older than 64 years; (2) being female; (3) being widowed, divorced or separated (not legally divorced, living in separate household with no expectation of unification); (4) having good cognitive functioning (able to rationally answer the questions) and (5) being materially deprived/facing economic exclusion. For material deprivation, the 9-item scale of Eurostat (2019) was used.

With reference to Table 5.1, most participants were aged 65 to 69 years. Around three quarters were widowed, with the remaining six participants being separated or divorced. One third of the sample lived in rural areas. Most participants had two children and more than half co-resided with children or grandchildren. More than half from Turkey possessed literacy issues, while half of Serbian participants completed high-school. Most participants married under the age of 18 years and around three quarters of the sample had a pension of their own or a pension from their husbands or fathers.

5.2.2 Data Analysis

After completion of all interviews, audio recordings were transcribed verbatim by the researchers. The framework method, efficient in multi-disciplinary research, which provides clear steps to follow and produces highly structured outputs (Gale et al. 2013) was used for the analysis. Following Ritchie et al. (2013), transcriptions were read, and themes were identified by the researchers separately. Themes identified by more than two researchers were included in the analysis. Using NVivo 12, transcriptions were coded and categorised by two researchers from each country. A framework matrix was developed for each country. Based on the matrices' similarities and differences between the countries and variance in lived experiences were identified.

Table 5.1 Characteristics of participants

	Number of participants		
	Turkey	Serbia	Total
Age			
65–69 years	9	2	11
70–74 years	5	2	7
75–79 years	1	1	2
80 years and more	1	6	7
Marital status			
Divorced	4	1	5
Widowed	11	10	21
Separated	1	0	1
Number of children			
No children	0	3	3
1	3	1	4
2	5	5	10
3	3	1	4
4	1	0	1
5 and more	4	1	5
Education			
No formal education	10	0	10
Less than primary school education	3	4	7
Primary school	0	1	1
High school	3	6	9
Type of settlement			
Rural	4	5	9
Urban	12	6	18
Living alone			
Yes	4	7	11
No	11	4	15
Unspecified	1	0	1

5.2.3 *Ethical Considerations*

The study received ethical approval from the Ethics Committee of the Municipal Institute of Gerontology and Palliative Care in Belgrade, Serbia, and the Ethics Committee of the Gebze Technical University, Turkey. While the consent of study participants was obtained in writing from the literate interviewees, oral consents were audio recorded for those who had literacy issues. The researchers were also careful not to raise any expectations amongst participants for the improvement of their circumstances.

5.3 Findings

Three main themes corresponding to the different phases of participants' lives emerged in interviews, namely: early life experiences, life during marriage, and life after marital disruption. Unless otherwise stated these themes were robust across widowed and separated/divorced participants in both countries.

5.3.1 Early Life Experiences

Except for a small number of participants in Turkey and Serbia, participants experienced multiple disadvantages during their childhood, namely financial insecurities, material deprivation and gender inequalities. Marrying early at the ages of 14–16 years and receiving little or no education are manifestations of these gendered inequalities. Turkish participants, particularly those with little formal education, talked about education in relation to gender inequalities and missed opportunities:

> 'Back then, women were to marry early…So they said there is no need for girls to go to school. Us, four sisters did not go …. My brothers went. We could not.' (TE04).

Faced with financial insecurities, participants raised the issue of working at an early age. Working as an unpaid household worker in the fields and orchards and engaging in domestic work were experiences shared by all participants in the rural and poorer areas in both countries. Some also provided care for younger siblings so that their mothers could work.

5.3.2 Life during Marriage

Within the scope of discussions during married life, participants mostly talked about their financial situation at the time and strategies they employed to cope with financial troubles.

5.3.2.1 Financial Situations

Although the degree and timing varied, most of the participants experienced economic exclusion. For instance, while one participant in Turkey stated that "I always had financial problems..." (TM09), another participant stated that financial problems started "when he [referring to husband] closed his shop after he got sick" (TM07). At times, these financial problems were accompanied by marital troubles such as economic abuse (*e.g.* denying access to financial resources), the husband's extra-marital relations or gambling. For instance, a divorcee housewife stated that her husband started acting out of the ordinary and held her responsible for financial problems. "My husband did not shop for the house, did not buy food, did not buy anything for the house and anything kids wanted" (TM12).

Participants living in impoverished neighbourhoods indicated that they had to work very hard to cope with economic hardships. Migrating to urban from rural settlements was also a marker of financial issues according to the respondents; "When we came to the city, our savings slowly melted away" (TM08). Precarious housing conditions at the start of the marriage was regarded as an indicator of low economic standing in both countries, and contrasted with the relative increase in standards of living experienced by some participants more recently: "It is good now, I have a bed, I have a bathroom, I was sleeping on the floor." (RSV2). Connected with material security, buying a house was a core objective in both countries.

5.3.2.2 Coping with Economic Exclusion During Marriage

Because of this experience of economic hardship during their married life, participants talked in detail about their coping strategies. The most dominant strategy employed in both countries to address, as well as cope with, economic exclusion concerned work and particularly increasing working-hours, with some individuals having to go to extensive lengths to reconcile work and family responsibilities:

> 'And how did I spend my life? One child on my back in the cradle, another in my arm, bag on my back and go walking one hour to the field, to work …I can't regret how I spent my life.' (RSV2).

When they received income, they spent it on children or domestic needs. In Turkey, almost all those working in their early married life worked in precarious jobs. Working in registered jobs with social security benefits was rare, even in later periods. Most participants did not have social security and access to pensions based on their work. While working conditions of the participants were not any better in Serbia, all participants contributed to a state pension fund to gain an entitlement to receive a pension in later life, albeit at the basic level.

In rural Serbia and Turkey, participants mostly worked in cleaning, agriculture and handcrafting industries. However in the cities (Serbia), clerical work and teaching were the dominant professions. To make ends meet, combining more than one job in a day was a strategy in both countries engaged in by several participants:

> 'I used to work three jobs a day. Sometimes I went to two houses to clean. Later, I went to wash dishes at a restaurant. If I was not tired late at night, I used to knit' (TM01).

When participants' husbands were sick, or when in some cases their husbands' neglected their familial responsibilities as the main bread earner in highly patriarchal societies, participants increased their efforts to earn money. However, some husbands in Turkey banned their wives from working.

In desperate times, converting assets to cash was another strategy employed by interviewees to cope with economic hardship. After migrating from a rural village, one Turkish participant had to sell her beloved rug: "I did not have much choice, either give up the rug or spend one more hungry night with my kids" (TI15).

Living with other relatives was another important coping mechanism. Some shared the same house with their parents, or parents-in-law. This typically meant an increased domestic workload, but also often enabled them to work outside the house as they had someone to take care of their children. In times of economic hardship, family members and relatives provided financial and in-kind support in both countries while support from friends and neighbours were limited and on an ad-hoc basis. Participants who were working as a domestic worker were able to diversify sources of support, getting help from their employers:

> 'The house owner was a doctor. He would help me whenever we needed to go to hospital. His friends would also help me' (TI14).

5.3.3 Life After Disruption of Marriage

5.3.3.1 Finances

All participants had a low income. In Serbia, the main source of income was participants' personal pension, or that of their late husband's where an interviewee was widowed – if the husband's pension was higher than a participant's, which was frequently the case, she sought to receive his pension instead of her own. The sources of income were more diverse in Turkey and included personal pensions, pensions from the husband or father, or social assistance such as widowhood and old-age allowances. As formal social security registration was not prevalent, many women were not entitled to a pension based on their own labour. "I couldn't register [for] social security. I could not get that kind of job" (TE04). In one case, a participant was working in a family shop, but the husband was registered with the social security.

Some participants in Turkey, who did not have any sources of income, applied to and received social assistance, like old-age or widowhood allowances. Participants living in more disadvantaged neighbourhoods received ad-hoc financial and/or in-kind aid from municipalities (food stuffs, and coal). On the other hand, while most Serbian interviewees were living on a small pension, no one received social assistance. All, except one, have never asked for such assistance. Only one urban participant applied for financial support because of disability and long-term disease.

While many had been trying to live within their financial means, debt was a significant issue of concern among Turkish participants. Many had drawn credit in the hope of securing better prospects. For instance, paying for college tuition or contributing to the development of a business for themselves or their children. In both countries, interviewees who were separated from their husbands at a young age, when the children were small, went through deeper economic struggles when bearing the responsibilities of raising children alone. This is especially true for some of the divorcees in the sample. For instance, a Turkish participant who divorced at 18 years, and who had a baby at the time, had to move back to her parents and had to work in two jobs to provide for her child.

5.3.3.2 Coping with Economic Exclusion After Marriage Disruption

Faced with low income, participants talked about family support, economic resourcefulness, lower levels of consumption, and self-sufficiency all as coping mechanisms.

First, children played an instrumental role in coping with economic and social hardships in both countries in later life. Co-residence was a mechanism for pooling resources. In some cases, financial support provided by children was the main income. “Subsistence was good with my husband. Now I depend on my son” (TM07). Children also facilitated access to services, providing transportation or handling basic administration and form filling, and supporting links to social life such as accompanying their older mothers when shopping, going to weddings and walking. Children were also considered to be a source of participants’ happiness, and thus children’s welfare was also sought. Provision of support by the participants in terms of financing and caring for adult children was also common.

> ‘If your child is comfortable, you are also comfortable…I drew credit for my son, for my daughter. When there is nothing, if I cannot give, I feel upset’ (TE02).

In Serbia, there were even cases where grandmothers looked after their grandchildren so that their daughters could go abroad and work to provide a better life. Other family members were also mentioned as providing support. “My sister took me in with my little one. We lived in separate houses in a single garden” (TE02). Furthermore, in Serbia, there were cases where older interviewees continue to live with their husband’s parents.

Second, and in terms of economic resourcefulness, most participants who were working before their marital disruption, continued to do so after the disruption had occurred, especially if they were young at that time. Providing for children was a strong incentive to work more. Even some participants in later life continued to demonstrate their economic resourcefulness in mitigating low income, either through income generation activities or subsistence farming (especially in the rural areas). For instance, one participant worked as a live-in helper. Others made tomato paste or knitted clothes.

Third, consuming less, buying only the fundamentals was another dominant coping strategy. Nearly all respondents talk about the need to be prudent.

> ‘It is all about being prudent. If there is some today, I save the half for tomorrow. I don’t spend all because it is coming. I clean, wash and wear the old. I don’t leave my kids hungry. It is all right if I have 5 cloths instead of 10’ (TE04).

Similarly, lowering expectations and concentrating on non-material aspirations, and abstinence was another coping strategy. "I am old woman, what do I need? Not so much." (RSV2). In both Serbia and Turkey, the most dominant wish was health, and secondly, for Turkey, peace: "Peace and health. Okay, nothing happens without money, but health is an absolute must" (TE03). Regardless of all the hardships, most participants in both countries were satisfied with their lives. "I am satisfied now, I do just what and how I want to do, to live." (RST4). As such, contentment surfaced as a coping mechanism connected with abstinence.

Fourth, self-sufficiency was a coping strategy spoken about by older women in both countries. While income was low and repeatedly referred to as insufficient, participants were grateful, especially for the perceived self-sufficiency and independence that their income provided:

> 'The income I receive, is it sufficient? No, not at all. But it is better than nothing. I don't need to go and ask [for] money from my son. I can go and buy needs by myself. I am not dependent on anyone' (TI13).

Another respondent who received a widowhood allowance stated that "at least I can buy my own medicine" (TE01). Fifth, for most, social life centred around meeting with their neighbours and relatives that lived in their immediate neighbourhoods, a low cost and convenient social activity. Participants living in rural areas or in the outskirts of the cities, gathered in front of their houses during summer. During winter, house visits were more frequent. While some went to weddings/or circumcision feats (Turkey), many refrained going there, either because it was too loud or crowded or due to mobility limitations: "Who wants to see an old woman, they are all young, my time is gone..." (RSV2). Some attended religious gatherings as a source of socialisation.

5.4 Discussion and Conclusions

Most participants experienced material deprivation and economic exclusion throughout their life, on a continuous or intermittent basis. Coping mechanisms and the extent to which they were employed generally varied. Participants who had previously combined various coping strategies early in life, continued to do so. While they might have needed support from their families, they did not feel needy. However, those who depended on their husbands or families, continued to depend on their children as a resource. In the main, there were few apparent differences between the divorced/separated and widowed participants in terms of coping mechanisms. Many divorcees, most of whom were separated from their husbands at young ages when their children were small, had to shoulder the lone responsibility for their children together with deep financial troubles from an early stage.

In line with the findings of Kok et al. (2018) for those of low socio-economic position, participants in this research demonstrated significant resilience. Among the participants, the most resilient individuals were typically those who had previously been more proactive in coping. This finding supports that of Browne-Yung et al. (2017) who highlighted how coping with adverse life events at various periods of life contributed to resilience. Also, Höltge et al. (2018) provided evidence that moderate adversity experienced in earlier life plays a role in generating a coping capacity for successful ageing.

The findings suggest that materially deprived widowed and separated/divorced older women in Serbia and Turkey employ similar mechanisms to cope with economic exclusion. Some are internal, where individuals exercise the mechanism themselves. Others are external, where individuals receive assistance and mobilise different kinds of resources. While economic resourcefulness, consuming less, and perceived independence are internal, support from family, friends, neighbours and the state are external.

In line with the international literature (Korkmaz 2014; Bennett et al. 2016) the study indicates that the family, especially children, play a central role in coping. Intergenerational support varies in each case and includes financial support (private transfers), accommodation support (through co-residence), transportation and accompaniment with outside tasks. While support with finances and housing is bi-directional, support relating to mobility and domestic chores is primarily given by the children. Friends and neighbours were not mentioned as providing financial support, but they constitute the main pillar of a low-cost social life that participants utilise (Cramm et al. 2012).

Consuming less or living within one's means is another dominant strategy, one of the most common strategies to mitigate economic difficulties (Fenge et al. 2012; Brünner 2019). Older participants in this study regarded prudence as a virtue and lived accordingly. They "choose" to spend just enough to meet fundamental needs. Within the scope of economic resourcefulness, engaging in income generation activities or semi-/subsistence farming are other strategies and, indeed, were widely employed (Davidova 2011). Consciously adopting low expectations and abstinence were other coping mechanisms.

Moreover, regardless of all the troubles experienced by participants, interviewees expressed satisfaction with life. This confirms the findings of Brünner (2019) for Danish state pensioners and King et al. (2012) for older adults with disabilities. Albeit needing support, perceived independence serves as a strong coping mechanism, and may in some ways be more important than objective assessments (Bennett et al. 2010) in how it contributes to a reservoir of resilience (Becker and Newsom 2005).

Participants in Serbia and Turkey differ in their use of social assistance (public transfers). While all participants are entitled to a state pension in Serbia, this is not the case in Turkey. One of the reasons for this gap is the differences in welfare regimes and their development level during participants' earlier adulthood. Nevertheless, financial and in-kind social assistance provided by the state, or the municipalities, were typically only a secondary form of coping. However, financial social assistance and pensions did provide a sense of self-sufficiency, independence and dignity, albeit often noted to be generally inadequate. Furthermore, there are differences in coping strategies employed before and after the disruption of marriage ties. Support from wider networks is rare and social assistance is more prevalent, at least in the Turkish case, at later life. This pattern coincides with the expansion of the welfare system in Turkey (Pelek and Polat 2019).

To conclude, this study contributes knowledge to a topic where there is a lack of understanding around the coping mechanisms of widowed and separated/divorced older women experiencing economic exclusion. However, a limitation of the study is that the sample does not include Turkish participants without children. Considering the central role children play in coping strategies, future research should investigate coping mechanisms of older materially deprived women without children in order to develop a more inclusive framework of understanding.

Editors' Postscript

Please note, like other contributions to this book, this chapter was written before the COVID-19 pandemic of 2020. The book's introductory chapter (Chap. 1) and conclusion (Chap. 34) consider some of the key ways in which the pandemic relates to issues concerning social exclusion and ageing.

References

Barnes, M., Blom, A. G., Cox, K., Lessof, C., & Walker, A. (2006). *The social exclusion of older people: Evidence from the first wave of the English Longitudinal Study of Ageing (ELSA)* (Final report). London: Office of the Deputy Prime Minister.

Becker, G., & Newsom, E. (2005). Resilience in the face of serious illness among chronically ill African Americans in later life. *The Journals of Gerontology Series B: Psychological Sciences and Social Sciences, 60*(4), S214–S223.

Bennett, K. M., Reyes-Rodriguez, M. F., Altamar, P., & Soulsby, L. K. (2016). Resilience amongst older Colombians living in poverty: An ecological approach. *Journal of Cross-Cultural Gerontology, 31*(4), 385–407. https://doi.org/10.1007/s10823-016-9303-3.

Bennett, K. M., Stenhoff, A., Pattinson, J., & Woods, F. (2010). "Well if he could see me now": The facilitators and barriers to the promotion of instrumental Independence following spousal bereavement. *Journal of Gerontological Social Work, 53*(3), 215–234. https://doi.org/10.1080/01634370903562931.

Browne-Yung, K., Walker, R. B., & Luszcz, M. A. (2017). An examination of resilience and coping in the oldest old using life narrative method. *The Gerontologist, 57*(2), 282–291. https://doi.org/10.1093/geront/gnv137.

Brünner, R. N. (2019). Making ends meet in financial scarcity in old age. *International Journal of Ageing and Later Life, 13*(1), 35–62. https://doi.org/10.3384/ijal.1652-8670.18391.

Calasanti, T. (2010). Gender and ageing in the context of globalization. In D. Dannefer & C. Philipson (Eds.), *The SAGE handbook of social gerontology* (pp. 137–149). Los Angeles: SAGE.

Cramm, J. M., Van Dijk, H. M., & Nieboer, A. P. (2012). The importance of neighborhood social cohesion and social capital for the well being of older adults in the community. *The Gerontologist, 53*(1), 142–152.

Davidova, S. (2011). Semi-subsistence farming: An elusive concept posing thorny policy questions. *Journal of Agricultural Economics, 62*(3), 503–524.

Eurostat. (2019). *Glossary: Material deprivation*. https://ec.europa.eu/eurostat/statistics-explained/index.php/Glossary:Material_deprivation. Accessed 10 Feb 2019.

Fenge, L. A., Hean, S., Worswick, L., Wilkinson, C., Fearnley, S., & Ersser, S. (2012). The impact of the economic recession on well-being and quality of life of older people. *Health & Social Care in the Community, 20*(6), 617–624.

Ferra, E. L. (2010). Family and kinship ties in development. In J.-P. Platteau & R. Peccoud (Eds.), *Culture, institutions, and development: New insights into an old debate* (pp. 107–124). London: Routledge.

Gale, N. K., Heath, G., Cameron, E., Rashid, S., & Redwood, S. (2013). Using the framework method for the analysis of qualitative data in multi-disciplinary health research. *BMC Medical Research Methodology, 13*(1), 117–125.

Georgas, J. (2006). Families and family change). In J. Georgas, J. W. Berry, F. J. Van de Vijver, Ç. Kagitçibasi, & Y. H. Poortinga (Eds.), *Families across cultures: A 30-nation psychological study* (pp. 3–50). Cambridge: Cambridge University Press.

Höltge, J., Mc Gee, S. L., Maercker, A., & Thoma, M. V. (2018). A salutogenic perspective on adverse experiences. *European Journal of Health Psychology, 25*, 53–69. https://doi.org/10.1027/2512-8442/a000011.

King, J., Yourman, L., Ahalt, C., Eng, C., Knight, S. J., Pérez-Stable, E. J., et al. (2012). Quality of life in late-life disability: "I don't feel bitter because I am in a wheelchair". *Journal of the American Geriatrics Society, 60*(3), 569–576.

Kneale, D. (2012). *Is social exclusion still important for older people?* (International longevity centre report). London: International Longevity Centre.

Kok, A. A. L., van Nes, F., Deeg, D. J. H., Widdershoven, G., & Huisman, M. (2018). "Tough times have become good times": Resilience in older adults with a low socioeconomic position. *The Gerontologist, 58*(5), 843–852. https://doi.org/10.1093/geront/gny007.

Korkmaz, N. K. (2014). Old age, family and the transfer of the capitals in the context of Pierre Bourdieu-Examples from two fieldworks in Turkey. In A. Klein, A. M. Chavez Hernandez, L. F. Macias Garcia, & C. Rea (Eds.), *Identidades, vínculos y transmisión generaciona* (pp. 115–126). Boenos Aires: Manantial.

Levitas, R., Pantazis, C., Fahmy, E., Gordon, D., Lloyd-Reichling, E., & Patsios, D. (2007). *The multi-dimensional analysis of social exclusion*. Bristol: Bristol Institute for Public Affairs, University of Bristol.

Myck, M., Ogg, J., Aigner-Walder, B., Kareholt, I., Kostakis, I., Motel-Klingebiel, et al. (2017). *'Economic aspects of old age exclusion: A scoping report' knowledge synthesis series*. ROSEnet Cost Action (CA15122) Reducing Old-Age Social Exclusion: Collaborations in Research & Policy.

Pelek, S., & Polat, S. (2019). *Exploring inter-household transfers: An assessment using panel data from Turkey*. Istanbul: Galatasaray University Economic Research Center 19–01.

Phillipson, C., & Scharf, T. (2004). *The impact of government policy on social exclusion among older people*. London: Office of the Deputy Prime Minister.

Ritchie, J., Lewis, J., Nicholls, C. M., & Ormston, R. (2013). *Qualitative research practice: A guide for social science students and researchers*. London: SAGE.

Rubin, H. J., & Rubin, I. S. (2012). *Qualitative interviewing (3rd ed.): The art of hearing data*. Thousand Oaks: SAGE. https://doi.org/10.4135/9781452226651.

Sataric, N., Milićević-Kalašić, A., & Ignjatovic, T. (2013). *Deprived of rights out of ignorance report on monitoring of the human rights of older people in residential care in Serbia*. Belgrade: Inpress.

Scharf, T. (2015). Between inclusion and exclusion in later life. In G. Carney, K. Walsh, & A. Ní Léime (Eds.), *Ageing through austerity: Critical perspectives from Ireland* (pp. 113–130). Bristol: Policy Press.

Sen, A. (2000). *Social exclusion: Concept, application, and scrutiny*. Manila: Asian Development Bank.

Sheppard, M. (2012). *Social work and social exclusion: The idea of practice*. Aldershot: Ashgate Publishing, Ltd.

Thoma, M. V., & Mc Gee, S. L. (2019). Successful aging in individuals from less advantaged, marginalized, and stigmatized backgrounds. *Clinical Psychology in Europe, 1*(3), e32578. https://doi.org/10.32872/cpe.v1i3.32578.
UNECE. (2016). *The active ageing index pilot studies for Turkey and Serbia*. Available at: https://statswiki.unece.org/download/attachments/76287849/Pilot%20study%20for%20Serbia%20and%20Turkey%20final.pdf?version=1&modificationDate=1473167139525&api=v2. Accessed 20 Sept 2019.
United Nations, D. o. E. a. S. A., Population Division. (2019). *World population ageing 2019: Highlights* (ST/ESA/SER.A/430).
Van Kessel, G. (2013). The ability of older people to overcome adversity: A review of the resilience concept. *Geriatric Nursing, 34*(2), 122–127.
Wagner, M., & Mulder, C. H. (2015). Spatial mobility, family dynamics, and housing transitions. *KZfSS Kölner Zeitschrift für Soziologie und Sozialpsychologie, 67*(1), 111–135. https://doi.org/10.1007/s11577-015-0327-4.
Walsh, K., Scharf, T., & Keating, N. (2017). Social exclusion of older persons: A scoping review and conceptual framework (journal article). *European Journal of Ageing, 14*(1), 81–98. https://doi.org/10.1007/s10433-016-0398-8.
Whitley, E., Benzeval, M., & Popham, F. (2018). Associations of successful aging with socioeconomic position across the life-course: The West of Scotland Twenty-07 prospective cohort study. *Journal of Aging and Health, 30*(1), 52–74.
Wiles, J. L., Wild, K., Kerse, N., & Allen, R. E. S. (2012). Resilience from the point of view of older people: 'There's still life beyond a funny knee'. *Social Science & Medicine, 74*(3), 416–424. https://doi.org/10.1016/j.socscimed.2011.11.005.

Section III
Exclusion from Social Relations

Chapter 6
Introduction: Framing Exclusion from Social Relations

Vanessa Burholt and Marja Aartsen

6.1 Introduction

In this section we focus on the domain of exclusion from social relations where social relations can be defined as comprising social resources, social connections and social networks. Other types of social engagement with formal civic, political and voluntary groups and organisations are not included in this section, but instead are incorporated in the domain of civic exclusion [see section VI]. Theorising on exclusion from social relations is facilitated by the ROSEnet Cost Action, which brought together experts in the field and led to the publication of a critical review and development of a conceptual model of exclusion from social relations for older people (Burholt et al. 2019). The model captured the complexity of exclusion from social relations through a subjective interpretation of the literature and took into account the interrelationships between systems in the critical human ecology framework (Fig. 6.1). The synthesis of the findings was endorsed by the working group on social relations comprising 45 members from 25 countries. The purpose of this introduction is to outline what exclusion from social relations involves, and to frame the three contributions within this section of the book in the broader research debates and scholarship on this topic.

V. Burholt (✉)
School of Nursing/School of Population Health, University of Auckland, Auckland, New Zealand

Centre for Innovative Ageing, Swansea University, Swansea, Wales, UK
e-mail: vanessa.burholt@auckland.ac.nz

M. Aartsen
NOVA-Norwegian Social Research, Oslo Metropolitan University, Oslo, Norway

K. Walsh et al. (eds.), *Social Exclusion in Later Life*, International Perspectives on Aging 28, https://doi.org/10.1007/978-3-030-51406-8_6

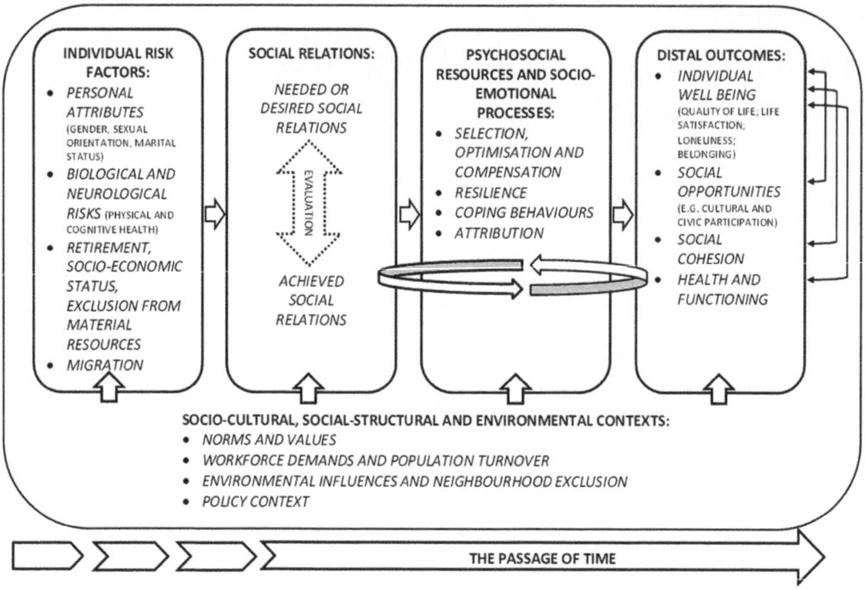

Fig. 6.1 Conceptual model of exclusion from social relations for older people

Source: Burholt et al. 2019

6.2 Exclusion from Social Relations

Social relations are key determinants of an individual's health, well-being and feelings of belonging, as they provide social and material resources and the value of attachment in its own right (Bowlby 1982). Hence, being excluded from social relations disrupts people from a fundamental aspect of human life and reduces possibilities of being healthy and happy in old-age. While empirical evidence for the beneficial effects of social networks is substantial, it is important to acknowledge also potential negative effects of social relations. Conflictual and/or abusive relations can be extremely stressful and may lead to negative health and well-being outcomes. Abusive relationships may be particularly difficult for older adults to terminate because of the increased risk of declining health and the need for support (Rook 2003).

It is important to define what we mean by exclusion from social relations, as the way it is defined determines our core understanding of it. Based on discussions in the ROSEnet Cost Action, we define exclusion from social relations as a situation in which people are disconnected from adequate levels and quality of intimate relationships, social networks, social support, and/or social opportunities to participate in the wider society. Although exclusion from social relations is often equated with loneliness, we consider it to be a different concept. Loneliness is defined as a negative feeling, which arises when the number and quality of social relations one has is smaller than one would like to have (Perlman and Peplau 1981). Loneliness is thus seen as just one of the possible outcomes of exclusion from social relations, but one that is highlighted by authors in this section of the book.

The conceptual model of exclusion from social relations articulates separately different elements of this form of exclusion. It describes risks for exclusion from social relationships as personal attributes such as age, gender, education, income, and socio-economic and marital status (De Jong Gierveld et al. 2009) and sexual orientation (Cronin and King 2010); biological and neurological characteristics (Aartsen et al. 2004; Lechner et al. 2007); and life experiences concerning, retirement, exclusion from material resources, and migration (Walters and Bartlett 2009). It makes a distinction between objective ratings and subjective assessments of social relations and how mismatches between these two elements lead to poor outcomes in terms of individual well-being (*e.g.* quality of life, life satisfaction, loneliness and belonging); health and functioning; social opportunities and social cohesion. The conceptual model takes into account the contexts that impact on the process of exclusion. This includes the role of psychological resources (Schoenmakers et al. 2015) and socio-emotional processes (Lang 2000). It also includes the immediate environment such as the walkability and level of safety of a neighbourhood [also see Drilling et al. this volume] and the quality and design of the house (Burholt et al. 2016) and policy contextual influences such as norms and attitudes towards older people, mandatory retirement age and pension systems (Palmore 2015; Gibney et al. 2017; and Ogg and Myck, this volume). Finally, the model illustrates a dynamic relationship between its constituent elements and how each element may change over time.

A helpful, but underutilised (Van Regenmortel et al. 2016) approach to further understand levels of exclusion from social relations is the life-course perspective (Elder 1994). This perspective implies that the degree of exclusion from social relations experienced in older-age is being shaped by conditions and decisions earlier in life. For example, the decision to study, to marry, to raise a family, and to divorce may not only have an immediate effect on the number of social relations people have, but it may have repercussions for the social network people have in later life. Moreover, developments in a person's life are interconnected with developments in other people's lives; for example, caring for a partner limits possibilities to participate in society. Life-course transitions are of particular importance, where for instance losing a spouse or retirement can disrupt a person's social relations. There may also be an accumulation of advantages and disadvantages that may result in inequities in later life for certain groups of older people *e.g.* ethnic minorities, migrants, LGBTQ+ groups, or women.

The life-course perspective further acknowledges that factors leading to exclusion from social relations may vary by time and place, norms, values, and policies, and hence, across societies. As individual lives change over time, so too do 'national cultures' and places, with these dynamics sometimes also contributing to exclusion from social relations. Structural changes such as improved communication or the mass media can influence changes in norms, beliefs, values, customs and traditions (Winter 2017) which in turn can influence older people's expectations concerning the ideal level of social relations. Industrial regional developments that influence local employment opportunities may directly affect population mobility or population turnover resulting in fewer proximal kin, or reduced neighbourliness (Skinner et al. 2014; Burholt and Sardani 2017) thus contributing to exclusion from social relations.

6.3 Outline of This Section

The three chapters in this section of the book provide an important contribution to the study of exclusion from social relations. They address gaps in evidence that contribute to the eco-bio-psychosocial understanding of differences in experiences of exclusion from social relations for older people. Each chapter in this section, has taken a different approach elucidating how biological manifestation of the body, psychological traits and the socio-cultural, social-structural, policy and physical environment fundamentally impact on the human experience of exclusion from social relations. The outcomes of the interaction are a result of adaption and negotiation that take place within particular cultural contexts. The multi-country approach, also taken in these chapters, is important, as the findings from the studies have greater credibility when they are found to apply beyond the confines of a single nation, and lead to an improved understanding of exclusion from social relations.

The first chapter in this section (Chap. 7 – Van Regenmortel et al.) explores cross-national similarities and differences in the experiences of exclusion from social relations between older people living in rural Britain and Belgium. The chapter expounds on the connections between exclusion from social relations and other domains of exclusion (*e.g.* economic exclusion and exclusion from services). The authors demonstrate the complexity of the interrelationships between the domains by developing and quantifying profiles of exclusion that are used to classify older people. The characteristics of the profiles demonstrate that older people may simultaneously experience exclusion in some domains but not in others.

Morgan et al., in Chap. 8, consider one of the outcomes of exclusion from social relations – loneliness. This chapter seeks to advance understanding of micro- and macro-level drivers of loneliness, and changes in loneliness over time in 11 European countries. The analyses confirms earlier results on micro-level drivers of loneliness, and provide innovative evidence for the influence of macro-level drivers of loneliness, such as perceived safety in the neighbourhood, normative levels of social connectedness and the average level of religiosity of people aged 55 years and over living in the country. Even more important than the level of micro-level factors are the changes therein. A two-year change in macro-level drivers did not lead to statistically significant changes in loneliness in a two-year period.

Waldegrave et al., Chap. 9, emphasise the importance of relationship conflict and quality, and the impact on outcomes in four countries (Norway, Israel, Italy and Finland). In this respect, non-supportive, harmful or abusive relationships contribute to exclusion from social relations and poor outcomes as they deviate from good and extensive social relations. In this chapter, each country level analysis adds another piece to the jigsaw concerning the holistic assessment of exclusion from social relations. Chapter 9 also addresses the impact of social values and discrimination on exclusion from social relations, with discriminatory attitudes serving to exclude groups or individual older people from opportunities to develop or maintain social relations.

Shortly after the chapters in this section were written, the COVID-19 pandemic broke out and many governments introduced physical distancing to slow the spread of the virus. Consequently, older people were frequently excluded from face-to-face contact and public discourse on the age-dependent value of life increased. The extent to which other forms of social contact (*e.g.* phone, video-calls), or shared experiential knowledge mitigated negative outcomes will be established by concurrent research. However, the academic community has a longer-term role to play in opposing ageist narratives and the 'legitimisation of ageism' in order to mollify discrimination and exclusion from social relations.

References

Aartsen, M. J., Van Tilburg, T., Smits, C. H., & Knipscheer, K. C. (2004). A longitudinal study of the impact of physical and cognitive decline on the personal network in old age. *Journal of Social and Personal Relationships, 21*(2), 249–266.

Bowlby, J. (1982). Attachment and loss: Retrospect and prospect. *American Journal of Orthopsychiatry, 52*(4), 664–678.

Burholt, V., & Sardani, A. V. (2017). The impact of residential immobility and population turnover on the support networks of older people living in rural areas: Evidence from CFAS Wales. *Population, Space and Place, 24*, e2132. https://doi.org/10.1002/psp.2132.

Burholt, V., Roberts, M. S., & Musselwhite, C. B. A. (2016). Older People's External Residential Assessment Tool (OPERAT): A complementary participatory and metric approach to the development of an observational environmental measure. *BMC Public Health, 16*, 1022. https://doi.org/10.1186/s12889-016-3681-x.

Burholt, V., Winter, B., Aartsen, M., Constantinou, C., Dahlberg, L., Feliciano, V., et al. (2019). A critical review and development of a conceptual model of exclusion from social relations for older people. *European Journal of Ageing, 17*, 3–19. https://doi.org/10.1007/s10433-019-00506-0.l.

Cronin, A., & King, A. (2010). Power, inequality and identification: Exploring diversity and intersectionality amongst older LGB adults. *Sociology, 44*, 876–892.

De Jong Gierveld, J., Broese van Groenou, M., Hoogendoorn, A. W., & Smit, J. H. (2009). Quality of marriages in later life and emotional and social loneliness. *Journal of Gerontology: Series B, 64*, 497–506.

Elder, G. H., Jr. (1994). Time, human agency, and social change: Perspectives on the life course. *Social Psychology Quarterly, 57*, 4–15.

Gibney, S., Delaney, L., Codd, M., & Fahey, T. (2017). Lifetime childlessness, depressive mood and quality of life among older Europeans. *Social Indicators Research, 130*(1), 305–323.

Lang, F. R. (2000). Endings and continuity of social relationships: Maximizing intrinsic benefits within personal networks when feeling near to death. *Journal of Social and Personal Relationships, 17*, 155–182.

Lechner, L., Bolman, C., & van Dalen, A. (2007). Definite involuntary childlessness: Associations between coping, social support and psychological distress. *Human Reproduction, 22*(1), 288–294.

Palmore, E. (2015). Ageism comes of age. *The Journals of Gerontology: Series B, 70*(6), 873–875. https://doi.org/10.1093/geronb/gbv079.

Perlman, D., & Peplau, L. A. (1981). Toward a social psychology of loneliness. In S. W. Duck & R. Gilmour (Eds.), *Personal relationships: 3. Personal relationships in disorder*. London: Academic.

Rook, K. S. (2003). Exposure and reactivity to negative social exchanges: A preliminary investigation using daily diary data. *The Journals of Gerontology: Series B, 58*(2), P100–P111.

Schoenmakers, E. C., van Tilburg, T. G., & Fokkema, T. (2015). Problem focused and emotion-focused coping options and loneliness: How are they related? *European Journal of Ageing, 12*, 153–161.

Skinner, M. W., Joseph, A. E., Hanlon, N., Halseth, G., & Ryser, L. (2014). Growing old in resource communities: Exploring the links among voluntarism, aging, and community development. *The Canadian Geographer, 58*(4), 418–428. https://doi.org/10.1111/cag.12087.

Van Regenmortel, S., De Donder, L., Dury, S., Smetcoren, A. S., De Witte, N., & Verté, D. (2016). Social exclusion in later life: A systematic review of the literature. *Journal of Population Ageing, 9*, 315–344.

Walters, P., & Bartlett, H. (2009). Growing old in a new estate: Establishing new social networks in retirement. *Ageing & Society, 29*(2), 217–236.

Winter, B. (2017). *Social exclusion among older people in rural areas: A multilevel and lifecourse perspective*. Swansea University. Swansea, Wales, UK.

Chapter 7
Exclusion from Social Relations Among Older People in Rural Britain and Belgium: A Cross-National Exploration Taking a Life-Course and Multilevel Perspective

Sofie Van Regenmortel, Bethan Winter, Angelika Thelin, Vanessa Burholt, and Liesbeth De Donder

7.1 Introduction

European countries are facing many challenges related to demographic changes and economic conditions. Recent evidence shows increasing socio-economic inequalities which are having a devastating effect on many people's lives (Joseph Rowntree Foundation and Bevan Foundation 2016). Such inequalities are also evident among older adults, with a significant proportion of this population experiencing disadvantage and social exclusion (Walsh et al. 2017). Social exclusion encompasses many forms: exclusion from socio-cultural participation, exclusion from services, exclusion from financial and material resources, exclusion from decent housing, ageism (Van Regenmortel et al. 2016; Walsh et al. 2017) but also exclusion from social relations which is a significant issue for older people within different countries (Winter 2018; Burholt et al. 2019).

As pointed out by Tsakloglou and Papadopoulos (2002) [and in the Introduction to this volume], social exclusion is "relative" implying that social exclusion does not manifest itself in the same way across countries. Not only prevalence, but also

S. Van Regenmortel (✉) · L. De Donder
Department of Adult Educational Sciences, Vrije Universiteit Brussel, Brussels, Belgium
e-mail: sofie.van.regenmortel@vub.be

B. Winter
Centre for Innovative Ageing, College of Human and Health Sciences, Swansea University, Wales, UK

A. Thelin
Linnaeus University, Växjö, Sweden

V. Burholt
University of Auckland, New Zealand, and Centre for Innovative Ageing, College of Human and Health Sciences, Swansea University, Wales, UK

K. Walsh et al. (eds.), *Social Exclusion in Later Life*, International Perspectives on Aging 28, https://doi.org/10.1007/978-3-030-51406-8_7

risk factors differ, leading to different national patterns (Pirani 2013). Some studies find, for instance, a higher risk of social exclusion in rural areas (Shergold and Parkhurst 2012; Spoor 2013; Vidovićová et al. this volume), while others find that urban dwelling individuals are at higher risk (Ogg 2005; Barnes et al. 2006; Nicholson and Cooper 2013). However, while a substantial body of literature on the social relations of older people exists, there is a paucity of cross-national comparative research on the topic of exclusion from social relations. This chapter attempts to address this gap by drawing upon two studies, conducted in rural Britain and Belgium, to explore similarities and differences in older people's experience of exclusion from social relations.

The chapter focuses on the following questions:

1. How does exclusion from social relations manifest among older people across rural Britain and Belgium?
2. What are the drivers that contribute to exclusion from social relations for older people within and across these countries?

This chapter will start with a definition of exclusion from social relations, and a summary of the outcomes and drivers of this form of exclusion documented in the international literature. In the following sections, a brief insight is given to the data and methods of the studies. Next, the results are presented: first the quantitative results, then the qualitative insights. Finally, the conclusions are summarised and limitations and paths for policy recommendations and further cross-national research are discussed.

7.2 Literature Overview

Drawing on a recent scoping review of social exclusion literature by Walsh et al. (2017), and as outlined by Burholt and Aartsen introducing this section, we conceptualise social relations as comprising social resources, social connections and social networks. This domain of exclusion is partially concerned with the ability of individuals to establish, develop and maintain relationships with family, friends and neighbours. The frequency, closeness and quality of these relationships are important factors to be taken into consideration (Barnes et al. 2006; Lubben 2006; Burholt et al. 2019).

In terms of outcomes, evidence suggests that good and extensive social relations with a range of people and groups including family, friends, neighbours and community groups foster social inclusion (Barnes et al. 2006; Gray 2009). Positive social relations have been found to be a significant source of satisfaction and meaning for older people (Gallagher 2012). Social relations can be a source of advice and support in a variety of ways, including providing care, transport or financial assistance, thus enabling older people to continue their lifestyle and maintain their independence (Scharf and Bartlam 2008). There is also good evidence that good social relations can help older people to maintain physical and psychological health and functioning (Gallagher 2012; Courtin and Knapp 2017; Shankar et al. 2017). Conversely, exclusion from social relations has been associated with greater levels of loneliness in the older population (de Jong Gierveld et al. 2006; Victor et al. 2008). Exclusion from social relations can lead to reduced social opportunities such as employment, volunteering, or other forms of social participation (Phillipson et al. 2004; de Espanés et al. 2015).

When looking at the drivers of social exclusion, we adopt a critical human ecological theoretical framework (Keating and Phillips 2008) and draw on three "systems" or levels within the ecological model to contextualise our approach. These are (i) the macro system which incorporates structural issues including ideology, political landscape, norms, values, and national policies; (ii) the exosystem which refers to structure and organisations that affect the immediate environment – that is, natural and physical elements of the environment, alongside services, amenities and employment opportunities in the local area; (iii) the microsystem which focuses upon individual characteristics, traits and attributes (Burholt et al. 2019). In addition to these three systems, the mesosystem comprises interactions between microsystems. While this is not explicitly labelled in this chapter, the interactions and interconnections between systems are referred to in each section.

At a macro level, cultural and policy effects exclusion from social relations. Normative expectations about sources of support and family forms have a bearing on the extent to which social relations can protect or buffer an older person from adverse outcomes. In more individualistic cultures, the state or the market are recognised as important actors in providing welfare for older persons in need. In more collectivistic cultures, private social networks and the civic sector are emphasised as important actors on this matter. The normative configuration of networks of family and friends differs between individualist and collectivist cultures and deviations from normative networks result in greater loneliness for older people (Burholt and Dobbs 2014; Winter 2018). Also (stereotypical) attitudes and beliefs towards older people and the ageing process (*e.g.* ageism), influence older adults' inclusion in social networks (Burholt et al. 2019).

In the exosystem the physical environment has an important influence on exclusion from social relations. For example, neighbourhood design, housing diversity, population density, mixed land use and open space are associated with walkability and social contact (Bowling and Stafford 2007; Byles et al. 2014; Lager et al. 2015; Burholt et al. 2016). The influence of the environment on social relations could be also considered in terms of settlement type, which may be defined using clusters of variables describing different types of rural/urban areas, or areas experiencing multiple deprivations or disadvantages [see Drilling et al. and Vidovićová et al. this volume]. While some authors have noted that exclusion from social relations is particularly pronounced for those living in deprived and remote rural areas (Milne et al. 2007), Scharf et al. (2005) found that older people living in deprived urban areas are more vulnerable to exclusion from social relations than those living in the UK as a whole. A close association has also been found between community change, notably inward-outward migration, population change and exclusion from social resources (Scharf and Bartlam 2008; Gray 2009). Population change for example may have a detrimental impact upon social relations of the indigenous local older people whose family networks may no longer be available, as well as on the networks of older people that have moved into an area and who do not have access to local support that has been established over time (Scharf and Bartlam 2008; Burholt and Sardani 2017).

At a micro level, studies reveal that certain individual characteristics or life events impact on exclusion from social relations including gender, marital status, health, retirement and socio-economic status [see Urbaniak et al. this volume]. While social isolation is more common for women than men (Wenger et al. 1996), the differences are largely due to differences in marital status with women more likely to be widowed and living alone. Older people who are living alone and those without children are most likely to experience difficulties with regards to social resources (Gray 2009). Poor health is also a risk for exclusion from social relations: poor health, impairment or pain impact on the ability to maintain usual lifestyles including customary levels of social interaction and can precipitate a decline in social relations (Bertoni et al. 2015; Hilaria and Northcott 2017). Research across a range of countries, reveals that material deprivation and poverty limits full participation in the social life of communities for older people, limiting opportunities to optimise and diversify social interaction, and contribute significantly to exclusion from social relations (Ajrouch et al. 2005; Ellwardt et al. 2014; see Sumil-Laanemaa et al. and Barlin et al. this volume).

7.3 Data and Methods

7.3.1 General Research Approach

To answer the research questions, the chapter draws upon two PhD studies on rural Britain (Winter 2018) and Belgium (Van Regenmortel 2017). Both studies show some similarities and differences. In terms of similarities, both used a theoretical framework informed by the life-course and exclusion literature. Both also examined social exclusion in general, with exclusion from social relations emerging as an important domain in their studies. Finally, both studies used a similar mixed method design: quantitative analyses of survey data and qualitative life story interviews. In terms of differences, the research in rural Britain was conducted between 2012 and 2017, and studied older people's experience of social exclusion underpinned by a transformative worldview (Winter 2018). The Belgian study of Van Regenmortel (2017) conducted between 2013 and 2017 was built upon a life-course perspective and environmental gerontology to study old-age social exclusion. In addition, the British study focused on rural-dwelling older adults in England and Wales, while the Belgian study included both rural and urban communities in the research.

7.3.2 Quantitative Phase

The quantitative phase of both cross-sectional studies examined the different categories of social exclusion through secondary analysis of existing datasets within each country: Grey and Pleasant Land study (2014) conducted in rural Britain (South West England and Wales) (Hennessy et al. 2014a); Belgian Ageing Studies (data collected in different municipalities between 2008 and 2014) in Belgium. In both studies, exploratory latent class analysis was used to develop classes of social exclusion that best fitted the data for older people living in rural Britain and Belgium.

The Belgian study operationalised social exclusion based on a systematic review conducted earlier (Van Regenmortel et al. 2016) and the data available in the large-scale quantitative Belgian Ageing Studies survey. This resulted in four sub dimensions for exclusion from social relations (for more detailed information on data collection and analysis, see Van Regenmortel et al. 2017). In the rural Britain study the best fit model used all relevant available data (for more detailed information on data collection and analysis, see Hennessy et al. 2014b). Table 7.1 shows how exclusion from social relations was operationalised in both quantitative studies.

Table 7.1 Operationalisation of exclusion from social relations in the rural Britain and Belgian studies

Exclusion from social relations	
Rural Britain	
Very lonely (emotionally & socially)	Loneliness was measured using the six-item de Jong Gierveld scale (de Jong Gierveld and Van Tilburg 2006) which measures loneliness through six indirect questions about emotional and social loneliness. The total loneliness score was the sum of the two scores (emotional & social) with scores ranging from zero (not lonely) through to six (extremely lonely) (de Jong Gierveld and Van Tilburg 1999).
Exclusion from social ties	An amended version of the Lubben Social Network Scale (LSNS-6) was used to measure exclusion from social relations. The scale consists of three questions that calculate kinship ties and three questions that assess non-kin ties. Lower scores indicated fewer social relations and higher scores indicated more social relations.
Belgium	
Very emotionally lonely	Loneliness was measured using the six-item de Jong Gierveld scale (de Jong Gierveld and Van Tilburg 2006). If respondents indicated for each of the three emotional loneliness indicators that they were lonely, they were assessed as very emotionally lonely.
Very socially lonely	Derived from the six item scale for loneliness (de Jong Gierveld and Van Tilburg 2006). If respondents indicated for each of the three social loneliness variables that they were lonely, they were assessed as very socially lonely.
Exclusion from social contacts	If respondents did not have at least once-a-month contact with family members, friends or neighbours they were considered as excluded from social contacts.
Exclusion from social support	If respondents could not count on support of family members, friends or neighbours they were considered as excluded from social support.

These measures that captured exclusion form social relations were taken together with a range of other social exclusion domains (*e.g.* exclusion from services, exclusion from participation) and latent class analysis was used to develop a model of social exclusion that "best fits" the sample of older people in each of the studies.

7.3.3 *Qualitative Phase*

The qualitative phase of both studies involved life history interviews with older people. In the rural Britain study, the sample was drawn only from Wales for the PhD study: ten older people in three rural case study areas (N = 30) were recruited, using purposive sampling, for life history interviews (Winter and Burholt 2018). Interviews focussed upon hardship and prosperity. An Interpretive Phenomenological Analytical approach (IPA) was used to analyse the data. This approach focuses upon understanding participants' subjective realities through personal interpretations of their lived experiences and the meanings they attach to experiences within a specific context (Smith 2004).

Qualitative data in the Belgian PhD study came from 19 life stories of older adults (60+ years) living on low income (for more detailed information on data collection and analysis, see Van Regenmortel et al. 2019). The qualitative study aimed to understand the experience and the narrated life course of financially excluded older adults, and consequently to give voice to groups of people that are often not reached by (longitudinal) surveys (Chamberlayne et al. 2000). The methodology leaned on narrative theory (Bluck and Habermas 2001) and used adapted life story interview guidelines of McAdams (2005, 2008) to conduct the study.

7.4 Results

The results section first presents the results of the quantitative phase, and then explores the qualitative material.

7.4.1 *Quantitative Results: Manifestations of Exclusion from Social Relations Among Older People Across Rural Britain and Belgium*

Table 7.2 provides the results from the Latent Class Analyses on the nature and level of social exclusion experienced by older people in rural Britain and Belgium.

Table 7.2 Categories of old-age social exclusion after latent class analysis

Rural Britain (N = 864 rural)	Belgium (N = 20,275 rural & urban)
Least Social Exclusion (76%): **high levels of social relations**, lowest levels of poverty, least difficulty accessing services and accessing leisure and cultural amenities, broadest civic engagement and participation in individual activities.	***Low Risk of Social Exclusion*** (45.7%)**: high levels of social relations**, low risk of exclusion from civic participation, financial resources, the neighbourhood, decent housing and services, low level of digital exclusion and ageism.
Moderate Social Exclusion (13%): **high levels of social relations**, moderate to low difficulty accessing services, leisure and cultural amenities, broad civic engagement and participation in individual activities, higher levels of poverty.	***Non- participating Financially Excluded*** (25.5%): high digital exclusion, high levels of exclusion from civic participation and financial exclusion / **higher levels of social relations**, inclusion in the neighbourhood, high levels of access to decent housing, services and less ageism.
Moderate Social Exclusion but Service Poor (7%): **high level of social relations**, broad participation in individual activities and moderate civic engagement, moderate to high difficulty accessing services, leisure and cultural amenities and higher levels of poverty.	***Environmentally Excluded*** (12.5%): **exclusion from social relations,** services, neighbourhood, decent housing and ageism.
Extreme Social Exclusion (4%): **lowest level of social relations**, greatest difficulty accessing services, leisure and cultural amenities, low civic engagement and participation in individual activities, higher levels of poverty.	***Severely Excluded*** (16.2%): **a higher probability of combined exclusion in all dimensions of old-age social exclusion.**

Analysis of the rural British data identified four latent classes. First, people classified in the "Least Social Exclusion" class were the largest group. They had high levels of social relations and the lowest levels of poverty. These older people had the least difficulty accessing services and accessing leisure and cultural amenities. They had the broadest involvement in civic engagement and the broadest participation in individual activities. Second, the "Moderate Social Exclusion" class was the second largest class. People classified in this group had high levels of social relations, moderate to low difficulty accessing services and moderate difficulty accessing leisure and cultural amenities. People in this class had broad involvement in civic engagement and broad participation in individual activities. They also had relatively high levels of poverty. Third, people in the "Moderate Social Exclusion but Service Poor" class had a high level of social relations, broad participation in individual activities and moderate involvement in civic engagement. However, they had moderate to high difficulty accessing services and moderate difficulty accessing leisure and cultural amenities. They also experienced relatively high levels of poverty. Fourth, people classified in the "Extreme Social Exclusion" group experienced the lowest level of social relations, the greatest difficulty accessing services and the greatest difficulty accessing leisure and cultural amenities [see Gallistl this volume for an exploration of the links between cultural participation and socio-economic status]. They had low involvement in civic engagement and low participation in individual activities. These people had relatively high levels of poverty.

The Belgian study also generated four different classes. The first class "Low Risk of Social Exclusion" had high levels of social relations and the lowest risk to be excluded from civic participation, financial resources, the neighbourhood, and decent housing. This category also had the lowest level of digital exclusion experiences or feelings of ageism. They had a considerably low chance of being excluded from services. Second, "Non- participating Financially Excluded" were older adults that combined the highest chance of digital exclusion [see Poli et al. this volume] with higher levels of exclusion from civic participation together with financial exclusion. They had, however, higher levels of social relations, and lower levels of exclusion from the neighbourhood, decent housing, and services and they experienced less ageism. Third, the "Environmentally Excluded" category were the most likely to have experienced exclusion from social relations and services. Furthermore, they experienced a higher probability of neighbourhood and housing exclusion. They also had a higher probability of feeling excluded due to their age (ageism). Fourth, the "Severely Excluded" experienced, compared to the total population, a higher probability of combined exclusion in all dimensions of old-age social exclusion.

It was striking how similar the characteristics of the latent classes were across both studies. One difference could be found in terms of social relations: in the rural Britain study exclusion from social relations was confined to one class which consisted of a small minority of the sample with only 4% comprising the "Extreme Social Exclusion" class. In contrast, exclusion from social relations affected a much larger proportion of older people in the Belgium study across two classes, namely the "Environmentally Excluded" (12.5%) and the "Severely Excluded" (16.2%). This may be because exclusion from social relations was operationalised differently in both studies, or because the areas selected (rural vs rural plus urban) experienced different levels of exclusion from social relations.

7.4.2 Qualitative Results: Manifestations and Drivers of Exclusion from Social Relations throughout the Life Course

First the results of the life story interviews in rural Britain are discussed. This is followed by the results of the life stories in Belgium. For both studies, manifestations of exclusion from social relations, and then the drivers of exclusion (in the microsystem, exosystem and macrosystem) will be discussed.

7.4.3 Rural Britain Study

In rural Britain (Wales only) the qualitative evidence suggested that relationships with family, friends and neighbours were a source of inclusion for the majority of participants during their childhood and working adult lives. For example, one male participant commented that:

> 'So, as I say it was a good place to be brought up in because you knew all your neighbours, friends and their parents as well.' (M 86 years)

These social relations were vital for several reasons. First, they were a source of emotional and instrumental support for participants and fostered a positive sense of community. Second, a number of participants linked their close family relationships to their limited material resources, explaining that living with extended family was a necessity because of poverty. This was especially true in the pre-Second World War period when state assistance was minimal. Some participants described how their family would care for family members suffering ill health, sometimes resulting in co-residence. Third, local people often worked and socialised together. Networks were important in terms of security and safety and created a sense of a close-knit community.

> 'You were in it together and no household was different to the other. It didn't matter about your status, your income or anything like… because people lived in the valley and they stayed in the valleys. They didn't move out.' (M, 95 years)

In rural Britain, exclusion from social relations was a problem for a small minority of participants during childhood and early adulthood. This was attributable to the remoteness of their homes: they lived either on farms or small holdings located a significant distance from others (family, friends and neighbours) as well as from services and activities. These participants explained that the experience of exclusion from social relations caused feelings of isolation and loneliness, especially during their childhood when they yearned to have friends to play with, as evidenced by the following quote from one participant:

> '[I was] a very remote and lonely child really, because I didn't have anyone to play with. I would play with the cats mostly […] and I had my dolls. But there were no children for me to play with.' (F 81 years)

Exclusion from relationships with family and neighbours became an increasing concern as participants aged, resulting in feelings of loneliness and isolation. This was the result of primary drivers of exclusion from social relations: older age (microsystem), bereavement (microsystem), remote and rural living (exosystem) and population change (macrosystem).

Bereavement had a significant impact on social relations for some participants resulting in feelings of loneliness and isolation. For example, one participant spoke at length about the effect that the death of his wife four years earlier from a short illness had on his life. He recollected that they were married for over 50 years and were extremely close, doing everything together and being a source of support to one another. He explained that currently, with his two sons living away and few friends in the locality, his social relations were dwindling.

Participants felt that population turnover had a negative impact on community cohesion and their sense of belonging. Out-migration was impacting negatively upon older people's social relations, in particular on the availability of family to provide physical and emotional support. For example, one participant who lived alone and whose son lived and worked abroad, expressed frustration at not having family nearby to ask for help with such tasks as household repairs. She also expressed deep sadness at the loss of emotional support and, during the interview, alluded to feeling lonely. At the same time in-migration had a negative impact on social relations of participants, especially neighbours. While a few participants spoke positively about their neighbours the majority were critical of those who had migrated to the area who, they felt, were not a source of support and did not contribute to the community. This is illustrated by the following quote:

> 'Um, I came to know everyone in the village and I could tell which house they were in. Everyone, I knew everyone, right? But now I don't know those that live on this road here. That's the difference. People have moved in you see. Strangers and they don't [help]……. the village has completely changed.' (F 81 years)

7.4.4 Belgian Study

In Belgium, social relations were an important element in the life stories of financially excluded older adults: both new social relations (*e.g.* childbirth, marriage) as well as exclusion from social relations (*e.g.* divorce and death of relatives and friends) were present. This shows the value that is given to social relations in one's life and how previous events and situations impacted on current experiences. When talking about their future lives social relations were emphasised as especially important. Many respondents wanted to live long enough to see (great) grandchildren growing up. Besides maintaining social relations, they also wanted to build new social relations in the future.

> 'I hope I may be around for many years. For my daughter. And for my grandchildren too. That I can be here for a long time.' (Leonie, F, 64 years)

Older respondents experienced exclusion because of social relations. Social relations were then drivers of old-age social exclusion. Marie, for instance, (F, 73 years) considered the bad way her mother treated her to be a major influence throughout her life, because it created an inferiority complex. Other respondents spoke about being scammed by their acquaintances or business partners, leading to financial difficulties and even bankruptcy. Taking custody of grandchildren had also led to financial difficulties and a significant decrease in participation in social and civic activities [see Waldegrave et al. this section for an in-depth discussion of conflicting social relations].

The older people interviewed did, however, not only problematise social relations but viewed them as a significant enabler for the future. This was especially the case if people had bad health or a disability. In many life stories, having (quality) social relations and social support could prevent (further) exclusion in different fields. For instance, Jos, an 81-year-old man, recounted that after a life full of misery and worries, the help of his wife was indispensable. Thanks to her, he went to the public service for local welfare and received help. For some older adults, the support of relatives mitigated financial or material difficulties slightly. This was illustrated by this account of Jos, whose son bought him a car.

> 'I drove fifteen years with that car. At the end, the car was worn out and I had no car anymore. My son said that I should have a car. We were in the garage and there was a little second-hand car for 2500 euros. My son bought me the car.' (Jos, M, 81 years)

Older respondents experienced exclusion because of the cumulative effects of particular drivers on the development of social relations over time. Important drivers were: divorce/widowhood (micro), financial difficulties (micro), regulations on social benefits (macro).

Divorce and widowhood were often significant life events or turning points causing exclusion from social relations [also see Barlin et al. this volume]. These events led to loneliness and influenced other dimensions of old-age social exclusion (*e.g.* financial loss).

Having a low income was clearly a driver of exclusion from social relations. Respondents talked about living on a low income and how this caused difficulties in their everyday lives, such as participating less in certain social and cultural activities. Both Roger's (M, 64 years) and Jos's (M, 81 years) social network for instance shrank after going bankrupt and subsequently facing financial difficulties.

A macro-level influence on social relations was the way in which financial social support provided by the government was organised. Some respondents receiving social benefits and having a relationship with someone with social benefits were prohibited to live in the same house, as this would mean a considerable loss for the financial support received.

It was clear from the life stories that there was a relationship between different drivers and the accumulation of turning points. For example, one male participant explained:

> 'That [depression] all started with my divorce, followed by losing my job and [then there were] all those bereavements. Everything piling up in one year.' (Jef, M, 76 years)

7.5 Conclusion

This chapter draws upon two studies conducted in rural Britain and Belgium which explored similarities and differences in older people's experience of exclusion from social relations. Although the research has demonstrated that in both rural Britain and Belgium social relations are vital for several reasons (*e.g.* health and care, practical support in times of poverty, safety), some older participants in both countries face exclusion from social relations (*e.g.* feelings of loneliness, isolation, 'bad' social relations). In both quantitative studies, exclusion from social relations were manifest in at least one type of old-age social exclusion. In Belgium, exclusion from social relations was more broadly operationalised which led to larger old-age social exclusion classes.

A second similarity between the studies is the strong interrelationship between exclusion from social relations with other domains of exclusion (*e.g.* economic and material exclusion). These interrelationships were also clearly demonstrated in the life story interviews (*e.g.* exclusion from social relations as a driver for other types of exclusion and vice versa).

In terms of drivers of exclusion from social relations the life stories revealed micro (*e.g.* marital status, gender), exo (*e.g.* being remote and rural living) and macro drivers of exclusion from social relations (*e.g.* the way in which financial social support provided by the government was organised, and population change).

Some limitations of the current research should be highlighted. Although the quantitative and qualitative research methods of both studies are very similar, differences posed challenges to this cross-national exploration. Not only do Britain and Belgium differ in language and socio-political organisation, but the way in which data were sampled and collected was not identical. These challenges should be taken into account when interpreting this cross-national exploration. The contribution of this chapter lays in the bringing together of existing quantitative and qualitative data sources for a cross-national explorative purpose in order to understand exclusion from social relations, and old-age social exclusion in general. Further cross-national explorative comparative research on the subject and with a common methodological approach is needed. We hope that such further research will find inspiration from the results of this and other already conducted explorative cross-national studies.

Based on our findings, two main recommendations can be identified. First, a multilevel approach targeting exo and macro factors is needed as not only individual factors (*e.g.* gender, age, education) influence the likelihood of being excluded from social relations. The fact that older adults tend to age in place (Wagner et al. 2010) and that they rely on resources and services available in the locality because of their reduced action radius (Krause 2004), promotes a focus on investing in the creation of age-friendly and prosperous environments to enable social inclusion (Scharlach et al. 2013; Drilling et al. this volume). Second, the life story interviews in both studies show that life events [see also Urbaniak et al. this volume] might influence exclusion from social relations in both the short and long-term. Consequently, policy tackling old-age social exclusion might usefully approach this form of exclusion from a life-course perspective, which means that fighting old-age social exclusion already starts with preventing and fighting exclusion at earlier life stages (Scharf et al. 2005). From this study, and earlier research, it is clear that disadvantages in different life stages are connected and therefore a life-course oriented social policy is needed.

Editors' Postscript

Please note, like other contributions to this book, this chapter was written before the COVID-19 pandemic of 2020. The book's introductory chapter (Chap. 1) and conclusion (Chap. 34) consider some of the key ways in which the pandemic relates to issues concerning social exclusion and ageing.

References

Ajrouch, K. J., Blandon, A. Y., & Antonucci, T. C. (2005). Social networks among men and women: The effects of age and socioeconomic status. *The Journals of Gerontology Series B: Psychological Sciences and Social Sciences, 60*(6), S311–S317.

Barnes, M., Blom, A., Cox, K., & Lessof, C. (2006). *The social exclusion of older people: Evidence from the first wave of the English longitudinal study of ageing (ELSA)*. London: Office of the Deputy Prime Minister, Social Exclusion Unit.

Bertoni, M., Celidoni, M., & Weber, G. (2015). Does hearing impairment lead to social exclusion? In A. Börsch-Supan, T. Kneip, H. Litwin, M. Myck, & G. Weber (Eds.), *Ageing in Europe – Supporting policies for an inclusive society* (pp. 93–102). DeGruyter.

Bluck, S., & Habermas, T. (2001). Extending the study of autobiographical memory: Thinking back about life across the life span. *Review of General Psychology, 5*(2), 135–147.

Bowling, A., & Stafford, M. (2007). How do objective and subjective assessments of neighbourhood influence social and physical functioning in older age? Findings from a British survey of ageing. *Social Science & Medicine, 64*(12), 2533–2549. https://doi.org/10.1016/j.socscimed.2007.03.009.

Burholt, V., & Dobbs, C. (2014). A support network typology for application in older populations with a preponderance of multigenerational households. *Ageing and Society, 34*(7), 1142–1169. https://doi.org/10.1017/S0144686X12001511.

Burholt, V., & Sardani, A. V. (2017). The impact of residential immobility and population turnover on the support networks of older people living in rural areas: Evidence from CFAS Wales. *Population, Space and Place, 24*, e2132.

Burholt, V., Roberts, M. S., & Musselwhite, C. B. A. (2016). Older People's External Residential Assessment Tool (OPERAT): A complementary participatory and metric approach to the development of an observational environmental measure. *BMC Public Health, 16*(1), 1022. https://doi.org/10.1186/s12889-016-3681-x.

Burholt, V., Winter, B., Aartsen, M., Constantinou, C., Dahlberg, L., Feliciano, V., et al. (2019). 156 A critical review and development of a conceptual model of exclusion from social relations for older people. *European Journal of Ageing, 17*, 3–19. https://doi.org/10.1007/s10433-019-00506-0.

Byles, J. E., Leigh, L., Vo, K., Forder, P., & Curryer, C. (2014). Life space and mental health: A study of older community-dwelling persons in Australia. *Aging and Mental Health, 19*(2), 98–106. https://doi.org/10.1080/13607863.2014.917607.

Chamberlayne, P., Bornat, J., & Wengraf, T. (2000). *The turn to biographical methods in social science: Comparative issues and examples*. London/New York: Routledge.

Courtin, E., & Knapp, M., (2017). Social isolation, loneliness and health in old age: A scoping review. *Health and Social Care in the Community, 25*, 799–812.

de Espanés, G. M., Villar, F., Urrutia, A., & Serrat, R. (2015). Motivation and commitment to volunteering in a sample of Argentinian adults: What is the role of generativity? *Educational Gerontology, 41*(2), 149–161.

de Jong Gierveld, J., & Van Tilburg, T. (1999). *Manual of the loneliness scale*. Amsterdam: Department of Social Research Methodology, Vrije Universiteit Amsterdam.

de Jong Gierveld, J., & Van Tilburg, T. (2006). A 6-item scale for overall, emotional, and social loneliness confirmatory tests on survey data. *Research on Aging, 28*(5), 582–598.

de Jong Gierveld, J., van Tilburg, T. G., & Dykstra, P. A. (2006). Loneliness and social isolation. In A. L. Vangelisti & D. Perlman (Eds.), *The Cambridge handbook of personal relationships* (pp. 485–500). Cambridge/New York: Cambridge University Press.

Ellwardt, L., Peter, S., Präg, P., & Steverink, N. (2014). Social contacts of older people in 27 European countries: The role of welfare spending and economic inequality. *European Sociological Review, 30*(4), 413–430. https://doi.org/10.1093/esr/jcu046.

Gallagher, C. (2012). Connectedness in the lives of older people in Ireland: A study of the communal participation of older people in two geographic localities. *Irish Journal of Sociology, 20*(1), 84–102. https://doi.org/10.7227/IJS.20.1.5.

Gray, A. (2009). The social capital of older people. *Ageing and Society, 29*(1), 5–31. https://doi.org/10.1017/S0144686X08007617.

Hennessy, C., Means, R., & Burholt, V. (2014a). *Countryside connections: Older people, community and place in rural Britain*. Bristol: Policy Press.

Hennessy, C., Means, R., & Burholt, V. (2014b). Countryside connections in later life: Setting the scene. In C. Hennessy, R. Means, & V. Burholt (Eds.), *Countryside connections: Older people, community and place in rural Britain* (pp. 1–30). Bristol: Policy Press.

Hilaria, K., & Northcott, S. (2017). "Struggling to stay connected": Comparing the social relationships of healthy older people and people with stroke and aphasia. *Aphasiology, 31*(6), 647–687. https://doi.org/10.1080/02687038.2016.1218436.

Joseph Rowntree Foundation, & Bevan Foundation. (2016). *Prosperity without poverty: A framework for action in Wales*. York: Joseph Rowntree Foundation.

Keating, N., & Phillips, J. (2008). A critical human ecology perspective on rural ageing. In N. Keating (Ed.), *Rural ageing: A good place to grow old* (pp. 1–10). Bristol: Policy Press.

Krause, N. (2004). Neighbourhoods, health and wellbeing in later life. In H. W. Wahl et al. (Eds.), *Annual review of gerontology and geriatrics* (pp. 22–49). New York: Springer.

Lager, D., Hover, B. v., & Huigen, P. P. (2015). Understanding older adults' social capital in place: Obstacles to and opportunities for social contacts in the neighbourhood. *Geoforum, 59*, 87–97. https://doi.org/10.1016/j.geoforum.2014.12.009.

Lubben, J. (2006). Abbreviated and targeted geriatric assessment. In B. Berkman (Ed.), *Handbook of social work in health and aging* (pp. 729–735). New York: Oxford University Press.

McAdams, D. P. (2005). Studying lives in time: A narrative approach. *Advances in Life Course Research, 10*, 237–258.

McAdams, D. P. (2008). *The life story interview.* http://www.sesp.northwestern.edu/foley/instruments/interview/. Accessed 15 Sep 2015.

Milne, A., Hatzidimitriadou, E., & Wiseman, J. (2007). Health and quality of life among older people in rural England: Exploring the impact and efficacy of policy. *Journal of Social Policy, 36*, 477–495.

Nicholson, L., & Cooper, S. A. (2013). Social exclusion and people with intellectual disabilities: A rural-urban comparison. *Journal of Intellectual Disability Research, 57*(4), 333–346. https://doi.org/10.1111/j.1365-2788.2012.01540.x.

Ogg, J. (2005). Social exclusion and insecurity among older Europeans: The influence of welfare regimes. *Ageing & Society, 25*(1), 69–90. https://doi.org/10.1017/S0144686X04002788.

Phillipson, C., Allan, G., & Morgan, D. (2004). Introduction. In C. Phillipson, G. Allan, & D. Morgan (Eds.), *Social networks and social exclusion: Sociological and policy perspectives* (pp. 1–6). Abingdon: Routledge.

Pirani, E. (2013). Evaluating contemporary social exclusion in Europe: A hierarchical latent class approach. *Quality & Quantity, 47*(2), 923–941.

Scharf, T., & Bartlam, B. (2008). Ageing and social exclusion in rural communities. In N. Keating (Ed.), *Rural ageing: A good place to grow old?* (pp. 97–108). Bristol: Policy Press.

Scharf, T., Phillipson, C., & Smith, A. E. (2005). *Multiple exclusion and quality of life amongst excluded older people in disadvantaged neighbourhoods*. London: Social Exclusion Unit.

Scharlach, A. E., Lehning, A. J., Warburton, J., Ng, S. H., & Shardlow, S. M. (2013). Ageing-friendly communities and social inclusion in the United States of America. *Ageing & Society, 33*(1), 110–136.

Shankar, A., McMunn, A., Demakakos, P., Hamer, M., & Steptoe, A. (2017). Social isolation and loneliness: Prospective associations with functional status in older adults. *Health Psychology, 36*(2), 179.

Shergold, I., & Parkhurst, G. (2012). Transport-related social exclusion amongst older people in rural Southwest England and Wales. *Journal of Rural Studies, 28*(4), 412–421. https://doi.org/10.1016/j.jrurstud.2012.01.010.

Smith, J. A. (2004). Reflecting on the development of interpretative phenomenological analysis and its contribution to qualitative research in psychology. *Qualitative Research in Psychology, 1*(1), 39–54.

Spoor, M. (2013). Multidimensional social exclusion and the 'rural-urban divide' in Eastern Europe and Central Asia. *Sociologia Ruralis, 53*(2), 139–157. https://doi.org/10.1111/soru.12008.

Tsakloglou, P., & Papadopoulos, F. (2002). Aggregate level and determining factors of social exclusion in twelve European countries. *Journal of European Social Policy, 12*(3), 211–225.

Van Regenmortel, S. (2017). *Social exclusion in later life: Measurement and drivers of social exclusion among older people* (Phd-dissertation). Zelzate: Open University Press.

Van Regenmortel, S., De Donder, L., Dury, S., Smetcoren, A.-S., De Witte, N., & Verté, D. (2016). Social exclusion in later life: A systematic review of the literature. *Journal of Population Ageing, 9*, 315–344. https://doi.org/10.1007/s12062-016-9145-3.

Van Regenmortel, S., De Donder, L., Smetcoren, A.-S., Lambotte, D., De Witte, N., & Verté, D. (2017). Accumulation of disadvantages: Prevalence and categories of old-age social exclusion in Belgium. *Social Indicators Research*. https://doi.org/10.1007/s11205-017-1817-8.

Van Regenmortel, S., Smetcoren, A., Marsillas, S., Lambotte, D., Fret, B., & De Donder, L. (2019). Exploring underexposed stories: The experienced lifecourse of financially excluded older adults. *Ageing and Society*, 1–22. https://doi.org/10.1017/S0144686X19001235.

Victor, C., Scambler, S., & Bond, J. (2008). *The social world of older people: Understanding loneliness and social isolation in later life*. London: McGraw-Hill Education.

Wagner, S. L., Shubair, M. M., & Michalos, A. C. (2010). Surveying older adults' opinions on housing: Recommendations for policy. *Social Indicators Research, 99*(3), 405–412.

Walsh, K., Scharf, T., & Keating, N. (2017). Social exclusion of older persons: A scoping review and conceptual framework. *European Journal of Ageing, 14*(1), 81–98.

Wenger, G. C., Davies, R., Shahtahmasebi, S., & Scott, A. (1996). Social isolation and loneliness in old age: Review and model refinement. *Ageing and Society, 16*(03), 333–358. https://doi.org/10.1017/s0144686x00003457.

Winter, B., 2018. *Disadvantage and advantage among older people in rural communities in Wales: A multi-level and life-course perspective*. PhD. Swansea University, Wales, UK.

Winter, B., & Burholt, V. (2018). Y Cymry Cymreig: Cultural exclusion among rural-dwelling older people, a critical human ecological approach. *International Journal of Aging and Later Life, 12* (2), 119–151. https://doi.org/10.3384/ijal.1652-8670.18399.

Chapter 8
Revisiting Loneliness: Individual and Country-Level Changes

Deborah Morgan, Lena Dahlberg, Charles Waldegrave, Sarmitė Mikulionienė, Gražina Rapolienė, Giovanni Lamura, and Marja Aartsen

8.1 Introduction

8.1.1 Background and Aim of the Chapter

The main focus of this chapter is on exclusion from social relations, and loneliness as an important outcome of this exclusion. Although exclusion from social relations is sometimes equated with loneliness, this is not the same. People can feel lonely in a crowd, while at the same time people who are socially excluded are not necessarily lonely (Weiss 1973). Nevertheless, [and as outlined in Burholt and Aartsen this section], loneliness is recognised as a critical outcome of exclusionary

D. Morgan (✉)
Centre for Innovative Ageing, Swansea University, Wales, UK
e-mail: d.j.morgan@swansea.ac.uk

L. Dahlberg
Dalarna University, Falun, Sweden

Aging Research Center, Karolinska Institutet, Solna, Sweden

Stockholm University, Stockholm, Sweden

C. Waldegrave
Family Centre Social Policy Research Unit, Lower Hutt, Wellington, New Zealand

S. Mikulionienė
Lithuanian Social Research Centre, Institute of Sociology, Vilnius, Lithuania

G. Rapolienė
Lithuanian Social Research Centre, Vilnius Lithuania

G. Lamura
Centre for Socio-Economic Research on Ageing, INRCA-IRCCS, National Institute of Health and Science on Ageing, Ancona, Italy

M. Aartsen
NOVA-Norwegian Social Research, Oslo Metropolitan University, Oslo, Norway

K. Walsh et al. (eds.), *Social Exclusion in Later Life*, International Perspectives on Aging 28, https://doi.org/10.1007/978-3-030-51406-8_8

processes within the social relations domain. The consequences of loneliness are severe, including poor physical and mental health (Wilson et al. 2007; Holt-Lunstad et al. 2015) and increased health care and societal costs (Cacioppo and Cacioppo 2018). Loneliness occurs at all ages, with a higher prevalence in older-age ranging from 10% in northern European countries to 30% in southern and Eastern European countries (Yang and Victor 2011).

Cross-sectional studies on loneliness in older-age have produced robust evidence for a number of individual correlates of loneliness (further presented below), and a growing number of longitudinal studies have also provided evidence that some of these correlates are in fact micro-level drivers of loneliness, that is, leading to increased feelings of loneliness. Cross-national studies so far provided insight on macro-level correlates with loneliness, but none of these studies had a longitudinal design. Hence, our understanding of micro and macro-level drivers of loneliness is still limited (Courtin and Knapp 2017). The aim of this study is to advance our understanding of micro- and macro-level drivers of loneliness in later life, by examining a number of the well-established micro-level factors, along with several theoretically plausible macro-level drivers. We base the selection of macro-level drivers on the theoretical conceptualisation of social exclusion by Walsh et al. (2017). This framework of old-age exclusion identifies six key domains: neighbourhood and community; services, amenities and mobility; material and financial resources; social relations; socio-cultural aspects of society; and civic participation. The conceptual framework on social exclusion illustrates how exclusion from one domain is associated with exclusion in other domains.

8.1.2 Micro-Level Drivers of Loneliness

Micro-level drivers of loneliness can be grouped into three broad domains: demographic, social relationships and health-related factors. A meta-analysis of 182 studies examining correlates of loneliness found that gender accounted for 0.6% of variance, with females reporting more loneliness than men. This association was stronger among those aged 80 years and over (Pinquart and Sörensen 2003). Longitudinal studies confirm the increased risk of loneliness in women, but the gender difference becomes usually non-significant when other variables are taken into account (*e.g.* Nicolaisen and Thorsen 2014; Dahlberg et al. 2015). A weak association between higher age and loneliness can be observed (Pinquart and Sörensen 2003), but this association becomes insignificant in multivariable analyses (*e.g.* Dahlberg et al. 2015; Pikhartova et al. 2016). Other longitudinal studies did not find age effects (*e.g.* Aartsen and Jylhä 2011; Nicolaisen and Thorsen 2014). A larger and supportive network, and having a partner is associated with lower levels of loneliness (Pikhartova et al. 2016; Böger and Huxhold 2018), and recent partner loss increases the risk of loneliness (*e.g.* Dahlberg et al. 2015; Pikhartova et al. 2016). Only a few studies explicitly examined an association between contacts with adult children and loneliness. These studies found no significant association between having children and loneliness (Cohen-Mansfield et al. 2016; Dolberg et al. 2016). Self-reported health, poor functional status, and mobility difficulties are associated with loneliness (*e.g.* Cohen-Mansfield et al. 2016; Hawkley and Kocherginsky 2018). To our knowledge, no previous longitudinal studies on risk factors for loneliness in older adults has considered the potential effects of visual impairments. However, longitudinal studies about hearing impairments and loneliness found that an association between self-reported hearing status and speech-in-noise test scores were predictive of adverse effects on social and emotional loneliness in specific subgroups (*i.e.* emotional loneliness and men; social loneliness and people living with a partner) (Pronk et al. 2011, 2014).

8.1.3 Macro-Level Correlates of Loneliness

Cross-national studies so far revealed variations in the prevalence of loneliness across countries (Gierveld and Tilburg 2010; Yang and Victor 2011; Fokkema et al. 2012; Swader 2018; Hansen and Slagsvold 2019), across welfare state regimes (Nyqvist et al. 2019), and across other typologies of countries (Swader 2018), suggesting the existence of macro-level drivers of loneliness. Indeed, research from nine countries of the former Soviet Union (Stickley et al. 2013) revealed that loneliness was associated with hazardous health behaviours in some countries (Armenia, Kyrgyzstan and Russia), which may indicate cultural habits concerning alcohol use. Another study found a modifying effect of the cultural context on associations between loneliness and different types of social relations, and the authors concluded that familial relationships seem to be more important for prevalence of loneliness, than friends in collectivistic societies, while confidants (*i.e.* people with whom to discuss personal and intimate matters) are more important in individualistic societies (Lykes and Kemmelmeier 2014). While the modifying effect of the cultural context in associations between micro-level factors and loneliness is also found in other cross-national studies in Europe (Swader 2018; Nyqvist et al. 2019), it does not seem to hold for severe forms of loneliness (Swader 2018). Higher levels of severe loneliness in eastern European countries, as compared to northern European countries, were associated with inequalities in socio-economic resources (Hansen and Slagsvold 2015). The cross-sectional nature of these studies limits conclusions on the direction of effects, and hence our understanding of macro-level drivers.

8.2 Methods

8.2.1 Study Design and Participants

Micro-level data come from SHARE (Börsch-Supan et al. 2013). SHARE is a multidisciplinary and cross-national panel database of microdata on health, socio-economic status, and social and family networks of more than 120,000 individuals aged 50 or older living in Europe. The first measurement took place in 2004. Every second year after that, a follow-up measurement took place, with the largest numbers of countries participating in the most recent waves of data collection. For the present study, we used data from wave five (W5, conducted in 2013) and wave six (W6, conducted in 2015) and included countries that participated in both waves. The countries comprised: Austria, Belgium, Czech Republic, Denmark, Estonia, France, Germany, Italy, Slovenia, Spain and Sweden. We excluded Israel, Switzerland and Luxemburg because of missing information on the macro-level variables. The total study sample was N = 52,562 at W5 of which N = 39,628 also participated in W6. SHARE W5 and W6 were reviewed and approved by the Ethics Council of the Max Planck Society. All participants provided written informed consent.

Macro-level data were derived from various databases: the World Bank for the GINI-index, the Eurobarometer for the level of ageism, the European Social Survey (ESS) for the proportion of people aged 55+ attending church once a month or more, and the percentage of people aged 55+ scoring five or higher on a religiousness scale from zero to ten. All other macro-level indicators were derived from tables of the Active Ageing Index (AAI) (UNECE, 2019). The AAI includes 22 indicators grouped into four domains (employment; participation in society; independent, healthy and secure living; capacity and enabling environment for active ageing). Data are available for all EU member states and some other European countries (Zaidi et al. 2013). Macro data for the years closest to the SHARE years included in this study come from 2012 and 2014.

8.2.2 Dependent Variable

Loneliness was measured with the short version of the Revised-University of California, Los Angeles (R-UCLA) scale (Russell et al. 1980; Hughes et al. 2004). The scale was based on three questions: How much of the time do you… (1) feel a lack of companionship, (2) feel left out, and (3) feel isolated from others [also see Myck et al. this volume for a discussion of the change in this loneliness measure over time and its relationship to material deprivation]. Answering categories are (1) often, (2) some of the time and (3) hardly ever or never. The R-UCLA score is the sum of the scores on these three variables and ranges from 3 to 9. The scores on the three questions were recoded so that a higher score reflects higher levels of loneliness.

8.2.3 Independent Variables at the Micro Level

Age reflects the year of birth of the respondent, and gender is dichotomised into 1 (men) and 2 (women). Three dummy variables were created to reflect *partner status*: never married; divorced; and widowed. Having a partner (inside or outside the household) was used as the reference category. *Frequency of contact with children* reflects the average number of contacts with children. Response categories range from daily (1) to never (7). *The number of grandchildren* reflects the number of grandchildren the respondent and his/her partner (if there is any) have altogether. *Limited hearing* [using hearing aids as usual] was assessed by asking "Is your hearing excellent" (1); very good (2), good (3), fair (4), and poor (5). *Limited eyesight* was based on the question "How good is your eyesight [using glasses or contact lenses as usual] for seeing things up close, like reading ordinary newspaper print", with answers ranging from excellent (1) to poor (5). The extent to which people are *health limitations* (*limited in activities because of health*) was measured via a categorical variable with answering categories severely limited (1) limited, but not severely (2) and not limited (3). *Changes in the contacts with children* and *number of (grand)children* reflect the raw difference between W5 and W6 and recoded into decline (−1) no change (0) and improvement (+1). *Change in hearing* and *change in eyesight* reflect the raw difference between W5 and W6, and coded as decline (−1) if there were two or more scale points decline, no change (0) if the change was 1 or 0 scale points, and improvement (+1) if there was a gain of two-scale points or more. *Change in health limitations* reflects the raw difference between W5 and W6 and coded as decline (−1) if there were one or more scale points decline, no change (0) if the change was 0 scale points, and improvement (+1) if there was a gain of one scale point or more. *Widowhood* reflects situations where people were widowed at W6, but not at W5. *Divorced* reflects situations where people were divorced at W6, but not at W5.

8.2.4 Independent Variables at the Macro Level

Macro-level variables were derived from the various datasets described previously and are listed in Table 8.1. These variables concern the population aged 55 and above (if not indicated otherwise).

A difference between 2012 and 2014 in country-level indicators was calculated by subtracting the 2012 indicator from the 2014 indicator.

Table 8.1 Description of macro-level variables

Variable	Description	Unit of measurement	Source	Domain of social exclusion (Walsh et al. 2017)
Access to health care services	People aged 55+ with no unmet need for medical and dental examination in the last year.	Per cent	Active Ageing Index (AAI), UNECE (2019).	Services, amenities and mobility
Use of ICT	People aged 55–74 using the Internet at least once a week in the last 3 months.	Per cent	Active Ageing Index (AAI), UNECE (2019).	
Relative median income	Ratio of the median equalised disposable income of people aged 65+ to the median equalised disposable income of those aged below 65.	Ratio	Active Ageing Index (AAI), UNECE (2019).	Material and financial resources
No poverty risk	People aged 65+ who are not at risk of poverty (people at risk of poverty are defined as those with an equalised disposable income after social transfers below the at-risk-of-poverty threshold, which is set at 50% of the national median equalised disposable income after social transfers).	Per cent	Active Ageing Index (AAI), UNECE (2019).	
No material deprivation	People aged 65+ who are not severely materially deprived.	Per cent	Active Ageing Index (AAI), UNECE (2019).	
GINI Index	Measures the extent to which the distribution of income among individuals or households within an economy deviates from a perfectly equal distribution.	Per cent	World Bank (2019).	
Social connectedness	People aged 55+ who meet socially with friends, relatives or colleagues at least once a week.	Per cent	Active Ageing Index (AAI), UNECE (2019).	Social relations

(continued)

Table 8.1 (continued)

Variable	Description	Unit of measurement	Source	Domain of social exclusion (Walsh et al. 2017)
Lifelong learning	People aged 55 to 74 who stated that they received education or training in the 4 weeks preceding the survey.	Per cent	Active Ageing Index (AAI), UNECE (2019).	Socio-cultural aspects
Ageism	People aged 15+ stating that discrimination based on being over 55 years old is widespread in the country.	Per cent	Eurobarometer, European Commission (2012, 2015).	
Safety in neighbourhood	People aged 55+ feeling safe or very safe in their area or neighbourhood after dark.	Per cent	Active Ageing Index (AAI), UNECE (2019).	Neighbourhood and community
Church attendance	People aged 55+ attending church once a month or more often, apart from special occasions such as weddings and funerals.	Per cent	European Social Survey, ESS Round 6 (2012); ESS Round 7 (2014).	Civic participation
Religiosity	People aged 55+ scoring 5 to 10 on a religiousness scale from 0–10, where 0 means "Not at all religious" and 10" Very religious".	Per cent	European Social Survey, ESS Round 6 (2012); ESS Round 7 (2014).	
Voluntary work	People aged 55+ engaged in unpaid activity through voluntary organisations at least once a week.	Per cent	Active Ageing Index (AAI), UNECE (2019).	
Political participation	People aged 55+ taking part in activities or meetings of trade unions, political parties or political action groups.	Per cent	Active Ageing Index (AAI), UNECE (2019).	

8.2.5 Analytical Approach

All analyses were conducted with SPSS version 26. The mean and the standard deviation for loneliness were calculated for each country separately. The rank order reflects the ranking of countries based on the loneliness score, with a lower number indicating a lower mean level of loneliness. Since the individual data is nested within the countries, we considered a multilevel regression model to estimate the associations between the micro- and macro-level variables. To test the relevance of the nested structure of the data, we first calculated the Variance Partition Coefficient (VPC), which was computed from a mixed effect linear model. The test shows that only 3.8% of the variance in loneliness can be attributed to differences between countries. We therefore decided to ignore the nested structure and conducted multivariable linear regression analyses instead with stepwise entering of blocks of independent variables. In the first block (M1), we entered the three dummy variables concerning the partner status. In the second block (M2), we additionally entered contact frequency with children and number of grandchildren; in the third block (M3) hearing, eyesight and health limitations were added. All macro-level variables were added in the last block (M4). Age and gender were included in all models. The extent to which micro- and macro-level factors, and changes therein, were associated with changes in loneliness was examined using the same approach as indicated above, but with loneliness at W5 included in the first step (M1). All changes in micro- and macro-level variables were added in M5 and M6 subsequently. Missing observations on any of the independent or dependent variables resulted in an exclusion of the case (list-wise deletion).

8.3 Results

The baseline (W5) and follow-up (W6) levels of loneliness, and its standard deviation per country are presented in Table 8.2, and the baseline characteristics of the independent variables at baseline are shown in Table 8.3. Loneliness differs for the 11 countries included at both waves, with the lowest levels of loneliness in Denmark, Austria and Sweden, and the highest levels in Estonia, Italy and Czech Republic at W5. The rank order of countries according to average level of loneliness is the same at W6.

At baseline (W5), the average age is 66.2 years (range 55–95 years), 55.6% are female, 66.7% have a partner inside or outside the household, 5.4% are never married, 8.4% are divorced, and 14% are widowed. The average level of contacts with children is 2.7 indicating a frequency of contact between weekly and monthly. People on average have 2.8 grandchildren, score between good and very good for hearing and eyesight, and are on average somewhat, but not severely, limited in their activities because of health. Note that the country-specific scores indicate large variations in these characteristics.

Table 8.2 Mean and standard deviation of loneliness (SD) at wave 5 and wave 6 and number of observations by country, 2012 and 2014

	Wave 5				Wave 6			
	N	M	SD	Rank order	N	M	SD	Rank order
Austria	4127	3.53	1.06	2	2847	3.50	0.99	2
Belgium	5473	3.92	1.47	8	4181	3.92	1.43	8
Czech Republic	5363	4.21	1.42	11	4163	4.20	1.38	10
Denmark	4009	3.40	0.96	1	3258	3.38	0.94	1
Estonia	5476	4.04	1.46	9	4246	4.04	1.50	9
France	4371	3.84	1.35	7	3044	3.88	1.35	7
Germany	5565	3.75	1.20	6	4156	3.74	1.17	5
Italy	4557	4.20	1.66	10	3417	4.27	1.65	11
Slovenia	2885	3.67	1.19	5	2295	3.81	1.18	6
Spain	6262	3.63	1.26	4	4556	3.73	1.34	4
Sweden	4474	3.59	1.08	3	3465	3.71	1.12	3
Total	52,562	3.82	1.34		39,628	3.85	1.33	

Table 8.4 presents the results of the multivariable linear regression of loneliness at W6 on individual characteristics and country characteristics at W5. All models had significant F-values, indicating that the regression models predicted loneliness significantly well. Higher age and female gender are related to higher levels of loneliness, and this effect cannot be explained by other micro- or macro-level characteristics. Compared to those who have a partner at W5, those who are divorced or widowed at W5 have higher levels of loneliness at W6. Being never married is also related to increased levels of loneliness. This association is partly explained by the absence of contacts with children, as adding contact frequency with children results in a smaller regression coefficient for never married. A higher contact frequency with children is associated with higher levels of loneliness 2 years later, while having grandchildren is not significantly related to loneliness 2 years later. Problems with hearing and eyesight and health limitations are related to higher levels of loneliness 2 years later.

Macro characteristics that led to reduced levels of loneliness 2 years later were a lower proportion of people with poverty risk, a lower proportion of people with material deprivation [see Myck et al. this volume for a more detailed analysis of this relationship], a higher proportion of people feeling physically safe in their neighbourhood, and a higher percentage of religious people. Surprisingly, a higher level of access to health care services and a higher level of social contacts in W6 were associated with increased loneliness scores. The lowest row in Table 8.4 presents the explained variances for each model. It shows that the individual factors explain approximately 10% of the variation in loneliness, whereas the selected country characteristics additionally explain 2.6%

Finally, we conducted a multivariable linear regression, in which change in loneliness from W5 to W6 was regressed on the micro and macro characteristics at W5, and change in all variables between baseline and follow-up. As presented in Table 8.5, loneliness at W5 is a strong predictor of loneliness 2 years later,

Table 8.3 Baseline characteristics of the micro-level variables

	Age, years	Female, per cent	With partner, per cent	Never married, per cent	Divorced, per cent	Widowed, per cent	Average contact with children (1 daily – 7 never)	Number of grand–children	Hearing (1 Excellent – 5 poor)	Eyesight (1 excellent – 5 poor)	Health limitations (1 severely limited – 3 not limited)
Austria	66.4	57.2	60.5	7.6	11.2	14.5	2.9	2.4	2.5	2.7	2.4
Belgium	65.3	55.0	65.2	5.4	11.2	13.2	2.9	2.9	2.6	2.6	2.4
Czech Republic	66.1	58.4	63.9	2.3	12.9	18.6	2.5	3.2	2.7	2.9	2.3
Denmark	64.4	53.5	66.8	5.9	10.0	10.6	2.8	2.9	2.3	1.9	2.5
Estonia	67.5	60.2	61.9	7.1	11.3	19.6	2.8	2.9	3.0	3.0	2.1
France	66.9	56.9	58.9	6.5	8.9	16.0	3.0	3.0	2.8	2.4	2.4
Germany	64.1	52.4	73.3	5.4	7.8	10.4	2.9	1.9	2.6	2.5	2.3
Italy	66.3	54.4	72.3	5.5	2.6	12.2	2.4	2.8	2.7	3.1	2.4
Slovenia	66.0	56.6	74.7	4.5	3.9	16.6	2.1	2.6	2.7	2.9	2.4
Spain	67.7	53.7	72.4	4.5	2.4	12.3	2.4	3.0	3.0	3.1	2.5
Sweden	67.5	53.3	63.5	6.1	9.7	9.2	2.8	3.1	2.5	2.2	2.5
Total	66.2	55.6	66.7	5.4	8.4	14.0	2.7	2.8	2.7	2.7	2.4

Table 8.4 Linear regression (stepwise selection) of loneliness at wave 6 on individual characteristics at wave 5 and country characteristics in 2013

	M1			M2			M3			M4		
	B	Beta	p	B	Beta	p	B	Beta	p	B	Beta	p
Constant	31.00		**	28.83		**	12.69		**	22.19		**
Individual characteristics												
Age	−0.01	−0.10	**	−0.01	−0.09	**	−0.01	−0.03	**	−0.00	−0.03	**
Gender (1 = men, 2 = women)	0.18	0.06	**	0.19	0.07	**	0.17	0.06	**	0.16	0.06	**
Partner status (ref. with partner)												
Never married	0.43	0.08	**	0.28	0.05	**	0.24	0.04	**	0.24	0.04	**
Divorced	0.38	0.09	**	0.35	0.08	**	0.32	0.07	**	0.33	0.08	**
Widowed	0.45	0.13	**	0.44	0.12	**	0.40	0.11	**	0.39	0.11	**
Frequency of contact with children				0.05	0.07	**	0.05	0.06	**	0.06	0.08	**
Number of grand children				0.00	0.01	0.26	0.00	0.01	0.21	0.00	0.01	0.30
Limited hearing							0.07	0.05	**	0.07	0.06	**
Limited eyesight							0.13	0.11	**	0.08	0.07	**
Health Limitations							−0.33	−0.17	**	−0.34	−0.18	**
Country characteristics[a]												
Access to health care services										0.02	0.06	**
Relative median income										0.00	0.00	0.72
No poverty risk										−0.04	−0.08	**
No material deprivation										−0.07	−0.17	**
Safety in neighbour hood										−0.02	−0.15	**
Social connectedness										0.02	0.16	**
Ageism										−0.00	−0.02	0.36
Religiosity										−0.01	−0.14	**
Explained variance			0.045			0.048			0.101			0.126

Note: ** $p < 0.001$, [a]Only the country-level variables that contributed significantly to the model fit were included in the final models

Table 8.5 Linear regression (stepwise selection) of changes in loneliness on individual characteristics at wave 5, country level variables in 2013 and changes in individual from wave 5 to wave 6 and changes in country level variables from 2013 to 2015

	M1			M2			M3			M4			M5			M6		
	B	Beta	p	B	Beta	p	B	Beta	p	B	Beta	p	B	Beta	p	B	Beta	p
Constant	1.87		**	18.20		**	17.04		**	9.58		**	14.59		**	8.17		**
Individual characteristics																		
Loneliness wave 5	0.55	0.54	**	0.53	0.53	**	0.53	0.53	**	0.50	0.50	**	0.49	0.48	**	0.48	0.47	**
Age				−0.01	−0.06	**	−0.01	−0.05	**	−0.00	−0.03	**	−0.00	−0.03	**	−0.00	−0.00	0.95
Gender (1 = men, 2 = women)				0.09	0.03	**	0.10	0.03	**	0.09	0.03	**	0.08	0.03	**	0.07	0.02	**
Partner status (ref. with partner)																		
Never married				0.16	0.03	**	0.09	0.02	*	0.08	0.02	*	0.08	0.02	*	0.09	0.02	*
Divorced				0.10	0.03	**	0.09	0.02	**	0.09	0.02	**	0.11	0.03	**	0.14	0.04	**
Widowed				0.12	0.04	**	0.12	0.04	**	0.12	0.04	**	0.12	0.04	**	0.18	0.05	**
Frequency of contact with children							0.02	0.03	**	0.02	0.03	**	0.03	0.04	**	0.04	0.05	**
Number of grandchildren							**	0.01	‘	**	0.01	‘	**	0.01	*	**	0.01	0.07
Limited Hearing										0.04	0.03	**	0.04	0.03	**	0.05	0.04	**
Limited Eyesight										0.07	0.05	**	0.04	0.03	**	0.05	0.04	***
Health limitations										−0.15	−0.07	**	−0.16	−0.08	**	−0.24	−0.12	**
Country characteristics[a]																		
Access to health care services													0.01	0.02	*	0.01	0.02	*
Relative median income													*	*	0.92	*	*	0.75
No poverty													−0.02	−0.04	*	−0.02	−0.04	*
No material deprivation													−0.04	−0.09	**	−0.04	−0.10	**

Safety in neighbourhood													−0.01	−0.06	*	−0.01	−0.06	*
Social connectedness													0.01	0.08	*	0.01	0.10	*
Ageism													*	0.0.2	0.51	*	0.01	0.80
Religiosity													−0.01	−0.05	0.05	−0.01	−0.07	*
Changes in individual characteristics																		
Widowed between W5 and W6																0.88	0.08	**
Divorced between W5 and W6																0.68	0.03	**
Change in number of grandchildren																−0.05	−0.02	*
Change in contact frequency with children																0.08	0.03	**
Change in hearing																0.15	0.04	**
Change in eyesight																0.07	0.02	*
Change in health limitations																−0.22	−0.09	**
Explained variance			0.296			0.304			0.305			0.315			0.323			0.339

Note: *p < .05; p > 0.01**, [a] Only the country-level variables and changes in country level variables that contributed significantly to the model fit were included in the final models indicating that loneliness is relatively stable (r = 0.47). Age is related to changes in loneliness, but this effect becomes insignificant after controlling for changes in the individual characteristics (M6). Women have a stronger increase in loneliness than men, and this effect remains significant after including other individual and country characteristics. People who are married at both waves have the lowest increase in loneliness. Becoming widowed or divorced between W5 and W6 leads to a substantial increase in loneliness. A higher contact frequency and an increase in contact frequency with children is related to an increase in loneliness. The effect of the number of grandchildren on loneliness is borderline significant and loses its significance in the final model. However, an increase in the number of grandchildren was related to increases in loneliness. Limited hearing, eyesight limitations, and health limitations are related to a stronger increase in loneliness. None of the changes in the macro-level variables explained variance in loneliness, and hence M5 was the final model. The much higher proportion of explained variance of changes in loneliness compared to the first model is mainly due to the inclusion of loneliness at W5. Almost 30% of the variation in loneliness at W6 is explained by the level of loneliness at W5.

8.4 Discussion

Unsurprisingly, loneliness at wave 5 explained most of the change in loneliness at wave 6, which underlines the persistence of loneliness over time and the challenge for service providers and policymakers. Today, loneliness is accepted as a substantial driver of ill-health (Holt-Lunstad et al. 2015; Steptoe et al. 2012) and clearly contributes to the perception and experience of social exclusion. Likewise ill-health can be a driver of loneliness (Cohen-Mansfield et al. 2016; Hawkley and Kocherginsky 2018). The micro-level variables that demonstrated significant effects on the level of and change in loneliness were largely in line with the literature noted at the beginning of this chapter (*e.g.* Pinquart and Sörensen 2003). Loneliness increased significantly for women, and when there was a decline in hearing ability or eyesight and an increase in health limitations. However, a greater frequency of contact with children was also related to an increase in loneliness. Although counterintuitive at first sight, a higher contact frequency may be indicative of a worsening of the older adults' personal situation that is associated with loneliness. If everything is fine, there is probably no need for an increased contact between the children and their parents.

Any significant effect of age disappeared when controlling for changes in the individual characteristics, which is basically what ageing is: a change in individual characteristics. While the number of grandchildren did not affect level of loneliness 2 years later, an increase in the number of grandchildren between W5 and W6 did, suggesting that a new grandchild leads to an immediate increase in loneliness but this effect fades after 2 years. This may relate to greater expectations of social interaction with children and grandchildren and disappointment when their children are more involved with their own children lessening contact with their parents. Having a partner leads to lower levels of loneliness and protects against becoming lonelier over time.

Macro-level factors leading to lower levels of loneliness were living in countries with low risks of poverty, low risks of material deprivation, safer neighbourhoods and higher levels of religiosity. Better access to health care services and a higher average level of social contacts were associated with increased levels of loneliness. While this is counter-intuitive, these results are probably country contextual. Loneliness is a subjective state. Living in a country where people generally have a high level of social contacts, may increase their own expectations, and normative orientations (Dykstra 2009), which makes it more likely to become lonely (Fokkema et al. 2012). In a similar vein, better access to health care services may raise people's awareness of health issues of which they would not be aware if they had not contacted health care professionals. Two other macro-level variables did not produce significant differences in loneliness, ageism and median income. The result for ageism is surprising, and in contrast with earlier findings by Sutin et al. (2015). While we do not know a reason for this, one technical explanation might be that the variable was derived from a different database, the Eurobarometer. A lack of effect of the country's median income may be too blunt a measure to identify the impact of income levels on loneliness, unlike the Active Ageing Index variables relating to poverty and material deprivation risk.

This study has focused on cross-national, longitudinal data on micro- and macro-level drivers in level and change of loneliness of older people with reference to specific domains of social exclusion. In the first series of regression models, estimating the effect of baseline micro- and macro-level drivers on level of loneliness 2 years later, indicated that 10% of the variation in loneliness was attributable to micro-level drivers, whereas macro-level drivers explained an additional 2.6%. This indicates that the country-level characteristics in this study have had only a modest influence on an individual's feelings of loneliness. From the second series of regression models it was concluded that change in loneliness can be explained in terms of micro- and macro-level drivers at baseline. However, change in macro-level drivers did not additionally explain variation in loneliness change. Given the significant correlations with loneliness for most country-level variables in the various models reported in the results, it suggests estimated variance effects in loneliness are small over a two-year period and a greater longitudinal period may produce more significant results. It may also imply that country-level data may present too blunt a measure when searching for effects on an individual factor like subjective loneliness.

The two-year period of this study is a limiting factor when considering the results. A longer period with more waves could be expected to produce more robust outcomes, especially with the country-level variables that were applied. They do, however, confirm that individual factors contribute to changes in loneliness. Social exclusion variables at country-level point to influences on loneliness, but the variables like neighbourhood safety and poverty risk may be better collected at the individual level to gain a more precise measure of their impact [see Van Regenmortel this section].

8.5 Conclusion

The purpose of this chapter was to explore loneliness as an outcome of exclusion from social relations. Micro- and macro-level factors were analysed over two waves, 2 years apart, providing a dynamic measure of change. Most of the individual variables from the demographic, social relationships and health domains that we considered would predict loneliness did in fact do so. The micro-level factors contributed to the estimated variance in loneliness, while the macro-level variables demonstrated a more modest influence. This might reflect a methodological problem of extracting country-level results that are precise enough to be correlated with individual loneliness scores and the short two-year time period. The results provide insights into loneliness and loneliness change, and is one of few longitudinal studies to consider both micro and macro drivers.

This study shows the need for longitudinal research over a greater time period that addresses both micro- and macro-level factors to particularly gauge the impact of the macro factors beyond the two time points used in this analysis. A greater time period would also further test the veracity of both the micro- and macro-level findings.

From a policy perspective and for the provision of services, the challenges of reducing loneliness are immense, as we found many factors at the individual and country level affecting loneliness and change in loneliness in older-age. This suggests that initiatives to reduce loneliness should not only take place at the country level, but their introduction needs to be carefully planned, and take into consideration the individual characteristics locally in health, well-being and social networks, given the substantial role these play in explaining late-life loneliness.

Editors' Postscript

Please note, like other contributions to this book, this chapter was written before the COVID-19 pandemic of 2020. The book's introductory chapter (Chap. 1) and conclusion (Chap. 34) consider some of the key ways in which the pandemic relates to issues concerning social exclusion and ageing.

References

Aartsen, M., & Jylhä, M. (2011). Onset of loneliness in older adults: Results of a 28 year prospective study. *European Journal of Ageing, 8*(1), 31–38. https://doi.org/10.1007/s10433-011-0175-7.

Böger, A., & Huxhold, O. (2018). The changing relationship between partnership status and loneliness: Effects related to aging and historical time. *The Journals of Gerontology: Series B*. https://doi.org/10.1093/geronb/gby153.

Börsch-Supan, A., Brandt, M., Hunkler, C., Kneip, T., Korbmacher, J., Malter, F., et al. (2013). Data resource profile: The survey of health, ageing and retirement in Europe (SHARE). *International Journal of Epidemiology, 42*(4), 992–1001.

Cacioppo, J. T., & Cacioppo, S. (2018). The growing problem of loneliness. *The Lancet, 391*(10119). https://doi.org/10.1016/S0140-6736(18)30142-9.

Cohen-Mansfield, J., Hazan, H., Lerman, Y., & Shalom, V. (2016). Correlates and predictors of loneliness in older-adults: A review of quantitative results informed by qualitative insights. *International Psychogeriatrics, 28*(4), 557–576. https://doi.org/10.1017/S1041610215001532.

Courtin, E., & Knapp, M. (2017). Social isolation, loneliness and health in old age: A scoping review. *Health & Social Care in the Community, 25*(3), 799–812. https://doi.org/10.1111/hsc.12311.

Dahlberg, L., Andersson, L., McKee, K. J., & Lennartsson, C. (2015). Predictors of loneliness among older women and men in Sweden: A national longitudinal study. *Aging and Mental Health, 19*(7), 409–417. https://doi.org/10.1080/13607863.2014.944091.

De Jong Gierveld, J., & Van Tilburg, T. (2010). The De Jong Gierveld short scales for emotional and social loneliness: tested on data from 7 countries in the UN Generations and Gender Surveys. *European Journal of Ageing, 7*(2), 121–130. https://doi.org/10.1007/s10433-010-0144-6.

Dolberg, P., Shiovitz-Ezra, S., & Ayalon, L. (2016). Migration and changes in loneliness over a 4-year period: the case of older former Soviet Union immigrants in Israel. *European Journal of Ageing, 13*(4), 287–297. https://doi.org/10.1007/s10433-016-0391-2.

Dykstra, P. A. (2009). Older adult loneliness: Myths and realities. *European Journal of Ageing, 6*, 91–100. https://doi.org/10.1007/s10433-009-0110-3.

ESS Round 6: European Social Survey Round 6 Data. (2012). Data file edition 2.4. Norwegian Social Science Data Services, Norway – Data Archive and distributor of ESS data. http://nesstar.ess.nsd.uib.no/webview/. Accessed 19 Aug 2019.

ESS Round 7: European Social Survey Round 7 Data. (2014). Data file edition 2.2. Norwegian Social Science Data Services, Norway – Data Archive and distributor of ESS data. http://nesstar.ess.nsd.uib.no/webview/. Accessed 19 Aug 2019.

European Commission. (2012). *Special Eurobarometer 393: Discrimination in the EU in 2012*. Factsheets in English, 2012: https://ec.europa.eu/commfrontoffice/publicopinion/index.cfm/Survey/getSurveyDetail/search/discrimination/surveyKy/1043. Accessed 30 Aug 2019.

European Commission. (2015). *Special Eurobarometer 437: Discrimination in the EU in 2015*. Factsheets in English, 2015: https://ec.europa.eu/commfrontoffice/publicopinion/index.cfm/Survey/getSurveyDetail/search/disczAIimination/surveyKy/2077. Accessed 30 Aug 2019.

Fokkema, M., De Jong Gierveld, J., & Dykstra, P. A. (2012). Cross-national differences in older adult loneliness. *The Journal of Psychology, 146*(1–2), 201–228. https://doi.org/10.1080/00223980.2011.631612.

Hansen, T., & Slagsvold, B. (2015). Late-life loneliness in 11 European countries: Results from the Generations and Gender survey. *Social Indicators Research*. https://doi.org/10.1007/s11205-015-1111-6.

Hansen, T., & Slagsvold, B. (2019). *Et Øst-Vest skille for eldres livskvalitet i Europa? En sammenligning av ensomhet og depressive symptomer i 12 land* (Vol. 33, pp. 74–90). Nordisk Østforum. https://doi.org/10.23865/noros.v33.1331.

Hawkley, L. C., & Kocherginsky, M. (2018). Transitions in loneliness among older adults: A 5-year follow-up in the National Social Life, Health, and Aging Project. *Research on Aging, 40*(4), 365–387.

Holt-Lunstad, J., Smith, T. B., Baker, M., Harris, T., & Stephenson, D. (2015). Loneliness and social isolation as risk factors for mortality: A meta-analytic review. *Perspectives on Psychological Science, 10*(2), 227–237. https://doi.org/10.1177/1745691614568352.

Hughes, M. E., Waite, L. J., Hawkley, L. C., & Cacioppo, J. T. (2004). A short scale for measuring loneliness in large surveys: Results from two population-based studies. *Research on Aging, 26*(6), 655–672.

Lykes, V. A., & Kemmelmeier, M. (2014). What predicts loneliness? Cultural difference between individualistic and collectivistic societies in Europe. *Journal of Cross-Cultural Psychology, 45*, 468–490. https://doi.org/10.1177/0022022113509881.

Nicolaisen, M., & Thorsen, K. (2014). Who are lonely? Loneliness in different age groups (18–81 years old), using two measures of loneliness. *The International Journal of Aging and Human Development, 78*(3), 229–257. https://doi.org/10.2190/AG.78.3.b.

Nyqvist, F., Nygård, M., & Scharf, T. (2019). Loneliness amongst older people in Europe: a comparative study of welfare regimes. *European Journal of Ageing, 16*(2), 133–143.

Pikhartova, J., Bowling, A., & Victor, C. (2016). Is loneliness in later life a self-fulfilling prophecy? *Aging & Mental Health, 20*(5), 543–549. https://doi.org/10.1080/13607863.2015.1023767.

Pinquart, M., & Sörensen, S. (2003). Risk factors for loneliness in adulthood and old age–A meta-analysis. In S. P. Shohov (Ed.), *Advances in Psychology Research* (Vol. 19, pp. 111–143). Hauppauge/New York: Nova Science Publishers.

Pronk, M., Deeg, D. J. H., Smits, C., van Tilburg, T. G., Kuik, D. J., Festen, J. M., & Kramer, S. E. (2011). Prospective effects of hearing status on loneliness and depression in older persons: Identification of subgroups. *International Journal of Audiology, 50*(12), 887–896. https://doi.org/10.3109/14992027.2011.599871.

Pronk, M., Deeg, D. J. H., Smits, C., Twisk, J. W., van Tilburg, T. G., Festen, J. M., & Kramer, S. E. (2014). Hearing loss in older persons: Does the rate of decline affect psychosocial health? *Journal of Aging and Health, 26*(5), 703–723. https://doi.org/10.1177/0898264314529329.

Russell, D., Peplau, L. A., & Cutrona, C. E. (1980). The revised UCLA Loneliness Scale: Concurrent and discriminant validity evidence. *Journal of Personality and Social Psychology, 39*(3), 472.

Steptoe, A., Shankar, A., Demakakos, P., & Wardle, J. (2012). Social isolation, loneliness, and all-cause mortality in older men and women. *Proceedings of the National Academy of Sciences, 110*(15), 5797–5801.

Stickley, A., Koyanagi, A., Roberts, B., Richardson, E., Abbott, P., et al. (2013). Loneliness: Its correlates and association with health behaviours and outcomes in nine countries of the former Soviet Union. *PLoS One, 8*(7), e67978. https://doi.org/10.1371/journal.pone.0067978.

Sutin, A. R., Stephan, Y., Carretta, H., & Terracciano, A. (2015). Perceived discrimination and physical, cognitive, and emotional health in older adulthood. *American Journal of Geriatric Psychiatry, 23*(2), 171–179. https://doi.org/10.1016/j.jagp.2014.03.007.

Swader, C. S. (2018). Loneliness in Europe: Personal and societal individualism-collectivism and their connection to social isolation. *Social Forces*, 1–29. https://doi.org/10.1093/sf/soy088.

UNECE (2019). *Active ageing index*. https://statswiki.unece.org/display/AAI/Active+Ageing+Index+Home. Accessed 4 Oct 2019.

Walsh, K., Scharf, T., & Keating, N. (2017). Social exclusion of older persons: A scoping review and conceptual framework. *European Journal of Ageing, 14*(1), 81–98. https://doi.org/10.1007/s10433-016-0398-8.

Weiss, R. S. (1973). *Loneliness: the experience of emotional and social isolation*. Cambridge: MIT Press.

Wilson, R. S., Krueger, K. R., Arnold, S. E., Schneider, J. A., Kelly, J. F., Barnes, L. L., et al. (2007). Loneliness and the risk of Alzheimer disease. *Archives of General Psychiatry, 64*, 234–240. https://doi.org/10.1001/archpsyc.64.2.234.

World Bank (2019). *LAC equity lab: Income inequality – Inequality trends*. https://www.worldbank.org/en/topic/poverty/lac-equity-lab1/income-inequality/inequality-trends. Accessed 4 Oct 2019.

Yang, K., & Victor, C. (2011). Age and loneliness in 25 European nations. *Ageing & Society, 31*, 1368–1388. https://doi.org/10.1017/S0144686X1000139X.

Zaidi, A., Gasior, K., Hofmarcher, M. M., Lelkes, O., Marin, B., Rodrigues, R., Schmidt, A., Vanhuysse, P., & Zolyomi, E. (2013). *Active ageing index 2012. Concept, methodology and final results*. Vienna: European Centre for Social Welfare Policy and Research. https://statswiki.unece.org/display/AAI/V.+Methodology. Accessed 21 Sep 2019.

Chapter 9
Conflicting Relations, Abuse and Discrimination Experienced by Older Adults

Charles Waldegrave, Marja Aartsen, Ariela Lowenstein, Marjaana Seppänen, Mia Niemi, Maria Gabriella Melchiorre, and Giovanni Lamura

9.1 Introduction

Social relationships are generally considered a major resource for older people's health and well-being. They provide social connection and social meaning, and can provide instrumental and emotional support in times of ill health and crises in later life. However, not all relations function equally well. Conflicting relations, abuse, and discrimination also exist, and these are associated with social isolation, limited support, and increased discomfort as they involve the denial of resources, rights, goods and services, and limit the ability to participate in normal relationships and civic society (Dong 2015; Rook 2015; Aartsen et al. 2018; Burholt et al. 2019; Jackson et al. 2019). Hence, conflicting relations, elder abuse, and discrimination are related to many aspects of social exclusion.

These three dimensions of negative social relations have not been brought together in a single study previously. They have been drawn together in this chapter because they each focus on fundamentally demeaning social interactions that by definition, reduce social inclusion and quality of life (Darbonne et al. 2013; Dong

C. Waldegrave (✉)
Family Centre Social Policy Research Unit, Lower Hutt, Wellington, New Zealand
e-mail: waldegrave.c@fc.org.nz

M. Aartsen
NOVA-Norwegian Social Research, Oslo Metropolitan University, Oslo, Norway

A. Lowenstein
Graduate Department of Aging Studies, Haifa University, Haifa, Israel

M. Seppänen · M. Niemi
Social Work, Faculty of Social Sciences, Helsinki Inequality Initiative (INEQ), University of Helsinki, Helsinki, Finland

M. G. Melchiorre · G. Lamura
Centre for Socio-Economic Research on Ageing, INRCA-IRCCS, National Institute of Health and Science on Ageing, Ancona, Italy

K. Walsh et al. (eds.), *Social Exclusion in Later Life*, International Perspectives on Aging 28, https://doi.org/10.1007/978-3-030-51406-8_9

2015; Jackson et al. 2019). Older people can find themselves in socially dysfunctional environments where the actions of others directly damage them. Elder abuse and discrimination, for example, have been shown to damage mental health and social relations. Known risk factors such as gender and socio-economic status [see previous chapters this section, and Barlin et al. this volume] can overlap with these (Dong 2015; Yunus et al. 2017). There is less research on conflictual relationships (Rook 2009), but that which does exist demonstrates harm to health and well-being.

Further, an in-depth consideration of cross-national evidence on these three dimensions is rare, with little analysis of how patterns relating to these phenomena, and their impacts, may differ across jurisdictions The cross-national evidence that does exist is largely confined to one of the dimensions, like abuse (Dong 2015; Yon et al. 2017) or discrimination (Kydd and Fleming 2015). This chapter brings together insights from a set of diverse research studies in five countries: Norway (Aartsen and Veenstra 2018), Finland (Seppänen and Niemi 2018), New Zealand (Waldegrave 2018), Israel (Lowenstein et al. 2009) and Italy (Melchiorre et al. 2012a) to show the importance of understanding these dysfunctional elements of relations in the conceptualisation of social exclusion in later life. The aim of this chapter is therefore to explore the complex nature of the conflicted, abusive and discriminative relations of older people and their differential exclusionary impacts across countries. We will consider each dimension in turn, commencing with conflicting relations, followed by elder abuse and then discrimination. In each section we will first review the international literature on these dimensions, and then draw on empirical evidence from the chosen studies to illustrate the impacts of such phenomena on the exclusionary experiences of older people. Finally, we present a discussion of our analysis and draw some conclusions.

9.2 Conflicting Relations

While the beneficial effects of being socially connected for health and well-being are widely acknowledged, social relations that are characterised by conflict may be equally disruptive to health and well-being. Conflicts in relations can refer to unpleasant social encounters that are characterised by criticism, rejection, competition, the violation of privacy, and the lack of reciprocity (Krause and Jay 1991). Family conflicts are particularly relevant as relationships with family members are difficult to terminate for older adults because of their increased dependency on family members and increased risk of declining health (Rook 2015).

However, research on the consequences of conflictual relations is limited (Rook 2009). The few studies that exist have observed that conflicts with other people are harmful for the health and well-being of the individual (Rook 2009; Darbonne et al. 2013). In addition, previous research suggests that there may be gender differences in the association between relationship conflicts and their outcomes, probably stemming from the different roles men and women fulfil within a couple (Iveniuk et al. 2014; see also Barlin et al. this volume).

This current section aims to contribute to this knowledge gap by describing the prevalence, the duration or stability of the conflicts and the health outcomes of relations that are characterised by conflicts. It takes into account the potential moderating effect of age and gender and examines whether physical and mental health enhance the likelihood of partner conflict. The data are derived from the Norwegian Life Course Ageing and Generation Study (NorLAG) (Slagsvold et al. 2012). NorLAG has three waves of data collection; 2002/3, 2007/8, and 2017. Data on partner conflict were collected in the first two waves. In this study, a particular relation (for example with the partner) is seen as conflictual, if the individual self-evaluates and perceives a relation as being conflictual.

9.2.1 Quantifying the Impacts of Conflicting Relations Between Partners: A Norwegian Study

In wave 1, 1251 people with a partner were asked whether they agree with the statement, "I often have conflicts with my partner". Slightly more than 10% (n = 129) of women and 7% (n = 88) of men answered that they slightly agreed, agreed, or fully agreed. The difference in prevalence between men and women is significant (Chi 2 = 4.14, df = 1, p = 0.04). The same question was repeated 5 years later, but with ten response categories. Recoding the responses into a five-category variable resulted in a higher prevalence of partner conflict, with 16.1% of men and 18.1% of women saying they often had conflicts with their partner. Gender differences were no longer statistically significant (Chi 2 = 1.54, df = 1, p = 0.22).

The results of a logistic regression in which partner conflict at wave 2 (T2) (1 = yes/0 = no) was regressed on partner conflict at wave 1 (T1), physical and mental health problems at T1, age, and gender are set out in Table 9.1. The Hosmer-Lemeshow test (Chi2 = 12,35, df = 8, p = 0,14) indicate a good model fit (Hosmer et al. 1980), and approximately 11% of the variation in conflicts with the partner at T2 is explained (Nagelkerke $R^2 = 10.8$).

Table 9.1 Logistic regression of partner conflict in 2007 on partner conflict, gender, age, and physical and mental health in 2002

	B	S.E.	Wald	Sig.	Exp(B)
Constant	0.21	2.17	0.01	0.92	1.23
Partner conflict T1	**2.21**	**0.69**	**10.27**	**0.00**	**9.13**
Gender (men = 0, women = 1)	–0.53	1.25	0.18	0.68	0.59
Age	0.00	0.01	0.00	0.99	1.00
Physical health T1	**–0.05**	**0.03**	**4.58**	**0.03**	**1.06**
Mental health T1	**–0.09**	**0.03**	**8.34**	**0.00**	**0.92**
Gender*Conflicts at T1	–0.20	0.44	0.20	0.66	0.82
Gender*Physical health T1	**–0.03**	**0.02**	**5.17**	**0.02**	**0.97**
Gender*Mental health T1	**0.04**	**0.02**	**4.61**	**0.03**	**1.04**

Physical and mental health were measured using SF12 (Ware at al. 1996), with higher scores indicating better mental and physical health

Partner conflict at T2 was best explained by partner conflict 5 years earlier. Gender and age did not predict partner conflict. Physical and mental health, as measured by the Short Form Health Survey 12 (SF12) (Ware et al. 1996) affected the odds of partner conflict 5 years later. Better physical and mental health was associated with a lower likelihood of partner conflict five years later. The effect of physical health on the odds of partner conflict was stronger for men than women, while the effect of mental health on the odds of partner conflict was stronger for women than men.

Finally, to explore the health consequences of conflictual relations with a partner, we conducted two linear regressions with mental and physical health at T2 as outcome variables. The results indicated that, after controlling for age and gender, partner conflict at T1 led to a significant decrease in mental health of two scale points on MCS12, an effect comparable to the gender difference in mental health. No significant effect of partner conflict on later physical health was observed.

A partner is often seen as the main source of support, and that is often justified. Sometimes, however, there is an inverse health effect, such as when a partner relationship is characterised by conflicts, as we described here. Even more devastating for health and well-being may be social relations that are characterised by violence, such as with abusive relations. That is the topic of the next section.

9.3 Elder Abuse

Elder abuse is an important human rights and public health issue (Yon et al. 2017). It is defined by the World Health Organisation (2018) as "a single, or repeated act, or lack of appropriate action, occurring within any relationship where there is an expectation of trust which causes harm or distress to an older person". It encompasses financial, physical, psychological and sexual exploitation, as well as intentional or unintentional neglect. Victims may suffer more than one type of abuse (Santos et al. 2019).

The lack of consensus in defining and measuring elder abuse has resulted in wide variations in reported prevalence rates. Cooper et al. (2008) reviewed 49 studies that examined prevalence in different countries. Reports ranged from 3.2% to 27.5%, reflecting differences in methodology, definitions, and cultures. Yon et al. (2017) used meta-analysis to synthesise the prevalence estimate for elder abuse and its subtypes. Fifty-two studies from 28 countries qualified for the analysis. They concluded that the pooled prevalence rate for overall elder abuse from 44 studies was 15.7%. In the subcategories, the pooled prevalence rate for psychological abuse was 11.6% from 44 studies, 6.8% for financial abuse (52 studies), 4.2% for neglect (30 studies), 2.6% for physical abuse (46 studies), and 0.9% for sexual abuse (15 studies).

The effects of elder abuse are complex and multidimensional. Studies identify a wide range of negative health outcomes (Fisher and Regan 2006), increased morbidity and mortality (Dong et al. 2013; Schofield et al. 2013) and psychological distress (Yunus et al. 2017). Systematic literature reviews show that elder abuse is associated with different aspects of exclusion from social relations such as social isolation (Murphy et al. 2013; Dong 2015), loneliness (Waldegrave 2015; Wong and Waite 2017), low social support (Dong et al. 2013), negative social well-being (Dong 2015), and interfamilial conflicts (Yan et al. 2002). Furthermore, it is associated with conditions that negatively impact on social relations such as poor mental health, psychological distress, anxiety, and suicidal thoughts (Lachs and Pillemer 2015; Yunus et al. 2017).

Three country studies make up the rest of this section on elder abuse. The studies in Israel and Italy show prevalence rates, types of abuse and important statistical associations as measured at a country level. The third study, from Finland, is of a qualitative design and explores social workers' records of elder abuse cases.

9.3.1 Quantifying the Impacts of Elder Abuse: An Israeli Study

The consensus in Israeli society had been that it was free from elder abuse. However, the number of older people who were referred to social work units has increased gradually. Thus, it was decided that a broad data base was needed: ESHEL (Association for Development of Social Services for Elders) and the Social Insurance Institute decided to conduct a large study on the topic. It was the first National Survey on Elder Abuse and Neglect in Israel and it challenged earlier perceptions (Lowenstein et al. 2009).

A random sample of 1045 adults aged 65+ participated, and findings showed that 18.4% experienced at least one type of abuse during the year preceding interview. Verbal abuse was the most prevalent (11.5%), followed by financial exploitation (6.6%) and physical and sexual abuse (2%). Neglect by a significant other, with older people unable to meet the primary activities for daily living, was common and more than a quarter (26%) experienced neglect in meeting both primary Activities of Daily Living (ADL) (basic self-care tasks like walking, eating, bathing and such) and secondary Instrumental Activities of Daily Living (IADL) (more complex tasks that require thinking and organisational skills like managing finances, shopping and meal preparation). Neglect of primary needs only was close to 18%. A small proportion (2.7%) suffered from limitation of freedom.

Regression analyses confirmed the earlier cited findings concerning health and different aspects of exclusion from social relations. Failing health was significantly associated with neglect and to a lesser extent with physical, sexual and verbal abuse, as set out in Table 9.2. Feelings of loneliness were strongly associated with verbal abuse and neglect, and to a lesser extent with limitation of freedom. Feelings of neglect were very strongly associated with neglect as would be expected, but also with financial exploitation.

The survey resulted in dynamic change regarding elder abuse and neglect, in research, policy, legislation, and social and health interventions. The Ministries of Health and Social Welfare for example, constructed a multidimensional, multi-systemic approach to policy on elder abuse that increased public awareness and developed special social and health services, including building a specialised-care system (Lowenstein and Doron 2013).

Table 9.2 Linear regressions for predicting abuse and/or neglect

	Physical & sexual abuse	Verbal abuse	Limitation of freedom	Financial exploitation	Neglect
Elders' attributes	Probability ratio	Probability ratio	Probability ratio	Probability ratio	Probability ratio
Gender (female)	NS	NS	NS	**0.36**^{t}	NS
Nationality (Jewish)	**0.16**^{t}	NS	NS	NS	NS
Level of income	NS	NS	**2.05**^{t}	NS	NS
Education	NS	**0.69*****	NS	NS	NS
Failing health	**1.79**^{t}	**1.25**^{t}	NS	NS	***1.38**
Feelings of neglect	NS	NS	NS	**1.40***	**2.5*****
Feelings of loneliness	NS	**1.38*****	**1.57***	NS	**1.4*****

^{t}<0.1; *p<0.05; **p<0.01; ***p<0.001; *NS* not significant

9.3.2 Quantifying the Impacts of Elder Abuse: An Italian Study

Similar results concerning health and different aspects of exclusion from social relations were found in Italy. Like the Israeli study, low socio-economic conditions including low income and low educational attainment were found to be significantly associated with elder abuse, albeit less strongly than in Israel.

The Italian component of the ABUEL (Abuse of the Elderly in the European region) cross-sectional survey found an overall prevalence rate for abuse of 13%. Psychological and financial abuse were the most common, reaching 11% and 3% of cases, respectively. Lower percentages were found for neglect (1%) and physical and sexual violence (1.5%) (Melchiorre et al. 2012a).

The perpetrators of psychological abuse were mainly relatives (spouses/partners or children) and friends of the family, often acting as carers of older persons with dementia and/or situations with high levels of carer-care-recipient co-dependency (Fondazione Caritas Ambrosiana 2011). However, a significant proportion of financial abuse was perpetrated by non-relatives (Ligabue 2010; Melchiorre et al. 2012b).

The findings showed social isolation and lack of social support to be two dimensions of exclusion from social relations that were significantly linked with elder abuse, confirming earlier studies cited above (Murphy et al. 2013; Dong 2015) and the Israeli research. Poor health (including older people experiencing anxiety, depression, and physical complaints) was also identified as a key risk factor confirming previous research. Low socio-economic status (including low levels of income and/or education, especially for divorced and separated individuals) and limited autonomy were further crucial risk factors that were identified (Melchiorre et al. 2014; Badenes-Ribeira et al. 2019).

9.3.3 *Elder Abuse Qualitatively Analysed: A Finnish Study*

The prevalence and complexity of elder abuse, as indicated in the Israeli and Italian studies, points to the need for gerontological social and health care professionals to have an understanding of the phenomenon, skills in its prevention and effective responses to its occurrence. A practice research approach implemented in a gerontological social work unit in Finland studied how social workers understand and describe elder abuse in family relations (Seppänen and Niemi 2018). The research employed a social reporting method developed at the city of Helsinki, based on Clinical Data Mining (Epstein 2010), that generates knowledge from direct social work practice. Clinical Data Mining utilises available agency data in its aims to identify service users' needs, connecting them to the macro-level context. The social reporting data were collected by social workers from social work service users' case records (n = 57) of elder abuse in 2017.

Content analysis identified numerous forms of abuse, such as physical, psychological (including violation of privacy, harassment, and disregard for self-determination), sexual and economic abuse, neglect, and the withholding of treatment, nutrition, or medication. Typically, client cases included many different forms of abuse.

Material and psychosocial interdependencies between family members, intergenerational marginalisation, and structural disadvantages increased the difficulty of disengaging from abusive relationships. Barriers to intervention were also identified, including the systemic failure to provide support and services for families with members in later life, particularly for the perpetrator relative. Analysis revealed that the abuse within families is often intertwined with structural factors and other individual and collective problems that affect families across the generations. Particular ethical considerations are required when assessing the client's need for safety alongside their need to maintain their family relationships.

Elder abuse is clearly a category of demeaning social interactions that reduces social inclusion and quality of life. Both it and conflictual relationships can be considered as dimensions of negative social relations. The third dimension we consider in this chapter is discrimination which follows in the next section.

9.4 Discrimination

Discrimination is generally defined as treating a person or particular group of people differently, especially to their disadvantage, because of their skin colour, sex, sexuality, age and other characteristics. Discrimination against older people has wide-ranging consequences: it harms older people's social inclusion, health, and well-being (Levy and Macdonald 2016; Jackson et al. 2019). Stereotyping older adults and ageist behaviour towards them leads to many ill-effects on older adults' lives, including lower levels of social integration, workforce barriers, abuse, and neglect (Lyons 2009; Vitman et al. 2013).

Alongside these negative impacts on well-being and social relations, age discrimination has wide-ranging impacts on older people's health. Perceived day-to-day age discrimination increased the odds of fair or poor self-rated health and a range of diseases compared with those who did not report discriminatory experiences, in a recent analysis of the English Longitudinal Study of Ageing (Jackson et al. 2019). A study of three waves of the US Health and Retirement Study suggested that perceived day-to-day discrimination may have broad health consequences through loneliness, especially for older adults with low education (Lee and Bierman 2018). Repeated exposure to chronic stressors associated with age stereotypes and discrimination is likely to increase the risk of chronic disease, mortality, and other adverse health outcomes (Allen 2015). A UK study found that older people with mental health problems were among the most socially excluded and stigmatised groups within mental health populations and the general population (Lievesley et al. 2009).

Six of these detrimental effects of discrimination were explored in two-waves of a New Zealand Study of older citizens. Associations between these dimensions and negative life impacts such as lower health, well-being, and social integration were analysed, and are summarised below.

9.4.1 Quantifying the Impacts of Discrimination: A New Zealand Study

The results from two waves of the New Zealand Longitudinal Study of Ageing (NZLSA) quantified the impacts of different forms of discrimination on the health, loneliness, depression, well-being, and social relationships of older people. A national random sample of 3,317 older New Zealand citizens aged 50–84 years was recruited, which reduced to 3,015 in wave two. Consistent statistical correlations were found between discrimination as measured by the Everyday Discrimination Scale (Williams et al. 1997; Williams 2012) and lower levels of both health and well-being, and higher levels of depression and loneliness (Waldegrave 2018).

In wave one (2010) almost 60% of respondents said they experienced some form of discrimination. This reduced to 53% in wave two (2012). Age discrimination (15%) was the most frequently experienced form of discrimination. Employment, and intra-family (3% each), and gender and race (2% each) were the next most frequently cited forms of discrimination. On the 6-point scale used across each dimension of discrimination, the two most common expressions were *"being treated with less courtesy and respect than other people*" and *"people acting as if they think you are not smart"*. Respectively 17% and 12% of respondents had experienced these at least a few times a year.

The study analysed both static cross-sectional results from each wave and dynamic results over the two waves. Six social and health scales that measure known indicators of social exclusion cited in the literature above, were chosen to explore associations with discrimination in wave 2. Significant negative relationships were found between discrimination and each of the well-being and health scales, demonstrating that higher levels of discrimination are closely associated with lower health and well-being scores. As expected, loneliness and depression demonstrated significant positive relationships with discrimination. The cross-sectional results for wave two (2012) are shown in Table 9.3. In this table the discrimination scale measured in wave two (2012) is the independent variable used to predict each of the six social and health scales in wave two (2012).

The two waves of NZLSA data were then used to develop a dynamic measure to predict the well-being and health outcomes associated with discrimination. Instead of simply using the discrimination scale measured in wave two (2012) to predict well-being and health outcomes, the measure of discrimination in wave one (2010) is used as the dependent variable to predict the outcomes in wave two (2012). A linear regression model was applied for each dimension of well-being and health outcomes rather than using the six in one model, as some dimensions were correlated with each other.

In this dynamic analysis, we further control for the baseline outcome by including the measure of each dimension in wave one (2010) as one of the independent variables to predict the outcome in wave two (2012). This enabled the researchers to measure the impact of discrimination on social and health outcomes over time. Age, gender, education levels, and ethnicity were also controlled for. The results are set out in Table 9.4.

The P-value results show a statistically significant relationship between discrimination and each of the social exclusion indicators over the 2 years. Respondents with higher discrimination scores in wave one had decreased well-being and health scores, and higher loneliness and depression scores in wave two, demonstrating an increasing negative effect over time. The β scores indicate that the impact is moderate, but consistent across the range of indicator variables.

Table 9.3 Linear regressions for predicting health and social variables in wave two (2012) using discrimination measured in wave two (2012)

Dependent variable	β	P-value
Well-being (WHOQoL-8)	−0.296	<0.01
Well-being (CASP-12)	−0.315	<0.01
SF 12 Physical Health	−0.114	<0.01
SF 12 Mental Health	−0.294	<0.01
Loneliness (de Jong Gierveld)	0.332	<0.001
Depression (CES-D)	0.318	<0.001

Source: Waldegrave and Nguyen FCSPRU (2018)

Table 9.4 Linear regression for predicting health and social variables in wave two (2012) using discrimination measured in wave one (2010)

Dependent variable	β	P-value	N
Well-being (WHOQoL – 8) in 2012	−0.075	0.001	2660
Well-being (CASP – 12) in 2012	−0.099	<0.001	2616
SF 12 Physical Health in 2012	−0.166	0.001	2296
SF 12 Mental Health in 2012	−0.200	<0.001	2296
Loneliness (de Jong Gierveld) in 2012	0.052	0.001	2492
Depression (CES-D) in 2012	0.083	0.001	2594

Source: Waldegrave and Nguyen FCSPRU (2018)

9.5 Conclusion

This chapter brought together three dimensions of negative social relations as they impinge on and are experienced by older people, which have not been addressed together in previous studies. The aim was to explore, through the literature and original research conducted by the authors, how socially dysfunctional experiences affect social relations, and in turn impact on exclusion from social relations. Each dimension: conflictual relationships, abuse and discrimination, is characterised by demeaning social interactions that are important to address when considering social exclusion in ageing societies.

The studies cited across the dimensions, consistently demonstrated negative health, well-being and social disconnection impacts. Those on conflictual relationships showed that such relationships are harmful to health and well-being (Rook 2009; Darbonne et al. 2013). The studies on elder abuse came to similar conclusions with respect to the devastating effects of abusive relationships on health and quality of life (Lowenstein et al. 2009; Melchiorre et al. 2014). Other studies showed the strong associations of abuse with social isolation (Dong 2015), loneliness (Wong and Waite 2017) and low social support (Dong et al. 2013). The research on discrimination against older people showed the significantly negative impacts it has on older adult experiences of social inclusion, health and well-being (Levy and Macdonald 2016; Lee and Bierman 2018; Jackson et al. 2019). Higher levels of discrimination were closely associated with lower health and well-being scores, and higher loneliness and depression results (Waldegrave 2018).

Abuse and discrimination, by definition, refer to actions designed to hurt and exclude, while partnership conflict where an individual self-evaluates and perceives a relation as being conflictual, refers to the loss of harmony or partnership in the relationship. Each lead to demeaning interactions that damage social relations and disrupt social connections. These are dysfunctional processes, particularly when they happen to older people, and as the studies in this chapter show, they diminish feelings of self-worth, reduce well-being and sever relationships.

All three dimensions are usually studied within their own boundaries and have not previously been linked as a single research focus. They have been brought together in this chapter to demonstrate the similar way each dimension reduces the quality of life and social inclusion of older people. They function as exclusionary mechanisms within the social relations domain and have an important place in a conceptual framework of old-age social exclusion. This lens on the similarities and interrelationships of the three dimensions has enabled a broader understanding of exclusionary mechanisms.

This chapter addresses a key policy gap in more positive ageing frameworks. Each of these dimensions is modifiable. Public education, responsible professional training, media foci and improved inter-generational linkages can contribute to reducing the acceptance of dysfunctional behaviour that disrupts social inclusion. A policy focus on the linkages and interrelationships between exclusionary mechanisms in the social relations domain can enable more comprehensive and effective policy formation than a focus on one dimension at a time. Furthermore, it provides a broader human rights platform for the development of high-quality social services and more comprehensive policy development.

Future research could usefully consider the interrelationship between these three dimensions in further developing our understanding of the mechanisms that lead to social exclusion. Studies that address the dynamic effects of these mechanisms with more waves over a longer period will provide further robust evidence. Qualitative research that will help us get behind the numbers and better understand the complex web of vulnerability, dependency and victimisation will enable more realistic and effective social inclusionary policy development and service provision.

Editors' Postscript

Please note, like other contributions to this book, this chapter was written before the COVID-19 pandemic of 2020. The book's introductory chapter (Chap. 1) and conclusion (Chap. 34) consider some of the key ways in which the pandemic relates to issues concerning social exclusion and ageing.

References

Aartsen, M. J., & Veenstra, M. (2018). *The social pattern of conflicting and low-quality social relations*. Paper presented at GSA 2018 Annual Meeting: The Purposes of Longer Lives, Massachusetts.

Aartsen, M., Valtorta, N., Dahlberg, L., Van Regenmortel S., Waldegrave, C., & Corrigan, T. (2018). *Exclusion from social relations in later life*. ROSEnet Briefing Paper Series: No. 1. CA 15122 Reducing Old-Age Exclusion: Collaborations in Research and Policy.

Allen, J. O. (2015). Ageism as a risk factor for chronic disease. *The Gerontologist, 56*(4), 610–614.

Badenes-Ribera, L., Fabris, M. A., & Longobardi, C. (2019). Elder mistreatment in an Italian population: Prevalence and correlates. *The International Journal of Aging and Human Development*. https://doi.org/10.1177/0091415019875454.

Burholt, V., Winter, B., Aartsen, M., et al. (2019). A critical review and development of a conceptual model of exclusion from social relations for older people. *European Journal of Ageing (online first)*.https://doi.org/10.1007/s10433-019-00506-0.

Cooper, C., Selwood, A., & Lingston, G. (2008). The prevalence of elder abuse and neglect: A systematic review. *Age and Aging, 37*, 151–160.
Darbonne, A., Uchino, B. N., & Ong, A. D. (2013). What mediates links between age and well-being? A test of social support and interpersonal conflict as potential interpersonal pathways. *Journal of Happiness Studies, 14*(3), 951–963.
Dong, X. (2015). Elder abuse: systematic review and implications for practice. *Journal of the American Geriatrics Society, 63*(6), 1214–1238.
Dong, X., Chen, R., Chang, E. S., & Simon, M. (2013). Elder abuse and psychological well-being: A systematic review and implications for research and policy-A mini review. *Gerontology, 59*(2), 132–142.
Epstein, I. (2010). *Clinical data-mining: Integrating practice and research*. Oxford: Oxford University Press.
Fisher, B., & Regan, S. (2006). The extent and frequency of abuse in the lives of older women and their relationship with health outcomes. *Gerontologist, 46*(2), 200–209.
Fondazione Caritas Ambrosiana. (2011). *Ferite invisibili. Il mal-trattamento psicologico nella relazione tra caregiver e anziano* (Invisible wounds. The psychological mistreatment in the relationship between caregiver and elder). Milano: Franco Angeli. (in Italian).
Hosmer, D. W., Hosmer, T., & Lemeshow, S. (1980). A goodness-of-fit tests for the multiple logistic regression model. *Communications in Statistics, 10*, 1043–1069.
Iveniuk, J., Waite, L. J., Laumann, E., McClintock, M. K., & Tiedt, A. D. (2014). Marital conflict in older couples: Positivity, personality, and health. *Journal of Marriage and Family, 76*(1), 130–144.
Jackson, S. E., Hackett, R. A., & Steptoe, A. (2019). Associations between age discrimination and health and wellbeing: cross-sectional and prospective analysis of the English Longitudinal Study of Ageing. *The Lancet Public Health, 4*(4), e200–e208.
Krause, N., & Jay, G. (1991). Stress, social support and negative interaction in later life. *Research on Aging, 13*, 333–363.
Kydd, A., & Fleming, A. (2015). Ageism and age discrimination in health care: Fact or fiction? A narrative review of the literature. *Maturitas, 81*(4), 432–443.
Lachs, M. S., & Pillemer, K. A. (2015). Elder abuse. *New England Journal of Medicine, 373*(20), 1947–1956.
Lee, Y., & Bierman, A. (2018). Loneliness as a mediator of perceived discrimination and depression: Examining education contingencies. *International Journal of Aging & Human Development, 89*(2), 206–227.
Levy, S., & Macdonald, J. (2016). Progress on understanding ageism. *Journal of Social Issues, 72*(1), 5–25.
Lievesley, N., Hayes, R., Jones, K., Clark, A. (2009). *Ageism and age discrimination in mental health care in the United Kingdom: A review from the literature.*. Centre for Policy on Ageing.
Ligabue, L. (2010). *Progetto DIADE: attività svolte ed elementi emersi dal progetto* (DIADE Project: activities and outcome). Conference 'DIADE Violenza agita e subita nella relazione di cura: ricerca, analisi, proposte per prevenirla ed affrontarla', Reggio Emilia. http://www.informanziani.it/docs/LL.pdf. (in Italian). Accessed 22 Jan 2019.
Lowenstein, A., & Doron, I. (2013). *Israel*. In A. Phelan (Ed.), *International perspectives on elder abuse* (pp. 97–121). London/New York: Routledge, Taylor and Francis Group.
Lowenstein, A., Eisikovits, Z., Band-Winterstein, T., & Enosh, G. (2009). Is elder abuse and neglect a social phenomenon? Data from the first national prevalence survey in Israel. *Journal of Elder Abuse and Neglect, 21*(3), 253–277.
Lyons, I. (2009). *Public perceptions of older people and ageing*. Dublin: National Centre for the Protection of Older People.
Melchiorre, M. G., Di Rosa, M., Lamura, G., Quattrini, S., Chiatti, C., Greco, C., & Soares, J. J. F. (2012a). Il maltrattamento delle persone anziane in Italia: alcuni risultati dallo Studio

Abuel (The mistreatment of the elderly in Italy: some findings from the Abuel Study). *Prospettive Sociali e Sanitarie, 3*, 16–19. (in Italian).
Melchiorre, M. G., Chiatti, C., & Lamura, G. (2012b). Tackling the phenomenon of elder abuse in Italy: A review of existing legislation and policies as learning resource. *Educational Gerontology, 38*(10), 699–712.
Melchiorre, M. G., Penhale, B., & Lamura, G. (2014). Understanding elder abuse in Italy: Perception and prevalence, types and risk factors from a review of the literature. *Educational Gerontology, 40*(12), 909–931.
Murphy, K., Waa, S., Jaffer, H., Sauter, A., & Chan, A. (2013). A literature review of findings in physical elder abuse. *Canadian Association of Radiologists Journal, 64*(1), 10–14.
Rook, K. S. (2009). Gaps in Social Support Resources in Later Life: An Adaptational Challenge in Need of Further Research. *Journal of Social and Personal Relationships, 26*(1), 103–112.
Rook, K. S. (2015). Social networks in later life: Weighing positive and negative effects on health and well-being. *Current Directions in Psychological Science, 24*(1), 45–51.
Santos, A. J., Nunes, B., Kislaya, I., et al. (2019). Elder abuse victimization patterns: Latent class analysis using perpetrators and abusive behaviours. *BMC Geriatr, 19*, 117.
Schofield, M. J., Powers, J. R., & Loxton, D. (2013). Mortality and disability outcomes of self-reported elder abuse: a 12-year prospective investigation. *Journal American Geriatric Society, 61*, 679–685.
Seppänen, M. & Niemi, M. (2018, 11 15). *Exclusion from supportive social relations—elder abuse in family.* Paper presented at GSA 2018 Annual Meeting: The Purposes of Longer Lives, Massachusetts.
Slagsvold, B., Veenstra, M., Daatland, S. O., Hagestad, G., Hansen, T., Herlofson, K., & Solem, P. E. (2012). Life-course, ageing and generations in Norway: the NorLAG study. *Norsk Epidemiologi, 22*(2), 95–102.
Vitman, A., Iecovich, E., & Alfasi, N. (2013). Ageism and social integration of older adults in their neighborhoods in Israel. *The Gerontologist, 54*(2), 177–189.
Waldegrave, C., (2015) *Measuring elder abuse in New Zealand: Findings from the New Zealand longitudinal study of ageing (NZLSA).* (Technical Paper, Office for Senior Citizens). Wellington: Ministry of Social Development, New Zealand.
Waldegrave, C., & Nguyen, G. (2018). *The impacts of discrimination and abuse on the health, well-being, and loneliness of older people.* Paper presented at GSA 2018 Annual Meeting: The Purposes of Longer Lives, Massachusetts.
Ware, J. E., Jr., Kosinski, M., & Keller, S. D. (1996). A 12-Item Short-Form Health Survey: Construction of scales and preliminary tests of reliability and validity. *Medical Care*, 220–233.
Williams, D. (2012). The everyday discrimination scale. In D. Williams (Ed.), *Measuring discrimination resource.* https://scholar.harvard.edu/files/davidrwilliams/files/measuring_discrimination_resource_feb_2012_0_0.pdf. Accessed 22 Apr 2020.
Williams, D. R., Yu, Y., Jackson, J. S., & Anderson, N. B. (1997). Racial differences in physical and mental health: Socioeconomic status, stress, and discrimination. *Journal of Health Psychology, 2*(3), 335–351.
Wong, J. S., & Waite, L. J. (2017). Elder mistreatment predicts later physical and psychological health: Results from a national longitudinal study. *Journal of Elder Abuse & Neglect, 29*(1), 15–42.
World Health Organization. (2018). *Elder abuse*. Geneva: World Health Organization. https://www.who.int/ageing/projects/elder_abuse/en/ Accessed 22 Apr 2020.
Yan, E., So-Kum, C., & Yeung, T. D. (2002). No safe haven: A review on elder abuse in Chinese families. *Trauma, Violence, & Abuse, 3*(3), 167–180.
Yon, Y., Mikton, C. R., Gassoumis, Z. D., & Wilber, K. H. (2017). Elder abuse prevalence in community settings: A systematic review and meta-analysis. *Lancet Global Health, 5*, 147–156.
Yunus, R. M., Hairi, N. N., & Choo, W. Y. (2017). Consequences of elder abuse and neglect: A systematic review of observational studies. *Trauma, Violence, & Abuse*. Advance online publication. https://doi.org/10.1177/1524838017692798

Section IV
Exclusion from Services

Chapter 10
Introduction: Framing Exclusion from Services

Veerle Draulans and Giovanni Lamura

10.1 Introduction

This section presents three specific examples of how old-age social exclusion can take place in the field of service provision. These contributions refer to the key areas of care, transportation and information and communication technology (ICT) based solutions, which represent some of the sub-domains of service-related exclusion in later life that are most frequently cited in the literature (Walsh et al. 2017; ROSEnet Services Working Group 2020). Given the current demographic trends, the availability of suitable services has become crucial to ensure social cohesion and inclusiveness. Governments, be it on national or community levels, social profit organisations and commercial companies offer a huge variety of services aimed at making people's lives easier and more comfortable. In order to better contextualise the contributions presented in this section, this chapter will provide an overview of old-age service exclusion in general, highlighting in particular macro- and micro-level considerations. It will then briefly introduce each contribution.

10.2 Old-Age Service Exclusion

Following Walsh et al. (2017), and paraphrasing the overall definition of social exclusion suggested by their scoping review, old-age related exclusion from services can be defined as the condition (and the processes leading to it) that involves

V. Draulans (✉)
Faculteit Sociale Wetenschappen, Centre for Sociological Research (CESO), KU Leuven, Belgium
e-mail: veerle.draulans@kuleuven.be

G. Lamura
Centre for Socio-Economic Research on Ageing, INRCA-IRCCS, National Institute of Health and Science on Ageing, Ancona, Italy

K. Walsh et al. (eds.), *Social Exclusion in Later Life*, International Perspectives on Aging 28, https://doi.org/10.1007/978-3-030-51406-8_10

the lack or denial of services in later life, to a larger extent than what might be considered as "normal" for the majority of people, with a negative impact both at individual and societal levels.

Exclusion from services in the health and/or social care sector represents one of the most frequently investigated dimensions (Walsh et al. 2017). This is clearly related to the fact that this sector represents a key area for meeting the needs of an increasingly ageing population. A large body of research, highlighting the risk factors for being excluded from the use of key care service infrastructure in late-life, have identified exclusionary mechanisms relating to geographic location, market-oriented care models, poverty and lack of sensitivity towards old-age specific needs (Srakar et al. 2015).

Another major area often reported in old-age related services exclusion is that of transport and mobility, which focuses on barriers such as lack of flexibility, costs, and environmental barriers and insufficient infrastructure, especially in rural regions (Siren and Gasparovic 2017). Service exclusion occurs, however, also in other fields characterised by a growing presence of older users requiring a more attentive approach in order to prevent marginalisation (Walsh et al. 2017). This includes, for instance, general area-based exclusion (Stoeckel and Litwin 2015), tourism (Eusebìo et al. 2015), and information and communication technologies (ICT) as a tool to access information (Kuerbis et al. 2017). With regard to the last sub dimension, in particular, it should be acknowledged that older people can experience less isolation and lower risks of loneliness as a result of using social media platforms enabling them to remain connected with family and friends (Hajek and König 2019). However, it is likely that the digital divide in terms of accessibility and usability, involving on average less digitally skilled older people, will grow considerably in the coming years, rendering this area key in preventing cross-cutting service exclusion in later life. It should be finally underlined that conceptual work in this area has been rather limited, with few exceptions (Simms 2004).

10.3 Considerations in Researching Service Exclusion in Later Life

Two issues emerge as crucial when considering how best to tackle exclusion from services in older-age. The first concerns the question of how to prevent and ameliorate exclusionary mechanisms impacting older adults within service systems. The second, given this challenge, regards the identification of the most effective strategies to target risk factors associated with old-age exclusion from services, without stereotyping "the" group of older users and the services that they most often use.

Investigating the relationship between old-age service exclusion and different social risks, such as poverty and material deprivation, gender and belonging to minority groups, requires a multidimensional and multidisciplinary perspective. For scientific research to assist in the formulation and implementation of appropriate policies, there must be a systematic consideration of the breadth of the key service infrastructures, such as health and social care services, general services, new technologies, and transport and mobility, but also cross-cutting issues concerning service restructuring, accessibility and affordability.

In addition, and closely related to the ways in which these issues can be propagated, attention should be paid to three distinctive levels: the macro level of political decision making; the meso level of organisations offering services; and the micro level of the immediate service agent-service user relationship. Actors within each of these levels not only serve to shape how older people make use of services, but also have a responsibility in ensuring the adequacy of services and that they meet the needs of older citizens. In the following section, we provide a brief overview of the macro and micro considerations, as these levels provide the analytical boundaries that shape the meso level (Serpa and Ferreira 2019).

10.4 The Macro Level and Government Responsibility

Lower individual level material deprivation is associated with higher state expenditure on services related to social protection and healthcare. Data from the fifth wave of the Survey of Health, Ageing and Retirement in Europe (SHARE) highlights the connection between unmet long-term care needs, social exclusion and welfare regimes (Srakar et al. 2015; also see Sumil-Laanemaa et al. and Grigoryeva et al. this volume). People who live in a context characterised by a comparatively high public expenditure on social protection and health care related services are generally more likely to report less problems in accessing services, as do people living in societies providing social housing, holding age-friendly social policies and offering accessible and affordable transport facilities.

Transport, in particular, is crucial in preventing exclusionary risks. In this regard, not only does the availability of transport facilities deserve attention, but so too does the impact of policies and legislation regarding age and driving licenses on late-life mobility and social exclusion (Haustein and Siren 2014). In this regard, additional factors, outside of immediate infrastructure, play a crucial role. Among them, having a driving license and/or having people around who are willing to drive has been reported as essential (Parkhurst et al. 2014). This risk of exclusion is highest in relation to discretionary travel, where research has demonstrated reductions in travel for leisure and/or social activities. This in turn compounds the challenges related to isolation and social exclusion, in a spiral that might be difficult to stop [see Siren this volume for a full discussion of transport as a cross-cutting mediator of social exclusion in later life].

10.5 The Micro Level: We Are All Different

A multitude of factors at the micro level can influence older people's access to services. Research demonstrates that many older women who are widowed or who live alone belong to one of the most disadvantaged groups, and those who live in rural or remote (mountain) areas are even more at risk (UNECE 2017). But, as the intersectionality approach (Crenshaw 1989; Thomsen and Finley 2019) suggests, it is often the combination of different dimensions of identity which make specific groups of the population more vulnerable, including to service exclusion.

Among the most relevant dimensions are gender, sexual orientation (LGTBQ+), ethnicity, race, migration, (dis)ability, physical or mental health, the spatial context that people live in, knowledge about and availability of (public) services, and personal access to transportation. In this regard, studies show that, for instance, older LGTBQ+ adults (King et al. 2019) or older people belonging to a racial or ethnic minority group (Torres 2015; De Tavernier and Draulans 2019) may meet more hurdles with regard to accessing services, since their specific needs might not be properly taken into account or respected by service providers. A group that deserves special attention in this regard is the (very heterogeneous) group of older homeless people (Warnes and Crane 2006). Dementia, as a health condition and as a socially constructed set of experiences, strongly influences vulnerability too. But here again an intersectional approach highlights the additional hurdles that some people can face, where for example older people living with dementia who belong to a migrant group may revert to their original mother tongue (Tipping and Whiteside 2015).

10.6 Outline of This Section

The three chapters included in this section of the book explore different facets of service exclusion in later life, including different service sectors, different risk factors and different levels.

In Chap. 11, Cholat and Daconto describe the risks of spatial- and mobility-related exclusion from services and social relations that might affect people living in mountain areas. The social and economic conditions of those who live in such remote areas, who may in some cases have a lower capacity for mobility, require as the authors argue a set of "reversed" mobilities. The concept of reversed mobility implies that products and services come to the person, provided by relatives, caregivers or mobile shops. By referring to the experience of two European Alpine territories (Isère in France and Bergamo in Italy), the authors aim to show how reversed mobilities may promote the inclusion of frail older people in mountain areas.

In Chap. 12, Széman, Golubeva and Patyán offer important insights on home care services provided in Central and Eastern European (CEE) countries and the Russian Federation. For a multitude of reasons, such as geographic distance and the absence of formal care facilities, a strong tradition of familialisation of care services, reflected by a central role of home-based informal care, is common practice in these countries. While this, on the one hand, might allow a more personalised delivery of care to those in need, on the other, it may increase the risk of social exclusion and social isolation.

In Chap. 13, Poli, Kostakis and Barbabella analyse what digital technologies can do to support health care provision, with a specific focus on the exclusionary dynamics occurring in this field. They highlight that the integration of digital technologies with ordinary care routines has been slower compared to the bank sector or e-commerce, due to specific challenges. Acknowledging that many older people are reluctant to use (newly developed) digital health services, Poli and colleagues investigate the main drivers of old-age social exclusion from digital health services, and illustrate how macro-, meso and micro decisions and experiences are of mutual influence.

While the three chapters certainly do not cover the wide spectrum of areas in which old-age service exclusion might take place, they offer in-depth insights into three fields representing core sectors of service delivery for an ageing population. They thus provide a valuable contribution to current debates on this topic. In this regard, it should be of course considered that they were written prior to the outbreak of the COVID-19 pandemic, and therefore they do not contain any direct reference to it. However, the topics they address have been so dramatically central in terms of both real life impact and measures adopted within the recent pandemic crisis, that their policy implications in this respect will be immediately evident to the reader.

References

Crenshaw, K. (1989). Demarginalizing the intersection of race and sex: A black feminist critique of antidiscrimination doctrine. *Feminist Theory and Antiracist Politics. University of Chicago Legal Forum, 1*, 139–167.

De Tavernier, W., & Draulans, V. (2019). Negotiating informal elder care, migration and exclusion: The case of a Turkish immigrant community in Belgium. *International Journal of Ageing in Later Life, 12*(2), 89–117.

Eusébio, C., Carneiro, M., Kastenholz, E., & Alvelos, H. (2015). Social tourism programmes for the senior market: A benefit segmentation analysis. *Journal of Tourism and Cultural Change, 15*(1), 1–21. https://doi.org/10.1080/14766825.2015.1117093.

Hajek, A., & König, H. (2019). The association between use of online social networks sites and perceived social isolation among individuals in the second half of life: Results based on a nationally representative sample in Germany. *BMC Public Health, 19*, 40. https://doi.org/10.1186/s12889-018-6369-6.

Haustein, S., & Siren, A. (2014). Seniors' unmet mobility needs – How important is a driving licence? *Journal of Transport Geography, 41*, 45–52. https://doi.org/10.1016/j.jtrangeo.2014.08.001.

King, A., Almack, K., & Jones, R. L. (2019). *Intersections of ageing, gender and sexualities. Multidisciplinary international perspectives*. Bristol/Chicago: Policy Press.

Kuerbis, A., Mulliken, A., Muench, F., Moore, A. A., & Gardner, D. (2017). Older adults and mobile technology: Factors that enhance and inhibit utilization in the context of behavioral health. *Mental Health and Addiction Research, 2*(2), 2–11. https://doi.org/10.15761/MHAR.1000136.

Parkhurst, G., Galvin, K., Musselwhite, C., Phillips, J., Shergold, I., & Todres, L. (2014). Beyond transport: Understanding the role of mobilities in connecting rural elders in civic society. In

C. Hennessey, R. Means, & V. Burholt (Eds.), *Countryside connections: Older people, community and place in rural Britain* (pp. 125–157). Bristol: Policy Press.

ROSEnet Services Working Group. (2020). Services exclusion in later life. In K. Walsh & T. Scharf (series eds.), *ROSEnet briefing paper series: No. 4. CA 15122 reducing old-age exclusion: Collaborations in research and policy.* ISBN: 978-1-908358-74-5. http://rosenetcost.com/wp-content/uploads/2017/01/cost_rosenet_actionpolicy4_web.pdf

Serpa, S., & Ferreira, C. (2019). Micro, meso and macro levels of social analysis. *International Journal of Social Science Studies, 7*(3), 120–124. https://doi.org/10.11114/ijsss.v7i3.4223.

Simms, M. (2004). A theory of age exclusion through closure: 'Chronological age' to 'clinical need'. *Journal of Aging Studies, 18* (4), 445–465.

Siren, A., & Gasparovic S. (2017). Transport related social exclusion. In Draulans V., Hlebec V., Maskeliunas R., Siren A. and Lamura G. (eds.) *Exclusion from services – Knowledge synthesis paper*. ROSEnet Services Working Group, Knowledge Synthesis Series: No. 3. CA 15122 Reducing Old-Age Exclusion: Collaborations in Research and Policy (pp. 13–17). http://rosenetcost.com/wp-content/uploads/2017/12/services-synthesis-paper-final.pdf.

Srakar, A., Hrast, M. F., Hlebec, V., & Majcen, B. (2015). Social exclusion, welfare regime and unmet long-term care need: Evidence from SHARE. In A. Börsch-Supan, T. Kneip, H. Litwin, M. Myck, & G. Weber (Eds.), *Ageing in Europe: Supporting policies for an inclusive society* (pp. 189–198). Berlin: de Gruyter.

Stoeckel, K. J., & Litwin, H. (2015). Accessibility to neighbourhood services and well-being among older Europeans. In A. Börsch-Supan, T. Kneip, H. Litwin, M. Myck, & G. Weber (Eds.), *Ageing in Europe: Supporting policies for an inclusive society* (pp. 39–48). Berlin: De Gruyter. https://www.degruyter.com/downloadpdf/books/.

Thomsen, C., & Finley, J. (2019). On intersectionality. A review essay. *Hypatia, 34*(1), 155–160. https://doi.org/10.1111/hypa.12450.

Tipping, S. A., & Whiteside, M. (2015). Language reversion among people with dementia from culturally and linguistically diverse backgrounds: The family experience. *Australian Social Work, 68*(2), 184–197. https://doi.org/10.1080/0312407X.2014.953187.

Torres, S. (2015). Expanding the gerontological imagination on ethnicity: Conceptual and theoretical perspectives. *Ageing and Society, 35*(5), 935–960. https://doi.org/10.1017/S0144686X14001330.

UNECE. (2017). *Older persons in rural and remote areas* (Policy Brief on Ageing No. 18, March). Geneva: UNECE Working Group on Ageing. https://www.unece.org/fileadmin/DAM/pau/age/Policy_briefs/ECE-WG1-25.pdf.

Walsh, K., Scharf, T., & Keating, N. (2017). Social exclusion of older persons: A scoping review and conceptual framework. *European Journal of Ageing, 14*(1), 81–98.

Warnes, A. M., & Crane, M. (2006). The causes of homelessness among older people in England. *Housing Studies, 21*(3), 401–421.

Chapter 11
Reversed Mobilities as a Means to Combat Older People's Exclusion from Services: Insights from Two Alpine Territories in France and Italy

Florent Cholat and Luca Daconto

11.1 Introduction

(Im)mobility and (in)accessibility play a key role in older people's exclusion from services. It can particularly happen in mountain areas, where we can find lower availability of services and higher transport constraints (slope gradients; lack of public transportation; weather conditions, etc.). Consequently, movement is necessary to reach and engage in relevant services. Older people's ability to move, the so-called motility or capital of mobility (Kaufmann et al. 2004), plays an important role in combatting exclusion from services, and social exclusion in general. It allows access to opportunities at specific locations, through which desires can be fulfilled, needs satisfied, and social networks maintained. While older people with a high capacity for mobility might easily adapt to the "mountain", accessing these opportunities is much more difficult for individuals with lower motility, such as frail and vulnerable older adults (Lord 2011), who may not be able to participate in relevant services (Church et al. 2000; Kenyon et al. 2002; Lucas 2012). In order to cope with the risks of spatial- and mobility-related exclusion from services, and social relations, people with a low capacity for mobility require and engage in a set of reversed mobilities (Cholat 2013). Reversed mobilities can be defined as different forms of indirect accessibility (Hine and Grieco 2003; Kellerman 2012) to relevant services based on the mobility of others, such as relatives, caregivers, social and health workers and mobile retailers.

F. Cholat (✉)
LabEx ITTEM, University Grenoble Alps, Gières, France

University of Milan Bicocca, Milan, Italy
e-mail: florent.cholat@univ-grenoble-alpes.fr

L. Daconto (✉)
Department of Sociology and Social Research, University of Milan Bicocca, Milan, Italy
e-mail: luca.daconta@unimib.it

K. Walsh et al. (eds.), *Social Exclusion in Later Life*, International Perspectives on Aging 28, https://doi.org/10.1007/978-3-030-51406-8_11

This adaptive strategy responds to a form of exclusion from services that is constituted across and impacts different spheres (spatial, transport, services and social relations) due to the interaction between environmental and individual level vulnerabilities. While reversed mobilities potentially represent a very important means of combatting older people's exclusion in mountain areas (Cholat 2013, 2018; Cholat et al. 2017), they may also shape and create further inequalities and compound exclusion for some individuals who do not have at their disposal the financial and relational resources needed to activate these strategies.

This chapter aims to stress how reversed mobilities may contribute to a better understanding of exclusion from services. In particular, we will analyze (1) the interaction between different factors in constructing service inaccessibility as an exclusionary process in the lives of mountain dwelling older people; (2) the key role played by reversed mobilities in combatting older people's experience of exclusion from services in mountain areas, as well as the environmental, economic and social costs and "new" inequalities that might be associated with this form of adaptation. As such, our analysis will address both exclusion from transport services, and exclusion from general services, and how these exclusions intersect, and how their impact are accentuated as a result of individual and environmental vulnerabilities.

Despite the potential role that reversed mobilities could play in combatting older people's social exclusion and guaranteeing the vitality of mountain areas, the topic has not been sufficiently considered by research, planning and public policy. This has consequences for our capacity to make informed decisions about the way to effectively support older people and promote their inclusion in these contexts.

To deepen our understanding of reversed mobilities, we will review the international literature on this topic, and draw on an exploratory analysis carried out in two European Alpine territories (Isère, France and Bergamo, Italy) to illustrate where such reversed mobilities may be needed and may be occurring. First, we review from a theoretical perspective the ways the relationship between older people and mountain environments may influence (in)accessibility to opportunities and lead to mutually reinforcing exclusionary processes. Next, we will explore the key role played by reversed mobilities in countering older people's exclusion from different domains in mountain areas and highlight challenges regarding the sustainability and inequalities of this form of adaptation. In conclusion, we will discuss the extent reversed forms of mobility offer a strategy for other socio-cultural environments in promoting older people's inclusion. We will also highlight some key research/policy gaps and required future directions.

11.2 (Im)Mobility and Service (in)Accessibility Related to Older Adults' Social Exclusion

Mobility is a very important dimension of well-being in later life (Metz 2000; Banister and Bowling 2004). Indeed, as for other groups, mobility is a facilitator of well-being and inclusion, as it allows older people to have access to opportunities and to participate in relevant services at specific locations. In addition, mobility is not just a means for participating in societies (as in the case of accessibility), but it is also an end in itself (Urry 2007). It can promote well-being directly such as in the form of: happiness and pleasure, felt during a trip with relevant others (*e.g.* relatives, grandchild, friends, neighbours) in an attractive environment (*e.g.* familiar places); and physical activity, as an active mobility central to healthy ageing (Swedish National Institute of Public 2007).

Despite the benefits of mobility in later life, studies (*e.g.* Colleoni 2016) generally show a lower likelihood among older people to be mobile, whatever the specific modal solution considered, compared to other social groups.[1] Generally, gerontological mobility research (OECD 2001; Risser et al. 2010; Nordbakke 2013) points out existing barriers to transport mobility in old-age (*e.g.* diseases or personal mobility difficulties; environmental barriers; physical obstacles; design/structure of public transport; lack of safety; accidents). However, more recent studies suggest the need to go beyond a simple transportation perspective of older adult mobility and to put more emphasis on emotional, motivational and social aspects of being mobile (Kaiser 2009; Lord et al. 2011). In this sense, Kaufmann et al. (2004) has introduced the concept of motility, and define it as the set of characteristics that enable people to move, *i.e.* a property of individuals shaped by biological, psychophysical, socio-cultural and environmental factors (De Witte et al. 2013).

Indeed, if older people's low motility is due to obstacles associated with age-related psychophysical health (Henrard 2007), a relevant role is also played by the relationship between this individual vulnerability and the characteristics of the environment. In these cases, the environment can act as a further determinant, able to enhance or limit individual functional ability. That is, the particular features of the built and social environment can improve or restrict personal capabilities, as conceived in the capability approach by Sen (1993) [see Tournier and Vidovićová, and Drilling et al. this volume for a discussion about older people's interactions with these aspects of the environment].

In this sense, mountain areas may further constrain older people's ability to move, as they are partly characterised by low availability of general services, lack of transportation and geographical and physical barriers (*e.g.* slope, road closures, seasonal

[1] However, senior mobility demand is highly differentiated. For instance, young older adults (65–74 years) have a profile very similar to that of the general adult population as regards the number of journeys and the high use of the car. The use of the car collapses in the older-age groups, unlike walking, which is the older people's privileged modal choice, in particular for women and those aged 75 years or more.

and weather conditions, etc.). In order to access opportunities and to participate in services relevant for social inclusion not available at the local scale (such as working, accessing goods and services, and maintaining social networks), the older mountaineers must be able to move and overcome the "mountain" constraints.

Consequently, the intersection between individual (low motility) and environmental (low transport and accessibility) vulnerabilities can result in limited accessibility to opportunities (Dijst and Kwan 2005) – not only goods, facilities and services but also the whole set of services which allow individuals to satisfy both elementary and more complex needs related to identity, relationships and social participation. Such limitations have been recognised as undermining older people's quality of life and potentially leading to their exclusion from different domains (SEU 2003) [also see Tournier and Lucie Vidovićová this volume for the discussion of person-environment fit as a relevant concept to this interaction of individual and environmental characteristics]. From this perspective, accessibility – described as "the ability of people to reach or take part in services or opportunities" (Farrington 2007 p. 321) – represents a condition necessary to exercise full citizenship (Madanipour et al. 1998) and so becomes a social indicator (Geurs and van Wee 2004) that is able to shed light on the ways to achieve social justice and inclusion (Martens 2016). For instance, it shows the mutually reinforcing exclusionary processes that may affect older people living in mountain areas resulting from the intersection of spatial, service, transport and individual dimensions. Furthermore, the notion of accessibility can help orient policy intervention towards more appropriate areas and populations.

In the context of "mountain" constraints, it is possible to observe new forms of inequalities linked to older people's different levels of motility. On the one hand, an older person with greater motility can respond to inaccessibility by choosing a mode of travel more suited to their needs, attitudes and preferences. On the other hand, transport poverty (Lucas et al. 2016), and lack of choice, and low capacity for mobility can lead to social exclusion and isolation. The intersection between environmental and individual vulnerability generates a circular set of dynamics: the low availability of services requires older people's mobility; high physical and transport barriers and low individual capacity for mobility lead to immobility and inaccessibility to relevant opportunities, which, in turn, bring an increased vulnerability to exclusion from services.

However, some scholars warn against this interpretation, which does not consider the vulnerable groups' expedients (Belton Chevallier et al. 2018) or coping strategies (Jouffe et al. 2015) in order to move, and access relevant opportunities. It is in this light, that these groups may turn to a set of reversed mobilities (Cholat et al. 2017), at least indirectly (Hine and Grieco 2003; Kellerman 2012) delivered by services or support networks (family, neighbours, etc.), to ameliorate risks of isolation and exclusion. For example, the weak motility of an older person may be compensated by the mobility of other people (professionals, family carers, neighbours or friends) that can meet his/her daily needs: if the older person no longer moves the goods and services will have to go to him/her. It is these reversed mobilities that we now consider.

11.3 Reversed Mobilities in Mountains: Types and Evidence

After outlining what reversed mobilities respond to and where they may be needed, in this section we propose a classification (Table 11.1) for the purpose of describing their actual use in the mountain regions of Isère (France) and Bergamo (Italy) based on previous work (Cholat 2013; Cholat et al. 2017). Reversed mobilities differ primarily in their purpose. For ageing mountain dwelling populations, these purposes focus primarily on ageing in place and mainly concern accessing health care and the main activities of daily living, such as shopping, socialisation and home maintenance/delivery services. Reversed mobilities therefore also vary according to the type of actor who moves. It is possible to distinguish at least three primary sources of reversed mobilities: family and local communities; public welfare institutions; and private sector companies.

Considering the healthcare purpose, a significant source of reversed mobilities in mountain areas is the Socio-Medical Home Assistance service provided by state institutions. For instance, in Bergamo, the proportion of older users of the Home Assistance service is greater in mountain areas, as is the per-capita expenditure for the delivery of meals, home laundry and social transport.[2] Access to goods and services is guaranteed by different actors. In a previous study (Cholat 2013; Cholat et al. 2017), conducted in these two mountain communities (Entraigues, Isère, France; Isola di Fronda, Bergamo, Italy), the private sector (*e.g.* mobile shops and home delivery) emerged as a main source of reversed mobilities, since family, relatives and friends live relatively close by in these areas. Considering dependent older adults, reversed mobilities constitute on average a distance of 293 Km per week in Isère and 121 Km per week in Bergamo. In Italy, territorial welfare policies aim to manage and harness reversed mobilities through the activation of the so-called Community "Butler" service, a figure who performs various services (*e.g.*

Table 11.1 Reversed mobilities: A classification of type and provider

	Family and local community	Public welfare	Private sector
Healthcare and home maintenance	- Support	- Socio-Medical Home Assistance	- "Badante"/ Caregiver
	-Socialisation and social care	- Personal assistance	
Goods	- Shopping	- Meal delivery	- Mobile shops
		- Laundry service delivery	- Home delivery
Services	- Running errands	- Social Transport	- Mobile shops
		- Community "Bulter"	- Home delivery

[2] In 2014, the total management cost of public services was €1,887,513 in the mountain domains of Bergamo (Source: Regional Health Fund 2014).

shopping; delivery; laundry; handling administrative paperwork; shipping and payment of utilities).

11.4 Mountain Territories and Indirect Accessibility by Reversed Mobility

The mountain is not a homogeneous territory and it is necessary to take into account the variation in the availability of services. This includes well-resourced and connected mountain settings, such as tourist zones and the "urban" and "metropolitan" mountain centralities, to more disconnected sites, such as remote villages and less desirable municipalities. The level of accessibility can also vary according to weather, seasons and climatic conditions (*e.g.* holiday/tourism period, snow cover, road closures, etc.). Furthermore, it is also necessary to consider the characteristics of the resident community (*e.g.* socio-economic conditions, identity and solidarity, share of frail/vulnerable population). Therefore, the intensity of reversed mobilities depends primarily on the "floating" availability and accessibility of sufficient goods and services at the local level. Then, the intensity of reversed mobilities is influenced by the older population's level of autonomy and motility. To illustrate these considerations in a very broad way, we draw on an empirical example from two mountainous regions.

11.4.1 Illustrating the Need for Reversed Mobility in Ageing Mountain Dwelling Populations

We analysed the spatial distribution of basic services and the older population[3] in two European alpine regions: *Département de l'Isère*, France and *Provincia di Bergamo*, Italy. These two territories, although each has a different geographic scale (Isère: 7431 Sq. Km, Bergamo: 2746 Sq. Km), are comparable in their territorial structures. From a geomorphological point of view, these two territories include both an agricultural plain, which lies north of Isere and south of the province of Bergamo, and a mountainous area close to important urban centres like the city of Grenoble (450,000 inhabitants) and the city of Bergamo (480,000 inhabitants). We use a geographic information system model (through a kernel density estimation (KDE- Daconto et al. 2017) to calculate and represent the percentage and spatial distribution of residents aged 75 years and over within the total municipal population, and to contrast this age structure concentration with the availability of basic

[3]The analysis of the resident population is based on open data provided by the national statistical agencies, namely INSEE for France via the 2016 population census and ISTAT for Italy via the 2011 census. In France, the data source is the SIRENE directory of INSEE (2017), while in Italy the same data are available via the 2011 census of industry and services (ISTAT). The collected data were inserted into a

services across these two regions. Services included in the analysis were selected on the basis of those identified within the literature as being critical for daily life and older adult inclusion (Krizek et al. 2012). These included: health services (*e.g.* pharmacies, physicians; hospital services; primary and community care clinics), supermarkets and shops, and places of sociability (bars/cafés).

At a first level of analysis, and with reference to Figs. 11.1 and 11.2, it is possible to identify the areas most exposed to the need for reversed mobilities where a low availability of services combines with a higher presence of potentially dependent older people, *e.g.* residents aged 75 years and older. In analysing the spatial distribution of basic services and the older population it is possible to argue that the availability of services is greater in urban and tourist areas and in the mountain resorts (Figs. 11.1 and 11.2).

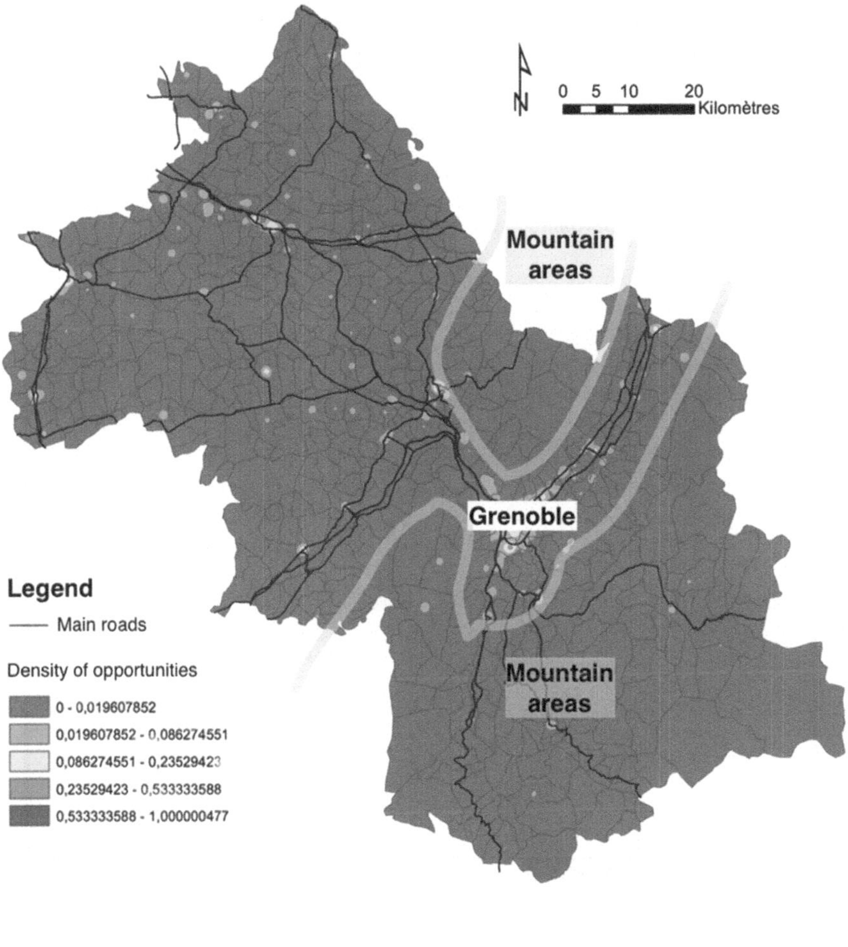

Fig. 11.1 The density of basic services in the department of Isère

Source: authors' elaboration on data INSEE, 2017, IGN, 2016

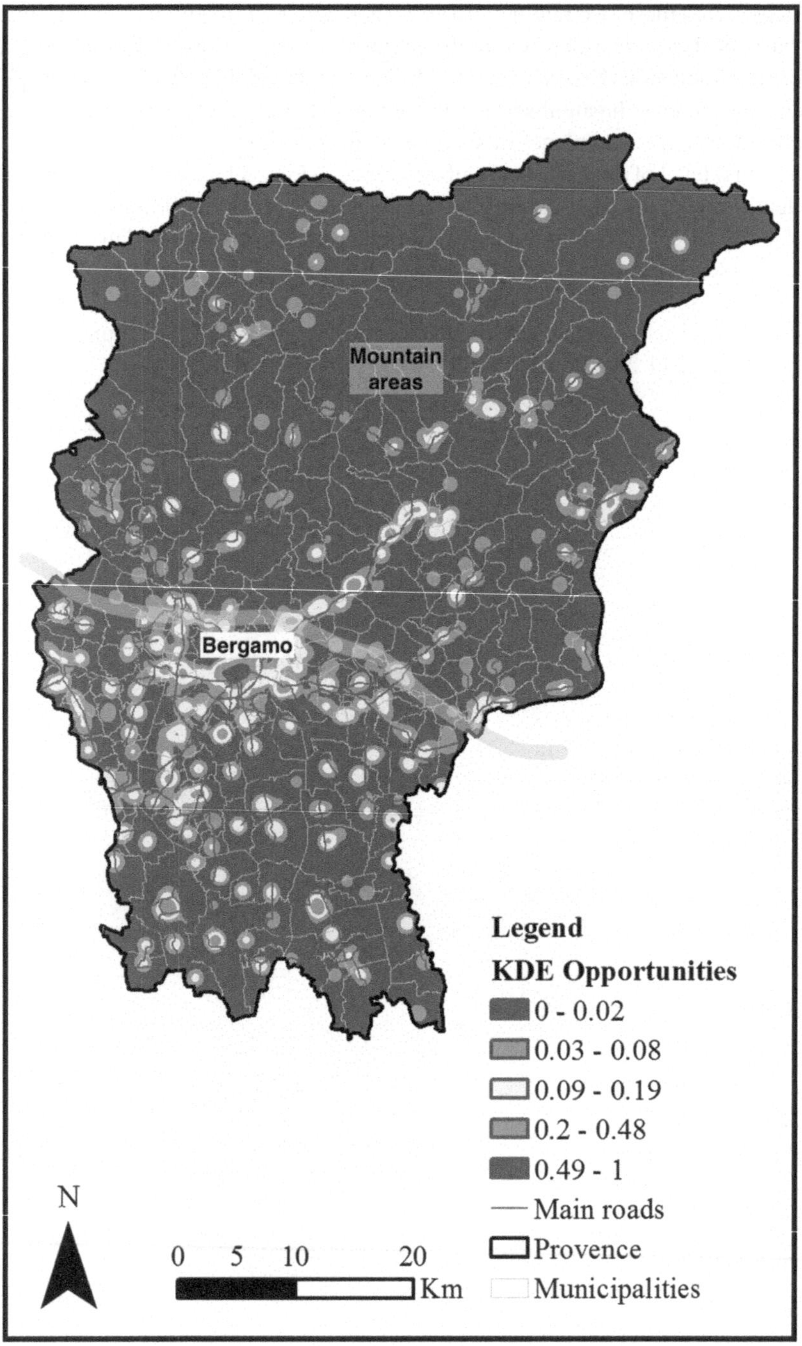

Fig. 11.2 The density of basic services in the province of Bergamo

Source: authors' elaboration on data ISTAT, 2011, OSM, 2017

Outside these areas, the availability of services, represented by a numeric scale, are lower, or even zero, in the non-peri-urban mountain. However, a higher offer of services in the mountain tourism areas is due to the seasonal presence (Winter-Summer) of tourists and temporary residents. For instance, shops often suspend their activity outside the tourist seasons. This leads to a changing configuration of these territories in terms of the opportunities they offer and, consequently, in terms of their need for reversed mobilities. Following this temporal perspective, it is also possible to put forward the hypothesis that, thanks to a greater presence of primary roads, tourist areas are less sensitive to the seasonal variation in accessibility due to the climatic hazards (climate conditions, snow, storms, etc.) and the closing of roads. The proportion of 75-year-old residents within the total municipal population (Figs. 11.3 and 11.4) allows us to show an over-representation of older people in mountainous areas, in comparison with the urban, peri-urban and rural territories. In

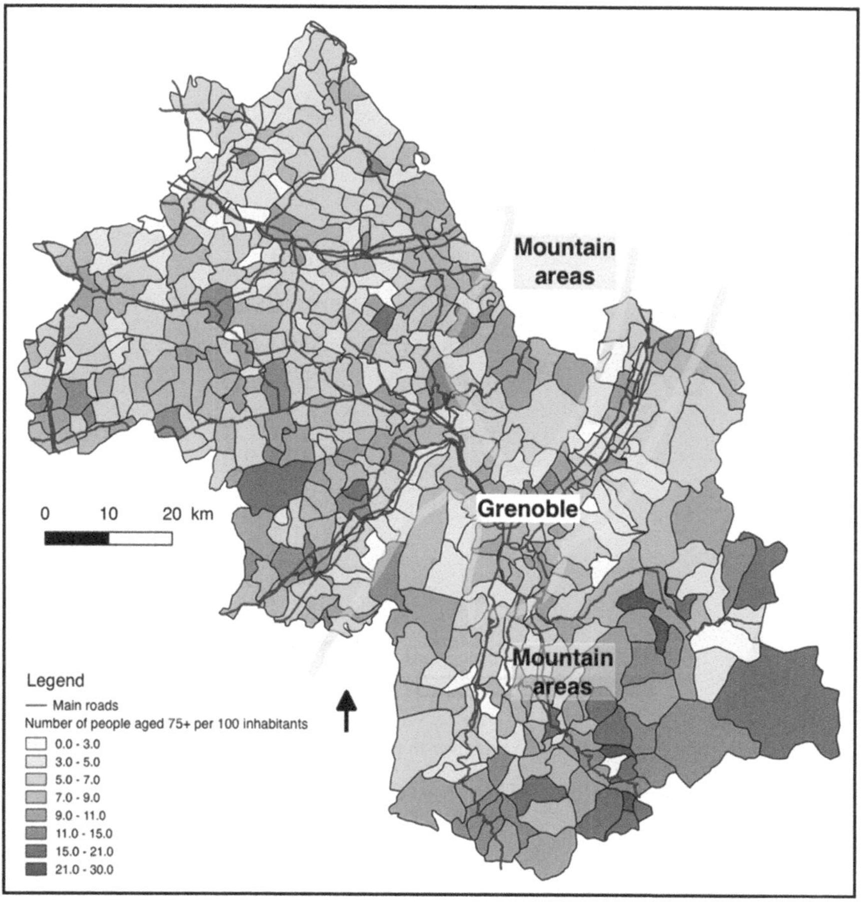

Fig. 11.3 Proportion of people aged 75 and over in the department of Isère

Source: authors' elaborations on data INSEE, 2017, IGN, 2016

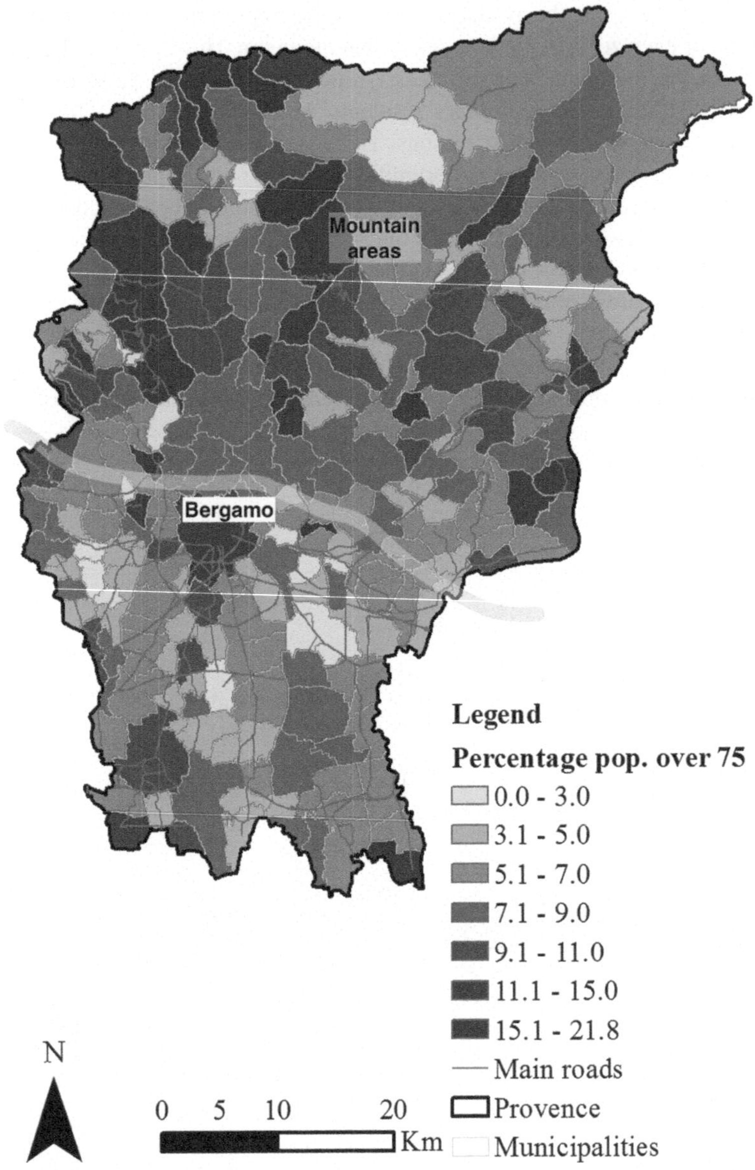

Fig. 11.4 Proportion of people aged 75 and over in the province of Bergamo

Source: authors' elaboration on data ISTAT, 2011, OSM, 2017

this sense, mountain areas emerge as the territories most exposed to service exclusion.

In these types of contexts, where service, spatial and individual vulnerabilities overlap, reversed mobilities may represent an adaptive strategy in order to cope with environmental (low availability and accessibility of services) and individual (low ability to move) vulnerabilities. In this sense, they can be considered as a response to the overlapping mechanisms of exclusion that can arise from spatial, transport and individual dimensions which function to undermine older people's access to key spheres of activity (*e.g.* healthcare, welfare, social networks, shopping, etc.). Therefore, from an individual perspective reversed mobilities allow older people to combat or ameliorate multidimensional exclusionary processes and to participate in daily life. From a societal point of view, they contribute to the liveability (employment, residential economy, etc.) of the mountain (Smit and Wandel, 2006) ensuring the habitability of territories affected by processes of abandonment and depopulation strongly related to the lack and inaccessibility of services.

This response and adaptation is not universal, however, as reversed mobilities require financial, cultural and relational resources, which are necessary, for instance, to acquire private delivery services (*e.g.* commerce, caregiver, nurse, etc.), including online services (*e.g.* e-commerce), and to activate support networks (*e.g.* relatives, neighbours, etc.).

11.4.2 Costs and Inequalities Related to Reversed Mobilities

In terms of the increasing concerns surrounding the sustainability of these sorts of communities, reversed mobilities present environmental, social and economic costs that scholars, professionals and policymakers must consider. First, from an environmental point of view reversed mobilities are highly car dependent (Dupuy 1999) in the current model of territorial development. This significantly increases travel times and requires also the ability to overcome environmental barriers (*e.g.* slope, weather conditions, etc.) to access these mountainous regions. In a similar way, public transport is not sustainable without a critical mass of demand, an absence of which frequently characterises these mountain territories. Hence, reaching these destinations, by means of other modal choices than the car is more difficult in mountain areas. This implies that in order to access opportunities and to participate in services relevant for social inclusion, the mountaineers must move by car.

Second, reversed mobilities have an economic cost: the direct and indirect costs linked to the increased public expenditure to compensate for the negative externalities of motorised mobility and inactive lifestyles. For example, a previous research study conducted in the French-Italian Alps (Isère and Bergamo) has quantified the increased cost of reversed mobility related to serving ageing in place populations to be up to €1800 per settlement per week in France and €800 in Italy (Cholat 2013).

Third, there is a social cost. This refers to the inequalities in the capacity of older people to make use of this form of adaptation. Reversed mobilities can depend on the economic capital of the person and/or household (*i.e.* the financial resources necessary for paying private services, such as delivery and home services). Then, services provided by reversed mobilities depend on the different capacities of individuals to build, maintain and activate the network of resources and social ties in which individuals rely on to harness reverse mobilities (Fol 2009). As argued by Ohnmacht et al. (2009), this type of support is based on the mobilisation of strong ties within older people's local communities, because it is at this scale that contacts can be easily activated, if necessary. In this sense, it is important to distinguish a grouped vulnerability from a dispersed vulnerability (Hine and Grieco 2003). In the latter case, the dispersed nature of relationship networks may make it more difficult to obtain support (Shergold and Parkhurst 2012). In other words, local support can be what Retière (2003) defines as an *autochthonous capital*, which encompass all the resources that belong to a local network of relations, which can help people, especially the most vulnerable, to access opportunities (Fol 2010).

In this sense, reversed mobilities emerge not only as a means to cope with exclusionary processes, but may serve as a further marker of inequalities in themselves, where older individuals are unable to respond to environmental and individual vulnerabilities through this strategy, compounding the disadvantage experienced by older people.

11.5 Conclusion

Reversed mobility is a form of adaptation for people who have a low capacity for mobility, especially older adults living in contexts where services are lacking, and accessibility to services is more difficult (like some mountain areas). Since they ensure an indirect access to key opportunities, reversed mobilities are a strategy adopted by older people in order to cope with the risks of exclusion from services, and different spheres of life, due to the interaction between environmental (lack of services and accessibility) and individual (low ability to move) vulnerabilities. Thus, they can in some circumstances strongly contribute to older people's inclusion and the habitability of the territories.

Despite the key role played by reversed mobilities, the topic has not been sufficiently considered by research and policy. To fill this gap, this chapter has stressed how reversed mobilities may contribute to combating exclusion that derives from the interaction of different forms of vulnerability (spatial, transport, individual), potentially leading to mutually reinforcing processes of disadvantage. But while reversed mobilities may be an effective way to promote older people's inclusion, this type of response to exclusionary processes may create further inequalities due to the resources needed to activate them. Then, they have an environmental and economic cost that must be taken into account in a context where sustainability has become an imperative.

Our analysis of reversed mobilities allows for the identification of useful directions for future research and policy. First, since reversed mobilities represent a key element for older people's habitability in mountain contexts, the issue at stake for policymakers concerns their optimisation through planning, which can guarantee older people's inclusion and the sustainability of these territories. An important set of considerations therefore includes optimising travel, sharing mobility, the management of logistics, mitigating environmental impacts (*e.g.* vehicle efficiency) and the social inequalities related to the differential ability to make use of this form of adaptation.

Second, research can inform policies by identifying the areas potentially exposed to service exclusion as a result of individual and contextual vulnerabilities intertwining. This is possible by cross-referencing different indicators of accessibility and population (*i.e.* mobility, social, economic capitals). Once these areas are identified, it is then possible to develop further qualitative research to understand at a micro scale the mechanisms at work and the ways to actually support older people in these contexts.

Editors' Postscript

Please note, like other contributions to this book, this chapter was written before the COVID-19 pandemic of 2020. The book's introductory chapter (Chap. 1) and conclusion (Chap. 34) consider some of the key ways in which the pandemic relates to issues concerning social exclusion and ageing.

References

Banister, D., & Bowling, A. (2004). Quality of life for the elderly: The transport dimension. *Transport Policy, 11*(2), 105–115. https://doi.org/10.1016/S0967-070X(03)00052-0.

Belton Chevallier, L., Motte-Baumvol, B., Fol, S., & Jouffe, Y. (2018). Coping with the costs of car dependency: A system of expedients used by low-income households on the outskirts of Dijon and Paris. *Transport Policy, 65*, 79–88. https://doi.org/10.1016/j.tranpol.2017.06.006.

Cholat, F. (2013). *Impact chrono-géographie de la perte d'autonomie liée à l'âgée*, Master Thesis, Grenoble: University of Grenoble.

Cholat, F. (2018). Les «mobilités inversées» comme clé de lecture de la dépendance dans les territoires de montagne. *Pour, 233*(1), 97–101. https://doi.org/10.3917/pour.233.0097.

Cholat, F., Gwiazdzinski, L., & Colleoni, M. (2017). Cartographier l'isolement. Une approche chronotopique de la vie quotidienne des personnes âgées. In G. Drevon, L. Gwiazdzinski, & O. Klein (Eds.), *Chronotopies. Lecture et écriture des mondes en mouvement* (pp. 110–121). Grenoble: Elya Editions.

Church, A., Frost, M., & Sullivan, K. (2000). Transport and social exclusion in London. *Transport Policy, 7*(3), 195–205. https://doi.org/10.1016/S0967-070X(00)00024-X.

Colleoni, M. (2016). La mobilità quotidiana delle popolazioni anziane. *Salute e società, XV*(1), 116–134. https://doi.org/10.3280/SES2016-001009.

Daconto, L., Colleoni, M., & Gwiazdzinski, L. (2017). L'accessibilità spaziale potenziale alle opportunità urbane. Un'analisi comparata tra la città metropolitana di Milano e la metropoli di Lione. *Archivio di studi urbani e regionali, XLVIII*(119), 73–91. https://doi.org/10.3280/ASUR2017-119005.

De Witte, A., Hollevoet, J., Dobruszkes, F., Hubert, M., & Macharis, C. (2013). Linking modal choice to motility: A comprehensive review. *Transportation Research Part A: Policy and Practice, 49*, 329–341. https://doi.org/10.1016/j.tra.2013.01.009.

Dijst, M. J., & Kwan, M. P. (2005). Accessibility and quality of life: Time-geographic perspectives. In K. Donaghy, S. Poppelreuter, & G. Rudinger (Eds.), *Social dimensions of sustainable transport: Transatlantic perspectives* (pp. 109–126). Aldershot: Ashgate.

Dupuy, G. (1999). *La dépendance automobile: Symptômes, analyses, diagnostic, traitements*. Paris: Anthropos.

Farrington, J. H. (2007). The new narrative of accessibility: Its potential contribution to discourses in (transport) geography. *Journal of Transport Geography, 15*(5), 319–330. https://doi.org/10.1016/j.jtrangeo.2006.11.007.
Fol, S. (2009). *La mobilité des pauvres: pratiques d'habitants et politiques publiques*. Paris: Belin.
Fol, S. (2010). Mobilité et ancrage dans le quartiers pauvres: les ressources de la proximité. *Regards Sociologiques, 40*, 27–43.
Geurs, K. T., & van Wee, B. (2004). Accessibility evaluation of land-use and transport strategies: Review and research directions. *Journal of Transport Geography, 12*(2), 127–140. https://doi.org/10.1016/j.jtrangeo.2003.10.005.
Henrard, J.C. (2007). *Les Défis du vieillissement*. Paris: Découverte.
Hine, J., & Grieco, M. (2003). Scatters and clusters in time and space: Implications for delivering integrated and inclusive transport. *Transport Policy, 10*(4), 299–306. https://doi.org/10.1016/S0967-070X(03)00055-6.
Jouffe, Y., Caubel, D., Fol, S., & Motte-Baumvol, B. (2015). Faire face aux inégalités de mobilité. Tactiques, stratégies et projets des ménages pauvres en périphérie parisienne. *Cybergeo: European Journal of Geography*. https://doi.org/10.4000/cybergeo.26697.
Kaiser, H. J. (2009). Mobility in old age: Beyond the transportation perspective. *Journal of Applied Gerontology, 28*(4), 411–418. https://doi.org/10.1177/0733464808329121.
Kaufmann, V., Bergman, M. M., & Joye, D. (2004). Motility: Mobility as capital. *International Journal of Urban and Regional Research, 28*(4), 745–756. https://doi.org/10.1111/j.0309-1317.2004.00549.x.
Kellerman, A. (2012). Potential mobilities. *Mobilities, 7*(1), 171–183. https://doi.org/10.1080/17450101.2012.631817.
Kenyon, S., Lyons, G., & Rafferty, J. (2002). Transport and social exclusion: Investigating the possibility of promoting inclusion through virtual mobility. *Journal of Transport Geography, 10*(3), 207–219. https://doi.org/10.1016/S0966-6923(02)00012-1.
Krizek, K., Horning, J., & El-Geneidy, A. (2012). Perceptions of accessibility to neighbourhood retail and other public services. In K. Geurs, K. Krizek, & A. Reggiani (Eds.), *Accessibility and transport planning: Challenges for Europe and North America* (pp. 96–117). London: Edward Elgar.
Lord, S. (2011). Le choix de vieillir à domicile: l'inévitable adaptation des modes de vie. Évolution de la mobilité quotidienne d'un groupe d'aînés de banlieue pavillonnaire. *Retraite et société, 60*(1), 197–213.
Lord, S., Després, C., & Ramadier, T. (2011). When mobility makes sense: A qualitative and longitudinal study of the daily mobility of the elderly. *Journal of Environmental Psychology, 31*(1), 52–61. https://doi.org/10.1016/j.jenvp.2010.02.007.
Lucas, K. (2012). Transport and social exclusion: Where are we now? *Transport Policy, 20*(0), 105–113. https://doi.org/10.1016/j.tranpol.2012.01.013.
Lucas, K., Mattioli, G., Verlinghieri, E., & Guzman, A. (2016). Transport poverty and its adverse social consequences. *Proceedings of the Institution of Civil Engineers – Transport, 169*(6), 353–365. https://doi.org/10.1680/jtran.15.00073.
Madanipour, A., Cars, G., & Allen, J. (1998). *Social exclusion in European cities: Processes, experiences, and responses*. London-Philadelphia: Jessica Kingsley Publishers.
Martens, K. (2016). *Transport justice: designing fair transportation systems*. New York-Abingdon: Routledge.
Metz, D. H. (2000). Mobility of older people and their quality of life. *Transport Policy, 7*(2), 149–152. https://doi.org/10.1016/S0967-070X(00)00004-4.
Nordbakke, S. (2013). Capabilities for mobility among urban older women: Barriers, strategies and options. *Journal of Transport Geography, 26*, 166–174. https://doi.org/10.1016/j.jtrangeo.2012.10.003.
OECD. (2001). *Ageing and transport*. Paris: Organisation for Economic Cooperation and Development.

Ohnmacht, T., Maksim, H., & Bergman, M. M. (Eds.). (2009). *Mobilities and inequality*. Farnham: Ashgate Publishing.

Retière. (2003). Autour de l'autochtonie. Réflexions sur la notion de capital social populaire. *Politix, 16*(63), 121–143.

Risser, R., Haindl, G., & Ståhl, A. (2010). Barriers to senior citizens' outdoor mobility in Europe. *European Journal of Ageing, 7*(2), 69–80. https://doi.org/10.1007/s10433-010-0146-4.

Sen, A. (1993). Capability and Well-being. In M. C. Nussbaum & A. Sen (Eds.), *The quality of life* (pp. 30–53). Oxford: Oxford University Press.

SEU. (2003). *Making the connections: Final report on transport and social exclusion*. London: Social Exclusion Unit - Office of the Deputy Prime Minister.

Shergold, I., & Parkhurst, G. (2012). Transport-related social exclusion amongst older people in rural Southwest England and Wales. *Journal of Rural Studies, 28*(4), 412–421. https://doi.org/10.1016/j.jrurstud.2012.01.010.

Swedish National Institute of Public. (2007). *Healthy ageing: a challenge for Europe*. Swedish National Institute of Public Health. http://www.healthyageing.eu/sites/www.healthyageing.eu/files/resources/Healthy%20Ageing%20-%20A%20Challenge%20for%20Europe.pdf. Accessed 9 Oct 2019.

Urry, J. (2007). *Mobilities*. Cambridge: Polity Press.

Chapter 12
Exclusion from Home Care Services in Central and Eastern European Countries: A Focus on Hungary and the Russian Federation

Zsuzsa Széman, Elena Golubeva, and László Patyán

12.1 Introduction

One of the challenges of care policies is to provide accessible and effective care that older adults can receive in their home. A report on long-term care (LTC) by the European Commission (2018) underlines that there is a clear trend on the part of the Commission and older people to prioritise home and community care provision. It also underlines that those in need of LTC in Southern (*e.g.* Cyprus, Greece, Malta, Portugal) and Eastern European countries (*e.g.* Bulgaria, Czech Republic, Estonia, Lithuania, Latvia, North Macedonia, Poland, Romania, Croatia, Slovenia, Slovakia), and in the UK, face insufficient availability of home care services. In recent years several countries within Central and Eastern Europe (CEE), among them Hungary, have restricted eligibility through austerity policies, while many others, such as the Russian Federation (Russia), remain focused on institutional care provision. Little evidence of intervention strategies relating to effective home care delivery in these contexts has been found within the international literature (Hirose and Czepulis-Rutkowska 2016). As much of the existing research focuses almost exclusively on Anglo-Saxon contexts and studies written in English, there are significant gaps in knowledge concerning home care provision, the potential of exclusion from this provision and regional variations across CEE countries. It is on this basis that this

Z. Széman (✉)
Institute of Mental Health, Semmelweis University, Budapest, Hungary
e-mail: szeman.zsuzsanna@public.semmelweis-univ.hu

E. Golubeva
Department of Social Work and Social Security Northern (Arctic) Federal University, Arkhangelsk, Russia

L. Patyán
Faculty of Health, Department of Gerontology, University of Debrecen, Nyíregyháza, Hungary

K. Walsh et al. (eds.), *Social Exclusion in Later Life*, International Perspectives on Aging 28, https://doi.org/10.1007/978-3-030-51406-8_12

chapter explores exclusion from home care services in Central and Eastern Europe,[1] focusing in particular on Hungary and Russia. The chapter concentrates on the presentation of research results available only in national languages. There are significant differences in relation to population size, territorial scope, culture and demographic structure. The proportion of those aged 65 and over in Hungary was 17.5% in 2014 (KSH 2014) while this figure was only 13.3% in Russia. By 2019 the figure increased to 19.3% (KSH 2019a) in Hungary while Russia will only reach a similar proportion (19.6%) by 2031 (WHO, 2013). However, they have a common feature in that both countries have a post-socialist background. Furthermore, little has been documented about the evolution of home care policy in the two countries after this shift away from socialism, and little is known about whether or not older people face exclusion from home care services.

The chapter begins with a short review of national studies within CEE countries on areas related to social exclusion and exclusion from health and home care services. It then focuses on the case of Hungary and the ways in which exclusion can arise within its home care system. The case of Russia is then examined, and the experiences of older people accessing home care provisions. Finally, conclusions emerging across these two cases are presented.

12.2 Exclusion from Home Care Services in Central and Eastern Europe

Exclusion from home care services is not always clearly conceptualised. As a result, research on care services in Central and Eastern Europe sometimes draws on general concepts and trends of social exclusion in later life based on secondary analysis of large-scale EU surveys, such as the European Quality of Life Survey (Hrast et al. 2013) and the Survey of Health, Ageing and Retirement in Europe (SHARE) (Srakar et al. 2015). Data from the European Quality of Life Survey has shown significantly higher levels of social exclusion in later life in CEE countries than in the rest of Europe, in relation to access to health care, health status, and material deprivation (Hrast et al. 2013). According to the fifth wave of SHARE, LTC needs are higher in Eastern than in Western and Central European nations, but because family support is generally reported as being strong, exclusion may be reduced (in absolute terms at least) through family help (Laferrère and Bosch 2015). An analysis of the same data does, however, indicate that there is a connection between unmet LTC needs, social exclusion and welfare regimes. In this regard, according to Sraker et al. (2015) Eastern European (*e.g.* Estonia/Baltic country, Czech Republic, Slovenia/

[1] We use the definition of the OECD for CEE countries comprising Albania, Bulgaria, Croatia, the Czech Republic, Hungary, Poland, Romania, Slovakia, Slovenia, and the three Baltic States: Estonia, Latvia and Lithuania.

Central Eastern European countries) welfare regimes lag comparatively behind other nations [also see Sumil-Laanemaa et al., Chap. 3, this volume].

There is also now a range of studies within the national scientific literatures of these countries that testify to the multifaceted exclusions of older people within CEE countries. A national exploratory study in Serbia noted the deterioration of the health and social status of women above 65 years (Petrusic et al. 2015). Konstantinova (2015) pointed out the increasing and unmet medical and social care needs of older people and people with disabilities in Bulgaria. A survey carried out by a charity service in the Ukraine found that the main concern of older people was their own health (Potischo 2015). In Romania, Ghenta and Mladen (2014) highlighted that the needs of Romanian older people for health and social services increased between 2009 and 2012, while key benefits designed to meet their needs had been decreased. To fill the gap, the role of non-governmental organisations was highlighted.

The observed social exclusion of older people in Slovenia included poor health and restricted access to health and social care, amongst other forms of disadvantage and deprivation. The limited availability of public services and spatially isolated locations result in lower access to services (Hrast et al. 2013). The low level of development of formal care settings in these contexts results in more pressure on family carers, while care allowances for caring families are generally low compared to national living standards. Available home care provision is also insufficient in CEE countries (Spasova et al. 2018) and policies barely emphasise the role of family caregivers and their support (Avram 2013; Hirose and Czepulis-Rutkowska 2016).

To further explore the challenges related to exclusion from home care services in Central and Eastern Europe, we will now compare and contrast the situations in Hungary and the Russian Federation.

12.3 Exclusion from Home Care Services in Hungary

In this section, we will first discuss current evidence concerning the general level of exclusion from care services in Hungary. We will then outline research concerning Hungarian care service legislation and the implications of the extant legislation and formal service provision for informal (family) caregivers.

Under the Social Welfare Act of 1993 local governments are obliged to provide social services for older people: home care, a maximum of four hours of daily help and meals on wheels. A per capita norm[2] at that time was assigned to carry out these services. This law established the nationwide system of home care services and opened a future pathway for older people to access formal care provision. Persons over 60 years were entitled to receive home care in the social sector. However, this allowance did not cover the full costs of home care services and this often resulted

[2] The "per capita" norm refers to the institution being financed based on the number of recipients (according to the task).

in unmet need. Certain settlements and regions, especially rural areas, remain unprovided for [also see Vidovićová et al., Chap. 17, this volume]. Despite the increase in the proportion of older people, healthy life years (HLY) lagged behind life expectancy. Even in recent years (2017) this gap persists: at age 65 years life expectancy was 14.4 years for men and 18.4 years for women (OECD 2019), while HLY was 6.9 years for men and 6.7 years for women (Eurostat 2019). Although the figures for HLY have improved slightly (to 6.9 and 7.4 years respectively in 2018) large numbers of both men and women still need some kind of help or care.

At the same time in 1995 one home carer cared for 3.6 old persons while this figure increased to 7.8 in 2012 (KSH 2012). It reached a peak of 9.5 in 2013 than slowly decreased back to 7.8 in 2018 (as the number of qualified carers slightly increased in 2018). Only 7% of people aged 65 years and over have access to home care services (Gyarmati 2019) with demand for home care services considered to be two to three times greater than current supply. This demand is likely to only increase with the ageing of the population, and the ageing of the care workforce and difficulties in recruiting formal carers due to low prestige and salaries. In recent years, research has focused therefore on home care services in Hungary.

Rubovszky (2014), using a quantitative survey, showed a high level of exclusion from basic social services (including home care services) among older Hungarians (Rubovszky 2014). Similarly, a regional study in a remote region in North-Eastern Hungary in 2014 found that isolated people have less information about the availability of care and therefore even if they are entitled to formal provision, they do not have access to such services. This highlights the imperative need to rethink regional and local policy concerning home care provision (Patyán 2014). Results of focus group interviews in the Hungarian capital and in an East Hungarian town clearly showed that the legislation on home care provision introduced in 2015 excluded those with lower levels of care need, even if they do not have family carers who could fill this gap (Széman and Tróbert 2017a, 2017b). Inadequate home care legislation, and the implementation of that legislation results in disadvantages for remote rural regions with small and low-density populations. Regardless of the high proportion of older people living alone in these settlements, increased costs of the delivery of public care services to these regions and a shortage of care professionals at a local level have combined to establish a pattern of public service withdrawal from these areas. This translates into significant spatial inequalities in provision. Geographical and urban-rural differences result in unequal access and older people living in remote areas being more likely to be excluded from care services (see Geurs and Van Eck 2001; and Vidovićová et al., Chap. 17, this volume). A representative survey of general practitioners in 2016 found that the majority of survey respondents identified the need for the introduction of a more formal social care system that would tackle issues around home care and address these sorts of gaps directly (Tróbert and Széman 2018).

Personal contributions by older people to home care service provision is limited and cannot exceed more than 20% of a person's pension.[3] However, recipients usually have low incomes and therefore request services for only a very limited time even when this is far from sufficient (Patyán 2018). This draws attention to the link between low income and service exclusion. In addition, official care regulations governed by state regulations do not always define an appropriate level and quality of home care and as a result provisions are often time-limited. Moreover, regulations do not allow for professionals to develop an individual care plan in specific care situations. This type of care demand can exclude very frail older people from care services or it can result in a lower level of care provision than an older person's needs would require. Formal carers find it difficult to cope with these problems and this often leads them to mix their professional and personal roles and provide care in their free time, *e.g.* at the weekend when they offer additional privately paid home care service (based on private contracts) for those who are able to pay.

Out of the total number of family carers within Hungary, which is estimated at 400,000-500,000 (many of whom are older persons), only 20,000 receive a carer's allowance (Gyarmati 2019), which is around 16% of the average net salary (KSH 2019b). Tróbert (2019) found that close to 50% of family carers between 51 and 60 years old faced a lack of support services and had reported increasing levels of care burden with a negative impact on their physical and mental state of health. Under the present legislation and service system many family carers (mainly older women) themselves face exclusion from social services. A qualitative research study involving 20 expert interviews within home care services recommends a care pattern which considers the capacity of a person's family carers to provide support at the beginning of care, and takes into account transportation, spatial inequalities and urban-rural differences (Patyán 2018). The new care pattern would result in appropriate levels of care provision and would decrease the care burden of family carers. Otherwise family carers would themselves be in need of significant health supports in the future in the absence of suitable financial and service assistance.

Summarising the results of these Hungarian studies: findings highlight the negative consequences of regulation, the unequal accessibility of services and the insufficiency of home care services. Evidence also highlights the consequences of service exclusion, particularly in relation to the growing pressure on family carers.

12.4 Exclusion from Home Care Services in the Russian Federation

Despite the fact that certain aspects of social exclusion of older people are widely considered within the Russian literature, there is no coherent approach to exclusion from home care services. Authors focus on peculiarities of regional exclusion

[3] https://net.jogtar.hu/jogszabaly?docid=99300003.tv

practices (Chernyshkova and Andriyanova 2011; Maksimova et al. 2015; Golubeva and Khabarova 2019), models of exclusion explored in different regions (Maksimova et al. 2018), and strategies for social inclusion of older persons (Grigoryeva and Chernyshova 2009; Grishina 2013). Grigoryeva and Sidorenko (2019) noted that the concept of exclusion from social services vis-a-vis older persons in Russia has to take account of two major factors: the significant size of Russia's territory and the reluctance of Russian people, particularly older Russians, to leave their place of birth.

To give an overview of the relevant literature, we again start by providing a general account of exclusion from home care services in Russia. We then highlight aspects of the Russian care service legislation and discuss the role of informal (family) caregivers. According to Russian law (Federal Law 442), there are three forms of social services: inpatient social services; day care social services; home care services. Emphasis is placed on prevention in service design and implementation, with a focus on the needs of each individual within service delivery. In addition, the number of state programmes aimed at providing social support to citizens has been increased. On the other hand, the progress of society itself led to the emergence in the system of new social care organizations such as socially oriented non-governmental organizations (NGOs), and private providers of social services. Since 2019, under the national project "Demography" there has been a phased introduction of a long-term care system aimed at developing and maintaining the functional abilities of the older population. This includes the incorporation of social and medical care at home, day care and inpatient care, as well as support for family carers.

According to the 2010 census, about 13% of Russian villages are designated as deserted and many others contain no more than ten inhabitants. This is due to outward migration of younger generations and younger people preferring to move to the urban areas in the central part of the country. About 80% of such villages are concentrated not in sparsely populated Siberia, but in the central regions of the country (Shcherbakova 2011). At the same time rural areas are considered to be characterised by a high level of integration of older people, which helps to create informal care networks (neighbours, friends), partially compensating for the insufficiency or absence of formal care services (Golubeva et al. 2017). The process of "ageing in place" (staying in one's own home and own local environment) is desirable for many older people, avoiding displacement and potential isolation in a new community. The situation regarding the accessibility of social care, including home and day care services for older people, in Russia is complicated due to the inaccessibility of key aspects of infrastructure, such as the low level of public transport in remote areas and restrictions in digital and mobile telecommunications access.

Only recently a new regulatory framework document "Evaluation of the effectiveness of state social assistance on the basis of a social contract" was adopted by the Ministry of Labour and Social Protection of the Russian Federation. The implementation of this policy, which allows for the assessment of service access by studying the "active measures of citizens" to overcome a "difficult life situation", can lead to changes or improve the material conditions of the family, including better access to services (Order 2016). Thus, when analysing home care services in the state system of social care in the Russian Federation, problems regarding insufficient monitoring of older people in need of social assistance should be resolved by application of this principle. In addition, most of the measures taken in the framework of the social protection of older people are largely aimed at eliminating factors and impediments of a difficult life situation, which do not allow an older person to perform everyday life activities (Grigoryeva and Sidorenko 2019).

Family care, as a part of informal care, plays a crucial role in home care service provision in Russia, but discussions on care policies are mainly focused on the responsibility of the state to provide support to carers in the family. Expanding family responsibility is becoming a key issue of care policy in Russia (Golubeva and Khabarova 2019). One of the traditional roles of the family in Russian society is to take care of its older members. Supported by cultural norms, religious beliefs, economic imperatives, and enshrined in informal sanctions, family care and care for older people is often one of the main mechanisms for caring for economically and socially weak, as well as physically dependent, family members (NAFI 2016). Almost every third Russian family includes an older individual who requires long-term care (30%), and in most cases they are cared for by relatives. This problem is most acute for residents of small cities, towns and villages (35–40%). The vast majority of Russians look after their older adult relatives on their own (94%). Only 4% of Russians use the social services of the state system. Another 2% of respondents seek the services of private patronage services (home carers) (NAFI 2016).

The Strategy for Action on Citizens of the Older Generation in the Russian Federation until 2025 highlighted a trend associated with the view that "it is necessary to shape public opinion aimed at the active interaction of the family and relatives of senior citizens in relation to care and social services" in the conditions of the atomization of society, which reduced the role of the family and has contributed to increased prevalence of social isolation and loneliness (Order 2016, see p. 21). Such issues can lead to the exclusion of the older generation from public life and directly contribute to a deterioration of well-being and health. In Russian cultural mentality, the practice of placing older parents in residential homes, if there are children or other close relatives, is not very widespread because the micro-community of friends and relatives can condemn children for such action.

The significance of loneliness amongst older people in remote and rural areas of Russia has led the state to produce innovations in home care services. The foster families programme is one of the Russian governments responses to ensure that older people are being offered an efficient form of family-type social support in the context of increasing demands on state capacities and resources. The foster family is understood as a joint residence, comprising the household of a person who needs home (social) care and a person who wishes to provide that care to the older person, who is not a relative. A tripartite agreement is signed by the person performing care (carer), the older person and the local social services office. This programme is particularly prevalent in rural and remote areas of northern Russia that are characterised by heavy depopulation, ageing and difficulties in accessing institutional care services. The programme is based on a focus on the needs of older people living in remote communities and an approach that acknowledges the benefits of "ageing in place" (UNECE, 2017). The innovation is directly connected to the Russian home (social) care services expanding the possibilities of social services and family working together in remote areas. The implementation of innovative care practices, such as foster families – based not only on the capabilities of the state but also on the values and traditions of the older population in relation to family and health – can contribute to and ensure greater accessibility of various types of services that lead to the reduction of most social risks in old-age.

12.5 Conclusion

This chapter highlights that in Hungary and Russia research rarely directly considers exclusion of older people from home care services, but more typically examines the challenges of the system in health and social care systems in general, *e.g.* issues of demand, system limitations, and legislation. The case of Hungary clearly shows that macro-level policy (the new legislation of 2015) has not diminished exclusion and has even in some cases resulted in an intensification of the exclusion of older people from home care services. In Russian Federation on the other hand a macro-level policy decision (Order 2016) may have commenced the start of a positive trend to improve home care services in the long run.

In both countries, it is a major task for families and informal helpers to substitute formal home care provision and mitigate exclusion of older people from home care services. Russian Federation implemented a macro-level response, the foster family initiative. This pilot programme may help reduce the most serious shortage of care services in particular regions. This model emphasises the importance of actions at the local level and the need for a reflective and flexible local care policy. On the other hand, in Hungary there is no such type of macro-level policy although formal carers of home care services proposed a new care model: the involvement of the family as a necessary, integrated part of home care service. In Hungary a similar idea to the Russian home care system is taking shape, that is, to combine informal and formal care in a unified home care system, but it is yet to be seen how this will evolve and to what degree it will be implemented.

It is of vital importance to mitigate social exclusion of older people from home care services. The analysis here indicates the value of state led solutions by applying suitable legislation, which can be further elaborated at the mezzo (local government, care centres) and micro levels (family carers, informal helpers). An innovative approach could ease social exclusion from home care services of older people. This requires a focus on reforms to home care services and should also consider individual needs of ageing, or already old family carers.

Editors' Postscript

Please note, like other contributions to this book, this chapter was written before the COVID-19 pandemic of 2020. The book's introductory chapter (Chap. 1) and conclusion (Chap. 32) consider some of the key ways in which the pandemic relates to issues concerning social exclusion and ageing.

References

Avram, S. (2013). *Social assistance in central and Eastern Europe: Features and characteristics*. Institute for Social and Economic Research, University of Essex https://www.iser.essex.ac.uk/research/publications/working-papers/iser/2013-19.pdf. Accessed 5 Dec 2019.

Chernyshkova, Y. V., & Andriyanova, Y. A. (2011). Potrebleniye meditsinskikh uslug pozhilym lyudyam v usloviyakh sotsial'nogo neravenstva [Consumption of medical services by elderly people in the context of social inequality (in the example of the Saratov region)]. *Saratovskiy nauchno-meditsinskiy zhurnal, 7*(1), 138–141.

European Commission. (2018). *Challenges in long-term care in Europe - A study of national policies 2018*. https://ec.europa.eu/social/main.jsp?catId=738&langId=en&pubId=8128&furtherPubs=yes. Accessed 9 Dec 2019.

EUROSTAT. (2019). *Healthy life years and life expectancy at age 65 by sex*. https://ec.europa.eu/eurostat/tgm/refreshTableAction.do?tab=table&plugin=1&pcode=tepsr_sp320&language=en. Accessed 5 Dec 2019.

Geurs, K. T., & van Eck, R. J. R. (2001). *Accessibility measures: Review and applications. Evaluation of accessibility impacts of land-use transport scenarios, and related social and economic impacts*. Biltoven: National Institution of Public and Health Environment.

Ghenta, M., & Mladen, L. (2014). *The partnership between public authorities and NGOs: An effective way of covering the need for social services in Romania*. ICESBA http://icesba.eu/RePEc/icb/wpaper/ICESBA2014_19GHENTA_P152-159.pdf. Accessed 4 Sep 2019.

Golubeva, E. Y., & Khabarova, L. G. (2019). Family care as a tool for mitigating the social risks of the elderly people in remote areas. *Advances in Gerontology, 9*(3), 373–378. https://doi.org/10.1134/S2079057019030056.

Golubeva, E. Y., Khabarova, L. G., & Soloviev, A. (2017). Priyemnaya semya kak novaya tekhnologiya sotsialnogo ukhoda v politike activnogo stareniya v otdalennyh severnyh territoriyah [Foster family as a new technology of social care in the policy of active ageing in remote northern areas]. *Ekologiya cheloveka, 11*, 42–46.

Grigoryeva, I. A., & Chernyshova, S. P. (2009). Novyye podkhody k profilaktike sotsial'nogo isklyucheniya pozhilykh [New approaches to prevention of the social exclusion of the elderly]. *Zhurnal sotsiologii i sotsial'noy antropologii XII*, (2), 186–196.

Grigoryeva, I. A., & Sidorenko, A. V. (2019). Eldercare in transition(s): The special case of Russia. *International Journal of Care and Caring, 3*(1), 59–73 (15). https://doi.org/10.1332/239788218X15411704353873.

Grishina, T. V. (2013). Kognitivnyye potentsial'nyye strategii issledovaniye sotsial'nogo vklyucheniya (illyustratsiya starshego vozrasta) [Cognitive potential strategies for the study of social inclusion (in the example of older age)]. *Nauchnyy potentsial, 3*(12), 84–88.

Gyarmati, A. (2019). Idősödés, idősellátás Magyarországon [Ageing and care for the elderly in Hungary], Budapest: Friedrich Ebert Stiftung, 7–10. http://library.fes.de/pdf-files/bueros/budapest/15410.pdf. Accessed 06 Dec 2019.

Hirose, K. & Czepulis-Rutkowska, Z. (2016). *Challenges in long-term care of the elderly in Central and Eastern Europe*. Budapest: ILO DWT and Country Office for Central and Eastern Europe. https://www.ilo.org/wcmsp5/groups/public/%2D%2D-europe/%2D%2D-ro-geneva/%2D%2D-sro-budapest/documents/publication/wcms_532427.pdf. Accessed 2 Oct 2019.

Hrast, F. M., Kopac, M. A., & Rakar, R. (2013). Social exclusion of elderly in Central and Eastern Europe. *International Journal of Social Economics, 40*(11), 971–989. https://doi.org/10.1108/IJSE-05-2012-0082.

Konstantinova, D. (2015). Mediko-sotsialni grizhi za vŭzrastni khora i khora s neudobstva chrez vizualizatsiya na meditsinski i sotsialni [Medico-social care for the elderly and people with disabilities as seen by medical and social care specialists]. *Naucsni Trudove na University Russenskija*, 8(3), 40–44. http://conf.uni-ruse.bg/bg/docs/cp15/8.3/8.3-6.pdf. Accessed 2 Oct 2019.

KSH, Központi Statisztikai Hivatal. (2012). Szociális Statisztikai Évkönyv (Social Statistical Yearbook). Budapest: Központi Statistikai Hivatal.

KSH, Központi Statisztikai Hivatal. (2014). Szépkorúak és vének. Október elseje az idősek világnapja. (Olds and Oldest olds. First of October is a day for Older Adults) *Statisztikai Tükör* (Social Statistical Mirror). 2014, (103). https://www.ksh.hu/docs/hun/xftp/stattukor/idosek_vilagnapja_14.pdf. Accessed 15 Jan 2020.

KSH, Központi Statisztikai Hivatal. (2019a). Magyarország népességének száma és életkor szerinti megoszlása 2019. január 1. [Population of Hungary and distribution by age on 1 January 2019]. https://www.ksh.hu/interaktiv/korfak/orszag.html. Accessed 9 Dec 2019.

KSH, Központi Statisztikai Hivatal. (2019b). Gyorstájékoztató. Keresetek 2019 január-szeptember [Flash Report. Earnings, January to September 2019]. https://www.ksh.hu/docs/hun/xftp/gyor/ker/ker1909.html. Accessed 6 Dec 2019.

Lafferrère, A., & Bosch, K. (2015). *Unmet need for long-term care and social exclusion*. https://pdfs.semanticscholar.org/581b/e670fbd5e4859fd8908d6a8c71c075f2fb64.pdf?_ga=2.245380228.107296117.1570280916-1104196352.1570280916. Accessed 4 Oct 2019.

Maksimova, S. G., Noyanzina, O. Y., Maksimova, M. M., & Shcheglova, D. K. (2015). Otsial'naya eksklyuziya lits starshikh vozrastnykh grupp: sotsial'no-ekonomicheskiye aspekty [Social exclusion of older age groups: Socio-economic aspects]. *Vestnik Altayskogo gosudarstvennogo agrarnogo universiteta, 5*(127), 180–184.

Maksimova, S. G., Noyanzina, O. E., & Omelchenko, D. A. (2018). A model of social exclusion of elderly people in Siberian regions. *Advances in Gerontology, 8*(1), 58–63. https://doi.org/10.1134/S2079057018010083.

OECD. (2019). *Data*. Life expectancy at 65. https://data.oecd.org/healthstat/life-expectancy-at-65.htm. Accessed 21 Feb 2020.

Order. (2016). Strategiya deistvii v interesah grazhdan starshego pokoleniya v Rossiiskoi Federatsii do 2025 [Strategy of action in the interests of the older generation in the Russian Federation until 2025]. *Order of the Government of the Russian Federation, 05*. 02.2016. - № 164-r. http://base.garant.ru/71322816. Accessed 20 Sep 2018.

Patyán, L. (2014). Időskorúak közszolgáltatáshoz való hozzáférésének és szolgáltatáshasználatának jellemzői az észak – alföldi régióban [The characteristics of elderly people's use of and access to public services in the North-East region]. *Esély, 1*, 62–78.

Patyán, L. (2018). Professzionális és családi gondozók viszonyrendszere az idősek otthoni gondozásában [The system of relationships between the professional and family caregivers in home care of the elderly]. Budapest: Eötvös Lóránd Tudományegyetem Társadalomtudományi Kar Szociológia Doktori Iskola. PhD dissertation. https://edit.elte.hu/xmlui/bitstream/handle/10831/41597/Disszert%E1ci%F3.pdf;jsessionid=1BB247616DA0F4DC2EBF255B5B16D0B3?sequence=1. Accessed 4 Oct 2019.

Petrusic, N., Todorovic, N., Vracevic, M., & Jankovic, B. (2015). Financial abuse of older women in Serbia. *Journal of Elder Abuse and Neglect, 27*(4–5), 410–421. https://doi.org/10.1080/08946566.2015.1094300. Accessed 1 Oct 2019.

Potischo, G. (2015). *Age, peerson and society*. http://www.tlu.org.ua/?p=2783. Accessed 26 Sep 2019.

Ruboszky, J. C. (2014). Házi segítségnyújtás talán egy kicsit másképp. [Home care – maybe a little bit differently]. *Esély, 1*, 4–30.

Shcherbakova, E. (2011). *The number of rural settlements and urban-type settlements continues to decline* (in Russian). Demoscope Weekly, 475–6. http://www.demoscope.ru/weekly/2011/0475/lisa01.php. Accessed 4 Oct 2019.

Spasova, S., Baeten, R., Coster, S., Ghailani, D., Casas-Pena, R., Vanhercke, B. (2018). *Challenges in long-term care in Europe. A study of national policies*. Brussels: https://ec.europa.eu/social/BlobServlet?docId=20225&langId=en. Accessed 4 Oct 2019.

Srakar, A., Filipovič Hrast, M., Hlebec, V., & Majcen, B. (2015). Social exclusion, welfare regime and unmet long-term care need: Evidence from SHARE. In A. Borsch-Supan, T. Kneip,

H. Litwin, M. Myck, & G. Weber (Eds.), *Ageing in Europe – Supporting policies for an ageing society* (pp. 189–198). Berlin: De Gruyter.

Széman, Zs, & Tróbert, A. M. (2017a). A szociális innováció lehetőségei az idősgondozásban. [Possibilities of Social Innovation in long-term care]. *Esély, 28*(6), 45–62.

Széman, Zs., & Tróbert, A. M. (2017b). Social innovation in the provision of Services in Long-term Care. *European Journal of Mental Health, 12*, 204–207.

Tróbert, A. M. (2019). Idős hozzátartozót gondozók leterheltsége [The burden of the caregivers taking care of elderly relatives]. PhD, Budapest: Semmelweis University http://semmelweis.hu/wp-content/phd/phd_live/vedes/export/trobertanettmaria.d.pdf. Accessed 4 Oct 2019.

Tróbert, A. M., & Széman, Zs. (2018). Háziorvosok és idősellátás egy kérdőíves kutatás tükrében [General practitioners and eldercare as reflected in a survey by questionnaire]. *Orvosi Hetilap, 159*(8), 312–319.

UNECE. (2017). *Policy brief on ageing*. Older persons in rural and remote areas, No.18. https://www.unece.org/population/ageing/policybriefs.html. Accessed 27 Sep 2019.

WHO. (2013). *Russian federation national report*. Study of global ageing and adult health (SAGE) Study 1. https://www.who.int/healthinfo/sage/en/. Accessed 10 Jan 2020.

Chapter 13
Receiving Care Through Digital Health Technologies: Drivers and Implications of Old-Age Digital Health Exclusion

Arianna Poli, Ioannis Kostakis, and Francesco Barbabella

13.1 Introduction

We are living in a world undergoing comprehensive digitalisation. Services, behaviours and lifestyles are deeply influenced by the availability and exploitation of digital technologies in most of the spheres of life, such as interpersonal communication, commerce, and public services (OECD 2016, 2017). The continual development and refinement of sophisticated, connected and ubiquitous digital technologies have opened the door for a revolution of how most services are conceived, designed and delivered to populations, including older people (Schnoll 2014; Olsson et al. 2017).

Digital technologies are conceived within this chapter as those devices, such as smartphones, tablets, wearable devices, sensors and computers, which allow users to perform different kinds of activities mainly by connecting to the Internet (Lupton 2014). 'Digital health technologies' is a broader concept which refers to the application of digital technologies to the health systems, for example, to the following services: electronic health records (EHRs) and personalised health records (PHRs); ePrescriptions; remote consultation, monitoring and care services (*e.g.* telehealth, telemedicine); mobile health (mHealth) solutions for self-management of health, chronic conditions and physical activity (*e.g.* mobile apps, smartwatches,

A. Poli
Division Ageing and Social Change (ASC), Department of Culture and Society (IKOS), Linköping University, Norrköping, Sweden

I. Kostakis
Department of Home Economics and Ecology, Harokopio University, Athens, Greece

F. Barbabella (✉)
Centre for Socio-Economic Research on Ageing, National Institute of Health and Science on Ageing (IRCCS INRCA), Ancona, Italy

Centre for Ageing and Life-Course Studies, Linnaeus University, Växjö, Sweden
e-mail: f.barbabella@inrca.it

K. Walsh et al. (eds.), *Social Exclusion in Later Life*, International Perspectives on Aging 28, https://doi.org/10.1007/978-3-030-51406-8_13

smart-wristbands); and health data analytics for clinical decision support systems (DSSs) (Bennett and Glasgow 2009; Barbabella et al. 2017; Sixsmith et al. 2017; World Health Organization 2017). In this chapter we focus on direct end-user technologies, based on the classification suggested by Weiss and colleagues (Weiss et al. 2018), targeting digital health. Direct end-user technologies are expected to be used by everyone, and thus by older people, for purposes of diagnosis, treatment, (self-) care, and communication with health and care professionals.

Health services are increasingly digitally-based in many European countries (Kummervold et al. 2008; European Commission 2018; Heart and Kalderon 2013), with direct effects on the behaviours of all patients and users. National and European policies promote and sustain such a trend, as the incorporation of digital health technologies is seen as a good strategy for improving the accessibility, quality and efficiency of current health systems which are challenged by an increased demand for care from an increasingly diverse and ageing population (Helbig et al. 2009; World Health Organization 2017; European Commission 2018).

It should be noted that digital health services are often, but not necessarily, linked to traditional health care providers. Usually these services are based on a health care infrastructure which consists of physical facilities and equipment, health professionals, patient information and further resources, which provide these digital health services with appropriate information, content and professional relationships with patients. For instance, telehealth services require (passive or active) remote monitoring by health professionals of an individual's condition and activity, and enable an interaction between the two (via connected devices or other equipment). Another possibility is that the digital health service is provided via a (quasi-) autonomous solution, *i.e.* an application or device that is used only by the patient without direct monitoring or correspondence with other health care staff. For instance, mHealth applications usually enable self-care for end users by providing notifications, reminders and advice on health status, lifestyle (*e.g.* diet, sleep) and physical exercise, on the basis of data reported manually or recorded automatically by the system. In this case, the digital health solution may or may be not connected to a specific health care facility within the framework of traditional health services.

Older people are one of the main user groups of health services (Robinson et al. 2015; Terraneo 2015), but also less likely to be engaged with these technologies (Peacock and Künemund 2007; Heart and Kalderon 2013; OECD 2017; König et al. 2018). Digital health technologies can improve the care of older people and its organisation, but also set some challenges with regards to old-age exclusion (Heart and Kalderon 2013; Czaja 2017; Olsson et al. 2017). The digital unpreparedness which characterises the circumstances of some older people can expose them to a higher risk of exclusion from the health services domain (Peacock and Künemund 2007). Hence, it is crucial to improve what is a limited understanding of the mechanisms of old-age digital health exclusion.

Despite the relevance and urgency of this topic, research in the field has not yet produced a coherent and systematic discussion of old-age digital health exclusion (Van Regenmortel et al. 2016; Van Regenmortel et al. 2018). The aim of this chapter is to conceptualise and discuss this phenomenon, contributing to a systematisation of the discourse in this area. The key research question addressed by this work is: what are the mechanisms, causes and implications of old-age digital health exclusion?

For this purpose, we adopt a definition of social exclusion in old-age as operationalised by Walsh et al. (2017), who adapted the classical definition by Levitas et al. (2007). Old-age digital health exclusion is considered indeed as a mechanism initiated by a lack or denial of health rights, resources, goods and services, which impacts health and social well-being of older people, as well as societal equity and cohesion [see Walsh et al. this volume for a more extensive discussion].

The chapter is structured in three main parts. First, the main causes of old-age digital health exclusion are defined and discussed according to structural, environmental, individual and socio-technical drivers. Second, the major implications for exclusion of older people are analysed in the context of a digital society. Third, we develop and describe a conceptual framework illustrating the process of old-age digital health exclusion. Finally, key issues, risks and challenges are addressed in relation to the current state and projected future progress on digital technologies.

13.2 Drivers of Old-Age Digital Health Exclusion

Research offers evidence that old-age exclusion in the field of digital health is based on complex social mechanisms, which mainly rely on four types of drivers and their combinations: (1) structural drivers, which include social norms, values and discourses, as influenced by policies and market evolution; (2) environmental drivers, such as the physical contexts where communities and older people live; (3) individual drivers, concerning personal, social and economic characteristics of older people (Helsper and Reaisdorf 2016; Olsson et al. 2017), as well as their awareness of, interest in and willingness to use digital technologies (Siren and Knudsen 2017); and (4) socio-technical drivers, which include the design, development and evaluation of digital health technologies, which may intrinsically facilitate or limit digital use (Fisk et al. 2009).

The first three types of drivers are factors which are well-known in old-age exclusion research (Scharf and Keating 2012), whereas the fourth – the socio-technical drivers – is a necessary complement to include and consider the actual object of technology and the interaction between it and older individuals.

13.2.1 Structural Drivers

By reallocating resources, directing investments and conveying social norms and values, policy and the market – and their interaction – influence inclusion-exclusion dynamics and individuals' life chances. In the context of promoting digital health, structural factors can redefine the ways in which older individuals have or do not have access to health and care and, thus, determine the prerequisites for benefitting from such services. Old-age exclusion from health services can result from a mismatch between prerequisites that are structurally defined and the resources on which an individual can count.

Digitalisation in the health sector has been largely promoted by European and national policies as a way to enhance health systems and make them more sustainable (European Commission 2018). Although the use of digital health services holds potential (Czaja 2017; Lindeman 2017), such policies introduce a deterministic view about the impact of a digital shift in the health sector – which relates to the concept of 'techtopia' (Turner 2010). As described by Peine (2019), policy discourse has mostly stressed the need to establish a 'technification of later life', which is meant to solve most issues of ageing societies. Within this perspective, digital health is promoted as an opportunity for users to be more in control of their own health, to receive more personalised care and to benefit from more accessible and efficient health systems (Lupton 2013; European Commission 2018).

However, such positive policy discourse seldom considers existing challenges for digital-based service provision for older people. Political action is lacking with regards to systematic investment in digitally-driven health systems, training of care professionals on how to deal with this digital shift, and improving technological infrastructure (Bennett and Glasgow 2009; Barbabella et al. 2017; Sixsmith et al. 2017; World Health Organization 2017). Moreover, limited attention is given to the digital inequalities which largely exist among older people. This reduces the efforts to ensure that the new services based on digital health technologies are inclusive, and that alternative services are provided where appropriate.

Positive discourse about ageing and new technologies are also market driven. The digital health solutions market has identified older people as a large consumer group to be targeted and as an opportunity for investment (Mostaghel 2016). Overall, the global digital health market is expected to grow from 140 to 380 billion USD in the period 2018–2024 (Capgemini 2018). Important technological advancements with the potential for improving health service provision are introduced, but it is crucial that market dynamics are not prioritised over individuals' needs and interests.

13.2.2 Environmental Drivers

The physical environment, be it the immediate home or wider community environment, is a key element in facilitating or preventing inclusion of older people (Mahmood and Keating 2012; see also section V, this volume). The appropriateness of places, transportation and services can support individuals' empowerment and participation. Two environmental drivers, linked to structural elements, are central to hindering the use of digital health technologies.

First, poor technological infrastructures generally constitute a major barrier to the access and use of digital services (König et al. 2018). Connectivity issues, which often characterise rural areas, are an example of a common limitation in infrastructure which limit the internet access in private and public spaces and reduce opportunities to access digital health services through digital health technologies (Berner et al. 2014; Salemink et al. 2017). In those areas where the poor connectivity combines with the lower socio-economic status of rural dwelling older individuals, the lower use of digital services is even more pronounced (Berner et al. 2014).

Second, the compatibility of digital health technologies with existing health care facilities is another key factor influencing social exclusion (Ross et al. 2016). Many local health systems and care organisations in Europe are progressively investing in and implementing solutions based on digital technologies, for example telehealth. Yet, these developments amidst great challenges and barriers that are often related to interoperability issues, lack of digital skills of or resistance by health professionals, unclear regulatory frameworks, and scarce financial resources (Bennett and Glasgow 2009; World Health Organization 2016; Barbabella et al. 2017; Sixsmith et al. 2017; World Health Organization 2017; Melchiorre et al. 2018a).

13.2.3 Individual Drivers

Individual drivers consist of those individual characteristics which make an older person more vulnerable to exclusion from digital health technologies. Several studies have investigated what predicts the use, non-use and low-use of digital technologies. Older people with lower levels of education and lower income are less likely to be digitally engaged, and more likely to have lower digital skills and perform a more limited range of activities when using digital technologies (Hunsaker and Hargittai 2018). Older people living alone are less likely to be digital users, presumably because of the lack, or absence, of help from family members or a partner in using new technologies (Friemel 2016). However, other studies found that living with children does not necessarily improve older people's digital engagement and digital skills, but rather it mostly increases the availability of digital technologies at home (Eynon and Helsper 2015).

Health status was found to be a relevant predictor, and both physical and cognitive impairments reduce the use of digital technologies among older people (Hunsaker and Hargittai 2018; Czaja et al. 2019). Overall, older people who are non-users are more likely to show a lack of motivation and interest in using digital technologies (Friemel 2016) and tend to report a lower perceived usefulness of new technologies, higher anxiety and lower self-efficacy regarding the use of digital technologies compared to their counterparts who are digitally-engaged (Czaja et al. 2006). Finally, the non-use of digital technologies, including digital health technologies can be also determined by individual preferences and choice (Wyatt 2003).

13.2.4 Socio-Technical Factors

The progressive introduction and rapid evolution of digital health technologies bring an additional level of complexity to the dynamics of old-age digital health exclusion. This relates to the characteristics of the technology itself and interactions (enabled or possible) with end-users. It also refers to the socio-material constitution of old-age (Peine et al. 2015; Peine 2019), as old-age is becoming increasingly permeated by digital objects and because major changes are occurring in older people's perceptions and experiences of technology in daily life.

In concrete terms, digital health technologies should facilitate interaction between technological objects and older users. Two main factors may contribute to exclusion of older people in this respect, leading to biased research and development (R&D) activity, selective implementation of digital health services, and limited opportunities for older people or groups with certain characteristics to use new technologies.

First, the paternalist design of technology can limit the choice and liberty of older people to decide how to use the digital health solution. Science and technology studies (STS) have been researching how technological objects are conceived, shaped and produced by designers and developers. In this sense, they try to imagine future users and inscribe a limited set of features and usage patterns within the socio-technical object (Akrich 1995). This means that, by default, any digital technology already offers a pre-fixed 'script' to end-users, which can be followed (ideally) or broken (non-desirable). In the case of older users, a design paternalism is usually imposed by technologies themselves (Peine 2019), as they embed certain ideas, visions and social roles of older individuals within technology. In this sense, older people would not be free to explore other uses, nor to learn by doing, failing and retrying.

Second, digitised service interfaces are often designed with a 'healthy' and 'active' person (user) in mind. There is growing concern that some groups of older people (typically the most disadvantaged) are systematically excluded from studies conducted within the field of digital health solutions. The oldest old, those with lower educational attainment, those with low digital skills and those with low familiarity with new technologies are more likely to be underrepresented in this kind of research, and hence their needs, attitudes and preferences are less often acknowledged and addressed in the design, development and evaluation process (Fisk et al. 2009; Poli et al. 2019).

13.3 Implications – Why Old-Age Digital Health Exclusion Matters

Old-age digital health exclusion has several significant implications at an individual, organisational and societal level. At an individual level, it leads to an increased risk of exclusion from access to health services which, in turn, can result in poorer individual health outcomes (Terraneo 2015). Indeed, if access to health services primarily depends on the use of digital health technologies, the health and care needs of older people who are non-users or low-users, either by choice or as a result of structural, environmental and individual circumstances, will not be fully addressed (Olsson et al. 2017) and can lead to the worsening of some older people's health. In addition, the feeling of not being able to benefit from available services provided by digital means can generate a sense of social exclusion, especially among those who perceive those services as useful (Seifert et al. 2018). On the other hand, the lack of availability of services based on digital health technologies in deprived areas (rural, mountain or remote areas) forces older adults to exploit directly administered health care resources, if available, which in turn can mean enduring significant travelling time and stress arising from difficulties in access [see Cholat and Daconto, this section].

Given that older people are one of the main user groups of health services (Tavares and Zantomio 2017) and are more likely to face challenges in accessing and using digital technologies, the growing allocation of resources into digital health provision might be less efficient than expected (Helbig et al. 2009). Previous studies found that e-government initiatives failed due to, among others, the limited adoption of the services and the return to the traditional services by many citizens (Janssen et al. 2013; Anthopoulos et al. 2016).

Moreover, if those older people who are less likely to use digital health technologies are also those who are most in need of care, the digital shift in health service provision can contribute to widening old-age inequalities (Robinson et al. 2015). Older people who have access and those who do not become increasingly dissimilar (Robinson et al. 2015). The former get more opportunities to address their health and care needs and possibly achieve better health outcomes; the latter are either prevented from accessing health services, if new services based on digital health technologies have replaced traditional variations, or have to choose among a more limited range of service options. Hence, some older people may benefit greatly from the incorporation of digital health technologies, but some others are at risk of being disadvantaged (Heart and Kalderon 2013).

13.4 Conclusion: Towards a Conceptual Framework on Old-Age Digital Exclusion

Health care provision in Europe is increasingly characterised by digital health. The use of digital health technologies has been promoted at European and national levels as a strategy for tackling the challenges facing health care systems (European Commission 2018) by a population which is ageing and increasingly more heterogeneous (Phillipson 2013). Digital health technologies are described as a way to make health care provision more efficient and sustainable, while guaranteeing good quality, equity and inclusiveness of services (European Commission 2018). Older people are expected to use such new digital-based services in order to address health and care needs (Helbig et al. 2009).

In general terms, the transition from traditional to digitised services can lead to new forms of digital health exclusion for older individuals (Helsper and Reaisdorf 2016; Olsson et al. 2017). The analysis of these mechanisms in relation to digital health should be framed within the more general concept of old-age social exclusion, as defined by Walsh et al. (2017) – see also Walsh et al. this volume.

By adopting this view, old-age digital health exclusion can be defined as a process in which older people are prevented, or limit themselves, from using digital health technologies and from benefitting fully from their use, due to a lack, or denial, of health rights, resources, goods and services.

On the basis of these dynamics, we present a conceptual framework which describes the process of old-age digital health exclusion in Fig. 13.1. We identify four types of drivers of old-age digital health exclusion, namely structural, environmental, individual and socio-technical, which combine and intersect with each other to

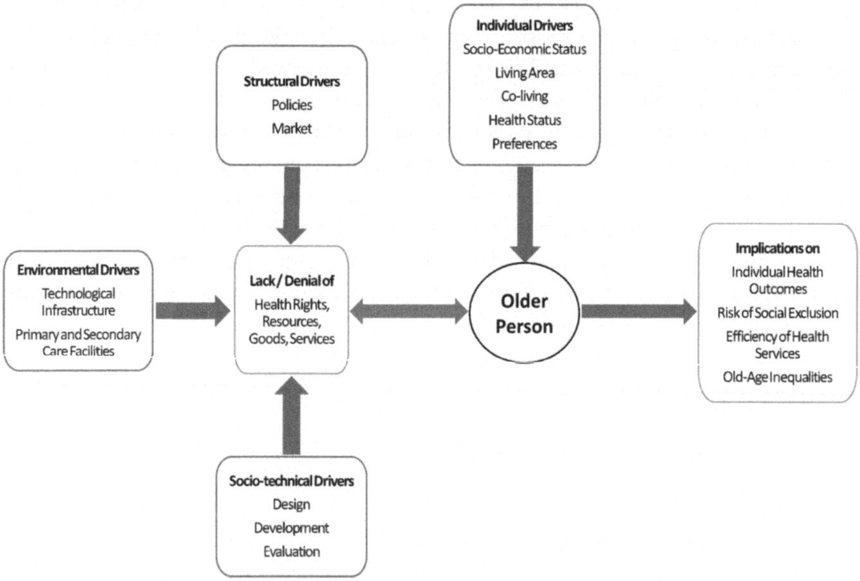

Fig. 13.1 A conceptual framework of old-age digital health exclusion

increase the vulnerability of older people to exclusion from health services. Structural, environmental and socio-technical drivers impact directly on digital health exclusion and are primarily only modifiable by organisational and high-level actors (*e.g.* policy makers, market players). Individual drivers influence the older person's preferences, capacities and behaviours towards digital health technologies, in accordance with their own will and social expectations. As a result of these multilevel and multifaceted drivers, implications of exclusion can be identified at individual, organisational and societal levels. Furthermore, older people's willingness to engage with digital technologies cannot be taken for granted. Non-use of digital technologies and, thus, of digital health services, can reflect individual decisions (Wyatt 2003).

The use of digital technologies and digital-based services should be promoted, explained and sustained by relevant institutional actors (Siren and Knudsen 2017). However, it is worth questioning how far digital health can be pursued and whether or not digital health can be the only option available for older people. The increased vulnerability of older people in relation to digital health must be addressed with research and policies aimed at disenabling drivers of social exclusion and making services based on digital technologies more inclusive. Research on digital health needs to have a stronger focus on the inclusiveness of digital health technologies. Older people should be involved in the studies which conduct design and evaluations of digital health technologies that are relevant to them (Östlund 2015). It is especially relevant that participation of older people in evaluations of digital technologies is not selective, and that study participants reflect the full heterogeneity of the target populations (Merkel and Kucharski 2018; Poli et al. 2019; Allemann and Poli 2020; Poli et al. 2020). Policies, in turn, should go beyond the mere promotion of digital health by actively shaping and impacting on key barriers and factors preventing full opportunities for older users (Melchiorre et al. 2018b). By doing so, the potential of digital health can be better exploited, and can actually contribute to enhancing current health care provision, for example, by reaching older people in underserved areas or by improving the care provided to people with complex conditions (Barbabella et al. 2017).

Digital health technologies can have exclusionary and inequality effects on older people (Poli et al. 2019; Poli et al. 2020). Such effects must represent a major concern for research, policy and practice, as digital health technologies are increasingly utilized in health systems and evolve rapidly. It is crucial to identify and address the mechanisms generating these exclusions and inequalities in order to turn digital health technologies into an available, relevant and impactful opportunity for most older adults, thus achieving inclusive digital ageing societies.

Editors' Postscript

Please note, like other contributions to this book, this chapter was written before the COVID-19 pandemic of 2020. The book's introductory chapter (Chap. 1) and conclusion (Chap. 34) consider some of the key ways in which the pandemic relates to issues concerning social exclusion and ageing.

References

Akrich, M. (1995) *User representations: Practices, methods and sociology*. Pinter.

Allemann, H., & Poli, A. (2020). *Designing and evaluating information and communication technology-based interventions? Be aware of the needs of older people*. London: SAGE Publications Sage UK.

Anthopoulos, L., Reddick, C. G., Giannakidou, I., & Mavridis, N. (2016). Why e-government projects fail? An analysis of the Healthcare.gov website. *Government Information Quarterly, 33*(1), 161–173. https://doi.org/10.1016/j.giq.2015.07.003.

Barbabella, F., Melchiorre, M. G., Quattrini, S., Papa, R., & Lamura, G. (2017). *How can eHealth improve care for people with multimorbidity in Europe*. Copenhagen: European Observatory on Health Systems and Policies. https://pubmed.ncbi.nlm.nih.gov/29144695/

Bennett, G. G., & Glasgow, R. E. (2009). The delivery of public health interventions via the internet: Actualizing their potential. *Annual Review of Public Health, 30*(1), 273–292. https://doi.org/10.1146/annurev.publhealth.031308.100235.

Berner, J., Rennemark, M., Jogréus, C., Anderberg, P., Sköldunger, A., Wahlberg, M., et al. (2014). Factors influencing internet usage in older adults (65 years and above) living in rural and urban Sweden. *Health Informatics Journal, 21*(3), 237–249. https://doi.org/10.1177/1460458214521226.

Capgemini (2018) *Digital health: Transforming healthcare*. https://www.capgemini.com/be-en/wp-content/uploads/sites/17/2018/10/Digital-health-final-paper-22.10.pdf. Accessed 13 Oct 2019.

Czaja, S. J. (2017). The potential role of technology in supporting older adults. *Public Policy & Aging Report, 27*(2), 44–48. https://doi.org/10.1093/ppar/prx006.

Czaja, S. J., Charness, N., Fisk, A. D., Hertzog, C., Nair, S. N., Rogers, W. A., et al. (2006). Factors predicting the use of technology: Findings from the center for research and education on aging and technology enhancement (create). *Psychology and Aging, 21*(2), 333–352. https://doi.org/10.1037/0882-7974.21.2.333.

Czaja, S. J., Boot, W. R., Charness, N., & Rogers, W. A. (2019). *Designing for older adults: Principles and creative human factors approaches*. Boca Raton: CRC press.

European Commission (2018) *Communication from the commission to the European parliament, the council, the European economic and social committee and the committee of the regions on enabling the digital transformation of health and care in the Digital Single Market; empowering citizens and building a healthier society*. Brussels: European Commission. https://ec.europa.eu/newsroom/dae/document.cfm?doc_id=51628.

Eynon, R., & Helsper, E. (2015). Family dynamics and internet use in Britain: What role do children play in adults' engagement with the internet? *Information, Communication & Society, 18*(2), 156–171. https://doi.org/10.1080/1369118X.2014.942344.

Fisk, A. D., Rogers, W. A., Charness, N., Czaja, S. J., & Sharit, J. (2009). *Designing for older adults: Principles and creative human factors approaches*. Boca Raton: CRC Press.

Friemel, T. N. (2016). The digital divide has grown old: Determinants of a digital divide among seniors. *New Media & Society, 18*(2), 313–331. https://doi.org/10.1177/1461444814538648

Heart, T., & Kalderon, E. (2013). Older adults: Are they ready to adopt health-related ICT? *International Journal of Medical Informatics, 82*(11), e209–e231. https://doi.org/10.1016/j.ijmedinf.2011.03.002.

Helbig, N., Ramón Gil-García, J., & Ferro, E. (2009). Understanding the complexity of electronic government: Implications from the digital divide literature. *Government Information Quarterly, 26*(1), 89–97. https://doi.org/10.1016/j.giq.2008.05.004.

Helsper, E., & Reaisdorf, B. C. (2016). The emergence of a "digital underclass" in Great Britain and Sweden: Changing reasons for digital exclusion. *New Media & Society, 19*(8), 1253–1270. https://doi.org/10.1177/1461444816634676.

Hunsaker, A., & Hargittai, E. (2018). A review of internet use among older adults. *New Media & Society, 20*(10), 3937–3954. https://doi.org/10.1177/1461444818787348.

Janssen, M., van Veenstra, A. F., & van der Voort, H. (2013). Management and failure of large transformation projects: Factors affecting user Adoption. In Y. K. Dwivedi, H. Z. Henriksen, D. Wastell, & R. De (Eds.), *Grand successes and failures in IT. Public and private sectors* (pp. 121–135). Berlin, Heidelberg: Springer.

König, R., Seifert, A., Doh, M. (2018). Internet use among older Europeans: An analysis based on SHARE data (Journal Article) 17(3), 621–633. https://doi.org/10.1007/s10209-018-0609-5.

Kummervold, P. E., Chronaki, C. E., Lausen, B., Prokosch, H.-U., Rasmussen, J., Santana, S., et al. (2008). eHealth trends in Europe 2005–2007: A population-based survey. *Journal of Medical Internet Research, 10*(4), e42–e42. https://doi.org/10.2196/jmir.1023.

Levitas, R., Pantazis, C., Fahmy, E., Gordon, D., Lloyd-Reichling, E., & Patsios, D. (2007). *The multi-dimensional analysis of social exclusion*. Bristol: University of Bristol. https://repository.uel.ac.uk/item/8666q.

Lindeman, D. A. (2017). Improving the independence of older adults through technology: Directions for public policy. *Public Policy & Aging Report, 27*(2), 49–52. https://doi.org/10.1093/ppar/prx011.

Lupton, D. (2013). The digitally engaged patient: Self-monitoring and self-care in the digital health era. *Social Theory & Health, 11*(3), 256–270. https://doi.org/10.1057/sth.2013.10

Lupton, D. (2014). Health promotion in the digital era: A critical commentary. *Health Promotion International, 30*(1), 174–183. https://doi.org/10.1093/heapro/dau091.

Mahmood, A., & Keating, N. (2012). Towards inclusive built environments for older adults. In T. Scharf and N. Keating (Eds.), *From exclusion to inclusion in old age: a global challenge* (pp. 145–162). Bristol: The Policy Press.

Melchiorre, M. G., Papa, R., Rijken, M., van Ginneken, E., Hujala, A., & Barbabella, F. (2018a). eHealth in integrated care programs for people with multimorbidity in Europe: Insights from the ICARE4EU project. *Health Policy, 122*(1), 53–63. https://doi.org/10.1016/j.healthpol.2017.08.006.

Melchiorre, M. G., Lamura, G., & Barbabella, F. (2018b). eHealth for people with multimorbidity: Results from the ICARE4EU project and insights from the "10 e's" by Gunther Eysenbach. *PLoS One, 13*(11), e0207292. https://doi.org/10.1371/journal.pone.0207292.

Merkel, S., & Kucharski, A. (2018). Participatory design in gerontechnology: A systematic literature review. *The Gerontologist, 59*(1), e16–e25. https://doi.org/10.1093/geront/gny034

Mostaghel, R. (2016). Innovation and technology for the elderly: Systematic literature review. *Journal of Business Research, 69*(11), 4896–4900. https://doi.org/10.1016/j.jbusres.2016.04.049.

OECD. (2016). *OECD science, technology and innovation outlook 2016*. Paris: OECD Publishing. https://doi.org/10.1787/sti_in_outlook-2016-en.

OECD. (2017). *OECD digital economy outlook 2017*. Paris: OECD Publishing. https://doi.org/10.1787/9789264276284-en.

Olsson, T., Samuelsson, U., & Viscovi, D. (2017). At risk of exclusion? Degrees of ICT access and literacy among senior citizens. *Information, Communication & Society*, 1–18. https://doi.org/10.1080/1369118X.2017.1355007

Östlund, B. (2015). The benefits of involving older people in the design Process. In J. Zhou & G. Salvendy (Eds.), *Human aspects of IT for the aged population. Design for aging* (pp. 3–14). Cham: Springer.

Peacock, S. E., & Künemund, H. (2007). Senior citizens and internet technology: Reasons and correlates of access versus non-access in a European comparative perspective. *European Journal of Ageing, 4*(4), 191–200. https://doi.org/10.1007/s10433-007-0067-z.

Peine, A. (2019). Technology and ageing—Theoretical propositions from science and technology studies (STS). In *Ageing and digital technology* (pp. 51–64). Springer.

Peine, A., Faulkner, A., Jæger, B., & Moors, E. (2015). *Science, technology and the 'grand challenge' of ageing—Understanding the socio-material constitution of later life*. Elsevier.

Phillipson, C. (2013). *Ageing*. John Wiley & Sons.

Poli, A., Kelfve, S., & Motel-Klingebiel, A. (2019). A research tool for measuring non-participation of older people in research on digital health. *BMC Public Health, 19*(1), 1487. https://doi.org/10.1186/s12889-019-7830-x

Poli, A., Kelfve, S., Klompstra, L., Strömberg, A., Jaarsma, T., Motel-Klingebiel, A. (2020). Prediction of (Non)Participation of Older People in Digital Health Research: Exergame Intervention Study. *J Med Internet Res, 22*(6):e17884. https://doi.org/10.2196/17884.

Robinson, L., Cotten, S. R., Ono, H., Quan-Haase, A., Mesch, G., Chen, W., et al. (2015). Digital inequalities and why they matter. *Information, Communication & Society, 18*(5), 569–582. https://doi.org/10.1080/1369118X.2015.1012532

Ross, J., Stevenson, F., Lau, R., & Murray, E. (2016). Factors that influence the implementation of e-health: A systematic review of systematic reviews (an update). *Implementation Science, 11*(1), 146. https://www.ncbi.nlm.nih.gov/pmc/articles/PMC5080780/pdf/13012_2016_Article_510.pdf.

Salemink, K., Strijker, D., & Bosworth, G. (2017). Rural development in the digital age: A systematic literature review on unequal ICT availability, adoption, and use in rural areas. *Journal of Rural Studies, 54*, 360–371. https://doi.org/10.1016/j.jrurstud.2015.09.001.

Scharf, T., & Keating, N. (2012). Social exclusion in later life: A global challenge. In T. Scharf & N. Keating (Eds.), *From exclusion to inclusion in old age: A global challenge* (pp. 1–16). Bristol: The Policy Press.

Schnoll, H. J. (2014). *E-government: Information, technology, and transformation.* Armonk: Routledge.

Seifert, A., Hofer, M., & Rössel, J. (2018). Older adults' perceived sense of social exclusion from the digital world. *Educational Gerontology, 44*(12), 775–785. https://doi.org/10.1080/03601277.2019.1574415.

Siren, A., & Knudsen, S. G. (2017). Older adults and emerging digital service delivery: A mixed methods study on information and communications technology use, skills, and attitudes (Article). *Journal of Aging and Social Policy, 29*(1), 35–50. https://doi.org/10.1080/08959420.2016.1187036.

Sixsmith, A., Mihailidis, A., & Simeonov, D. (2017). Aging and technology: Taking the research into the real world. *Public Policy & Aging Report, 27*(2), 74–78. https://doi.org/10.1093/ppar/prx007.

Tavares, L. P., & Zantomio, F. (2017). Inequity in healthcare use among older people after 2008: The case of southern European countries. *Health Policy, 121*(10), 1063–1071. https://doi.org/10.1016/j.healthpol.2017.08.011.

Terraneo, M. (2015). Inequities in health care utilization by people aged 50+: Evidence from 12 European countries. *Social Science & Medicine, 126*, 154–163. https://doi.org/10.1016/j.socscimed.2014.12.028.

Turner, F. (2010). *From counterculture to cyberculture: Stewart brand, the whole earth network, and the rise of digital utopianism.* University of Chicago Press.

Van Regenmortel, S., De Donder, L., Dury, S., Smetcoren, A.-S., De Witte, N., & Verté, D. (2016). Social exclusion in later life: A systematic review of the literature. *Journal of Population Ageing, 9*(4), 315–344. https://doi.org/10.1007/s12062-016-9145-3

Van Regenmortel, S., De Donder, L., Smetcoren, A.-S., Lambotte, D., De Witte, N., & Verté, D. (2018). Accumulation of disadvantages: Prevalence and categories of old-age social exclusion in Belgium (journal article). *Social Indicators Research, 140*(3), 1173–1194. https://doi.org/10.1007/s11205-017-1817-8.

Walsh, K., Scharf, T., & Keating, N. (2017). Social exclusion of older persons: A scoping review and conceptual framework. *European Journal of Ageing, 14*(1), 81–98. https://doi.org/10.1007/s10433-016-0398-8.

Weiss, D., Rydland, H. T., Øversveen, E., Jensen, M. R., Solhaug, S., & Krokstad, S. (2018). Innovative technologies and social inequalities in health: A scoping review of the literature. *PLoS One, 13*(4), e0195447. https://doi.org/10.1371/journal.pone.0195447

World Health Organization. (2016) *From innovation to implementation: eHealth in the WHO European Region*. Copenhagen. http://www.euro.who.int/__data/assets/pdf_file/0012/302331/From-Innovation-to-Implementation-eHealth-Report-EU.pdf.

World Health Organization. (2017). *Global diffusion of eHealth-making universal health coverage achievable: Report of the third global survey on eHealth*. World Health Organization. https://apps.who.int/iris/bitstream/handle/10665/252529/9789241511780-eng.pdf

Wyatt, S. M. (2003). Non-users also matter: The construction of users and non-users of the internet. In N. Oudshoorn & T. Pinch (Eds.), *How users matter: The co-construction of users and technology* (pp. 67–79). Cambridge: MIT Press.

Section V
Community and Spatial Exclusion

Chapter 14
Introduction: Framing Community and Spatial Exclusion

Isabelle Tournier and Lucie Vidovićová

14.1 Introduction

This section focuses on the community and spatial aspects of social exclusion. For this introduction, we define the community aspect of exclusion as the unintended reduction of participation in local life and spatial aspects of exclusion as the unintended reduction of mobility outside and inside of a person's home. Fighting against social exclusion of older adults is a priority due to the negative effects of exclusion on older adults' quality of life as well as on the equity and cohesion of an ageing society as a whole (adapted from Levitas et al. 2007 in Walsh et al. 2017, p. 83). Place, as a socio-spatial phenomenon, can shape older adults' lives and their experiences of social exclusion. It encompasses dimensions such as social and relational aspects of place, amenities and built environment, place-based policy and experiential belonging. The purpose of this chapter is to briefly introduce some allied concepts related to older people's relationship with their place and environment, and broadly illustrate the relevance of this relationship to old-age social exclusion. The chapter closes with a short introduction to each contribution within this section.

I. Tournier (✉)
Info-Zenter Demenz, Luxembourg City, Luxembourg
e-mail: isabelle.tournier@i-zd.lu

L. Vidovićová
Faculty of Social Studies, Masaryk University, Brno, Czech Republic

K. Walsh et al. (eds.), *Social Exclusion in Later Life*, International Perspectives on Aging 28, https://doi.org/10.1007/978-3-030-51406-8_14

14.2 To Age in a "Good Place"

The majority of older adults wish to age-in-place and avoid having to move to other neighborhoods or particularly to care institutions (Rioux 2005). Defined as the ability of older people to live in their own home and community safely, independently, and comfortably, ageing-in-place has become a priority policy agenda for many countries (WHO 2015). However, when considering the challenges of community and spatial exclusion, it may be more relevant to focus on ageing in a "good place".

The risk of social exclusion in older-age is increased due to physical, psychological, cognitive and social changes that might threaten an older person's capacity to adapt to their environment. As highlighted by the ecological theory of ageing (Lawton 1983), autonomy and well-being are linked to a good person-environment fit or, in other words, when older adults' competencies correspond with the demands of their environment. Consequently, experiences in later life can be dependent upon the quality of an older person's immediate social and physical surrounding. When environmental demands overwhelm an individual's biopsychosocial resources, a person's capacity to age-in-place is reduced (Greenfield 2012). Despite this, the role of the environment, as well as the importance of processes of belonging to place, remains relatively overlooked in gerontological research (Wahl et al. 2012).

14.3 Spatial Aspects of Social Engagement During Ageing

The idea of contributing to society is emphasised by the concept of *active ageing*, whereby older people can remain active contributors to their families, peers, communities and nations. Active ageing is the "process of optimizing opportunities for health, participation and security in order to enhance quality of life as people age" (WHO 2002, p. 12). Adapted physical environments and safe housing are two main aspects to promote active ageing and reduce the risk of social isolation.

To better illustrate the intersection of multilevel spatial environments and the needs of older adults with respect to engagement and inclusion, we propose the model of life-space locations (Webber et al. 2010) which allows for a better understanding of the different scales of life-space that constitute the physical environment. Vidovićová et al. (2013) proposed a modification to this original model to incorporate seven (plus one) life-space locations of older adults. It is presented as a system of overlapping circles from the smallest, most immediate of environments, such as a room, through a graduated environmental scale of the home, the outdoors, the neighborhood, the surrounding areas and the world, all wrapped in an online world (Vidovićová and Tournier 2020). This model can serve as an inventory of different levels of policies which are needed to address major challenges with respect to person-environment interactions, and the sort of exclusions that may occur within or as a result of those interactions (Fig. 14.1).

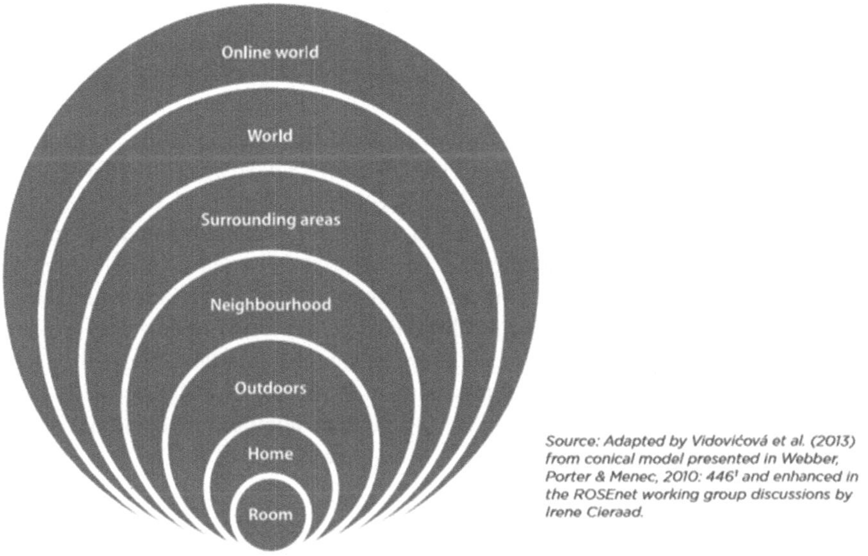

Fig. 14.1 Adapted framework model of life-space locations

The level of the "world" may serve, for example, as a reminder that the environmental issues of sustainable development and the related challenge of climate change need global action, while their impact is very local and is differentiated by age (Pillemer et al. 2011; Pope et al. 2016). The surrounding areas and neighbourhood levels raise questions about supported mobility, travel and accessible transport (*e.g.* frequency, timing of connections and barrier-free vehicles), as well as social cohesion and connectivity (*e.g.* safety and the absence of crime; dense social networks). Policy makers also face a challenge in fostering processes that enhance a sense of belonging to place through community-building policies (Barrett and McGoldrick 2013; Buffel et al. 2014).

The outdoors' level encompasses the need for policies to address walkability, greenery, aesthetics and surveillance zones (*e.g.* respect for pleasant views from houses when revitalising or building new neighbourhoods), comfortable benches, and accessible and centrally located public toilets (Tournier et al. 2016).

Additionally, there are policies which need to have a more direct effect on the homes of older people, combating housing related risks of exclusion in older-age by addressing challenges in home maintenance, heating/cooling costs, affordability, and sustainability (Kneale 2016; Martin-Matthews and Cloutier 2017). The room level indicates the importance of this environment in relation to addressing exclusion around care provision, in the case of increased frailty, or where, for example, injuries and falls may be prevented.

The overarching "online world" expresses the (not so) new impact of technologies and communication devices in altering our living spaces and how we use them. Although not physical in the original meaning of the term, it represents a place, derived from enabled connections across spatial environments, where both social relations are established and maintained and care provided (Blackman et al. 2007).

The centric circles and their variant sizes are especially relevant for older adults because everyday routines tend to become more and more centered around their immediate locale, leading to a reduction of their life-space mobility, with their radius of action more centered around their home (Rantakokko et al. 2015). This also affects their sense of belonging, which according to Wahl et al. (2012) refers to environment-related experiences linked to subjective evaluations and interpretations of place (*e.g.* place attachment). The potential for a sense of belonging to increase with age (due to the accumulation of ties and long-term tenure within environments), together with a physical "shrinking" of the action radius, may explain why old, and particularly very old, adults are hesitant to undertake repeated relocations, show high stability and regularity in their out-of-home-related activities (*e.g.* preferred places and travel patterns), and value their familiar home and neighborhood environment, even if they present inherent risks (Wahl et al., 2012, p. 309).

14.4 Outline of this Section

The three chapters in this section, through theories and case studies, examine various aspects of how community and space impacts older adults' lives within their environments and influences their overall experiences of exclusion in later life.

Drilling et al. (Chap. 15) present a model of "Age, Space and Exclusion - ASE-Triangle" as a multifaceted concept for the analysis of situations of social exclusion and their causes. In this model, the authors rely on Lefebvre's (1991) work according to whom space is designed as a product of dynamic relations between materialisations (spatial practice/perceived space), conceptions (representations of space/conceived space) and experiences (representational spaces/lived space). Drilling et al. present two case studies, from Ireland and Cyprus, to illustrate how their ASE-triangle is supported by empirical work and can help explain real-world interactions between age, space and exclusion. As a result, authors stress the need to include all stakeholders in the planning process, including older adults, to ensure that spatial and local civic exclusion does not occur.

The second chapter presented by Urbaniak et al. (Chap. 16) relies on empirical cases from data collected in Poland, Germany and Ireland to illustrate how place, social exclusion and life transitions are closely interrelated. The authors focus on bereavement and retirement (two types of life-course transitions considered as normative in old-age) to explore how the person-environment exchange processes of agency and belonging have the potential to mediate social exclusion that might result from life-course transitions. Urbaniak et al. conclude with a focus on the importance of policy and practice to enable older adults to exert spatial agency and develop a sense of belonging within a community in the context of key life transitions.

The final chapter approaches the question of ageing in rural environments. Vidovićová et al. (Chap. 17) remind us that rurality is seldom mentioned in national ageing policies despite the fact that a large proportion of older adults are living in rural places. Through the example of three neighboring countries (Czech Republic, Germany and Poland), this chapter addresses to what extent social exclusion in later life is linked to the organization of care in rural areas, underlining the multifaceted nature of various exclusionary processes. The authors highlight the necessity for state, non-governmental, civil society and private actors of the older adult care sector to learn from each other in order to develop more inclusive approaches to provision in heterogenous rural contexts.

These topics resonate also with the effects the global COVID-19 responses in various ways. The call addressed in many countries specifically to older adults to "stay at home" and "to cocoon" has directly affected their use of space and community involvement. These safety measures might have aggravated the exclusion of especially those living alone, disrupting their access to care and social relationships by building both physical and symbolic barriers, and negatively affecting both their mental (United Nations 2020) and physical health (Pelicioni & Lord 2020).

14.5 Improving Social Inclusion of Older Adults Through Spatial and Community Aspects

To conclude this introductory section, let us stress once again, that the places where (older) people live influence the risk of social exclusion, by being a threat or a significant resource to their participation within society. As emphasised earlier, place, as a socio-spatial phenomenon, can fundamentally shape older adults' lives. The maintenance and quality of communities and relational connections are essential components of everyday life that directly impact numerous spheres such as emotional well-being, quality of life or even the maintenance of cognitive skills during ageing (Mendes de Leon et al. 2003; Ylvisaker et al. 2005). Despite current efforts of communities to become more age-friendly, older adults with specific needs can be at high risk of social exclusion. For example, people living with dementia, that represent approximately 21 per cent of the 85–89 age group, and more than 40 per cent of the 90 years and over age group (Alzheimer Europe 2019), face several specific obstacles (*e.g.* cognitive and behavioral changes, social isolation, stigma) that threaten the continuity of their participation in local environments. Like in other groups who can experience forms of spatial displacement and disconnection, for them the lack of connectivity to local neighbourhoods and communities can be a complex and under attended challenge (Schölzel-Dorenbos et al. 2010). This needs to be more extensively addressed to foster more inclusive communities for all older people.

References

Alzheimer Europe. (2019). *Estimating the prevalence of dementia in Europe. Dementia in Europe Yearbook 2019*. https://www.alzheimer-europe.org/Publications/Dementia-in-Europe-Yearbooks. Accessed 31 Mar 2020.

Barrett, G., & McGoldrick, C. (2013). Narratives of (in)active ageing in poor deprived areas of Liverpool, UK. *International Journal of Sociology and Social Policy, 33*(5), 347–366. https://doi.org/10.1108/IJSSP-09-2012-0084.

Blackman, T., Van Schaik, P., & Martyr, A. (2007). Outdoor environments for people with dementia: An exploratory study using virtual reality. *Ageing and Society, 27*(6), 811–825. https://doi.org/10.1017/S0144686X07006253.

Buffel, T., McGarry, P., Phillipson, C., De Donder, L., Dury, S., De Witte, N., Smetcoren, A.-S., & Verté, D. (2014). Developing age-friendly cities: Case studies from Brussels and Manchester and implications for policy and practice. *Journal of Aging & Social Policy, 26*, 52–72.

Greenfield, E. A. (2012). Using ecological frameworks to advance a field of research, practice, and policy on aging-in-place initiatives. *The Gerontologist, 52*, 1–12.

Kneale, D. (2016). Connected communities? LGB older people and their risk of exclusion from decent housing and neighbourhoods. *Quality in Ageing and Older Adults, 17*(2), 107–118. https://doi.org/10.1108/QAOA-04-2015-0019.

Lawton, M. P. (1983). Environment and other determinants of well-being in older people. *The Gerontologist, 23*, 349–357.

Lefebvre, H. (1991). *The social production of space*. Oxford: Blackwell.

Levitas, R., Pantazis, C., Fahmy, E., et al. (2007). *The multi-dimensional analysis of social exclusion*. London: Cabinet Office.

Martin-Matthews, A., & Cloutier, D. S. (2017). Household spaces of ageing. When care comes home. In M. W. Skinner, G. J. Andrews, & M. P. Cutchin (Eds.), *Geographical gerontology: Perspectives, concepts, approaches* (pp. 162–173). Routledge.

Mendes de Leon, C. F., Glass, T. A., & Berkman, L. F. (2003). Social engagement and disability in a community population of older adults: The New Haven EPESE. *American Journal of Epidemiology, 157*, 633–642.

Pelicioni, P. H., & Lord, S. R. (2020). COVID-19 will severely impact older people's lives, and in many more ways than you think! *Brazilian Journal of Physical Therapy*. https://doi.org/10.1016/j.bjpt.2020.04.005.

Pillemer, K., Wells, N. M., Wagenet, L. P., Meador, R. H., & Parise, J. T. (2011). Environmental sustainability in an aging society: A research agenda. *Journal of Aging and Health, 23*(3), 433–453. https://doi.org/10.1177/0898264310381278.

Pope, R., Wu, J., & Boone, C. (2016). Spatial patterns of air pollutants and social groups: A distributive environmental justice study in the phoenix metropolitan region of USA. *Environmental Management, 58*(5), 753–766. https://doi.org/10.1007/s00267-016-0741-z.

Rantakokko, M., Iwarsson, S., Portegijs, E., Viljanen, A., & Rantanen, T. (2015). Associations between environmental characteristics and life-space mobility in community-dwelling older people. *Journal of Aging and Health, 27*(4), 606–621. https://doi.org/10.1177/0898264314555328.

Rioux, L. (2005). The well-being of aging people living in their own homes. *Journal of Environmental Psychology, 25*, 231–243.

Schölzel-Dorenbos, C. J. M., Meeuwsen, E. J., & Olde Rikkert, M. G. M. (2010). Integrating unmet needs into dementia health-related quality of life research and care: Introduction of the hierarchy model of needs in dementia. *Aging and Mental Health, 14*, 113–119.

Tournier, I., Dommes, A., & Cavallo, V. (2016). Review of safety and mobility issues among older pedestrians. *Accident Analysis and Prevention, 91*, 24–35.

United Nations. (2020). *Policy brief: The impact of COVID-19 on older persons*. United Nations, May 2020. https://www.un.org/development/desa/ageing/wp-content/uploads/sites/24/2020/05/COVID-Older-persons.pdf. Accessed 24 Jun 2020.

Vidovićová, L., Galčanová, L., Petrová Kafková, M., & Sýkorová, D. (2013). *Stáří ve městě, město v životě seniorů*. Praha: Sociologické nakladatelství.
Vidovićová, L. & Tournier, L. (2020). Community and spatial aspects of exclusion in later life. In K. Walsh & T. Scharf (series Eds.) ROSEnet Briefing Paper Series: No. 2. CA 15122 Reducing Old-Age Exclusion: Collaborations in Research and Policy. ISBN 978-1-908358-72-1.
Wahl, H.-W., Iwarsson, S., & Oswald, F. (2012). Aging well and the environment: Toward an integrative model and research agenda for the future. *The Gerontologist, 52*, 306–316.
Walsh, K., Scharf, T., & Keating, N. (2017). Social exclusion of older persons: A scoping review and conceptual framework. *European Journal of Ageing, 14*, 1–18.
Webber, S. C., Porter, M. M., & Menec, V. H. (2010). Mobility in older adults: A comprehensive framework. *The Gerontologist, 50*(4), 443–450. https://doi.org/10.1093/geront/gnq013.
WHO. (2002). *Active ageing: A policy framework*. Geneva, Switzerland: World Health Organisation.
WHO. (2015). *World report on ageing and health*. Geneva, Switzerland: World Health Organization.
Ylvisaker, M., Turkstra, L. S., & Coelho, C. (2005). Behavioral and social interventions for individuals with traumatic brain injury: A summary of the research with clinical implications. *Seminars in Speech and Language, 26*, 256–267.

Chapter 15
Towards a Structural Embeddedness of Space in the Framework of the Social Exclusion of Older People

Matthias Drilling, Hannah Grove, Byron Ioannou, and Thibauld Moulaert

15.1 Introduction

Social exclusion can be viewed as a component, expression or manifestation of a process by which individuals and groups become isolated from major societal mechanisms providing resources (Chakravarty and D'Ambrosio 2006). Scholars have asserted that exclusion is the outcome of the failure of specific systems that promote civic, economic, social and interpersonal participation in mainstream society, particularly in older-age (Hodge et al. 2002, Walsh et al. 2017). Thus, exclusion in older-age is multidimensional, relational, and dynamic (Atkinson 1998; Barnes et al. 2006) [also see Walsh et al. this volume for a full discussion of the attributes of exclusion in later life]. When highlighting the spatial dimension in the debate around exclusion, we must acknowledge that this spatial dimension is itself multidimensional: Older adults can be excluded from different spatial arrangements – institutions, social groups, specific local benefits, or even particular events in specific places. Social exclusion is relational because it is not just about looking at a number of spatial arrangements individually (*e.g.* old-age residential housing units, a dementia village), but rather looking at their interlinkages between, as well

M. Drilling (✉)
University of Applied Sciences and Arts, School of Social Work, Institute for Social Planning, Organizational Change and Urban Development ISOS, Muttenz, Switzerland
e-mail: matthias.drilling@fhnw.ch

H. Grove
Department of Geography, Maynooth University, Maynooth, Ireland

B. Ioannou
Department of Architecture, Frederick University, Nicosia, Cyprus

T. Moulaert
PACTE Social Sciences Laboratory, Université Grenoble Alpes, & CNRS, Sciences Po Grenoble, Grenoble, France

K. Walsh et al. (eds.), *Social Exclusion in Later Life*, International Perspectives on Aging 28, https://doi.org/10.1007/978-3-030-51406-8_15

as their embeddedness, in the dominant model of society (like "successful ageing" or "active ageing") from which exclusion occurs (Silver 1994). Finally, exclusion is dynamic because it is a process that is highly conditional on time and place. As different places have different histories, cultures and institutions, they shape norms, values and, therefore, different approaches and access to resources. In conclusion, using the multidimensional concept of social exclusion put forward in this edited volume suggests that we need to think in more complex and interwoven ways, and more theoretically, about spatial exclusion of older people (Moulaert et al. 2018).

This chapter aims to address this challenge. We first introduce relevant writings that can be used to relate spatial aspects to older people's social exclusion more comprehensively; and accordingly adapt these thoughts to a model which we call the "Age, Space and Exclusion ASE-Triangle". We then identify new pathways for empirical research and present two case studies (Greater Dublin – Ireland, and Nicosia – Cyprus) to explore the possibilities and limits of applying the ASE-Triangle to empirical work. The conclusion then situates our model within existing literature.

15.2 Triadic Thinking – Trans-Disciplinary Theorizing of Spatial Exclusion

The debate about age, space and exclusion is usually tied to the epistemological objectives of a discipline. Human geography has the longest tradition of exploring spatial concepts, and the 'humanistic turn' in the 1970s freed the discipline from its basic positivist attitudes towards an understanding of 'space' from a subjective and micro-geographical perspective (Drilling and Schnur 2019). At almost the same time, French-speaking sociology intensified its debate around 'space', orientating itself to Lefebvre who maintained "that space must be understood not simply as a concrete, material object, but also as an ideological, lived, and subjective one." (Warf and Arias 2009, p. 3). These discussions were supported by other disciplines such as philosophy. Casey (2000/1987) bridged the gap to 'place'-concepts, when he differentiated between 'locus' and 'place', describing the latter as selective for memories and related to the body. "In the end, we can move into place, indeed *be* in a place …" (Casey 2000/1987, p. 189). In the following years the focus of these new pathways in space-related research varied enormously and embraced studies on space and identity, on places as centres of meaning constructed out of lived experience, or on space as a process that forms and shapes itself along perceptions and attributions, filled with opinions that can run across objective concepts such as life situations, milieus or age groups (detailed in Drilling and Schnur 2019). In geography, a sub-discipline of geographical gerontology arose, defining places as "the context in which we live, settings, to which we feel attached but which also shape our experience of social processes, such as the provision of health care, the process of ageing, or social and economic restructuring." (Wiles 2005, p. 101).

The call for gerontology to be the key interdisciplinary frame to guide age-related questions to become more spatial is still relevant. Despite that "place is now a central concept within national and international ageing policy" (Urbaniak and Walsh 2019, p. 1), scholars like Moulaert or Wanka still state that gerontology "tends to ignore longstanding traditions of researching spatial exclusion in other disciplines…" (Moulaert et al., p. 11) and "often shares a positivistic understanding of space" (Wanka et al. 2018, p. 25).

But how to combine a relational theory of space with a concept of social exclusion in later life? We propose a starting point in the vision of space as a simultaneity of the material, the social and the symbolic as developed by Henri Lefebvre. In Lefebvre's work, cities and neighbourhoods are understood as constantly changing human relational structures that are regulated by political, social and economic conditions (Lefebvre 1991). The space is thus designed as a product of dynamic relations between materialisations (spatial practice/perceived space), conceptions (representations of space/conceived space) and experiences (representational spaces/lived space).

- Spatial practice (perceived space) derives, for example, from non-reflexive daily routines that are affected by the built neighbourhood and infrastructures, all of them located in specific sites. These structures that can be physically touched, navigated to or frequented, lead to specific individual perceptions and actions. How older people with differing lifestyles and concepts of life perceive environments and other people and how they act in their environments is influenced by age stereotypes that are inherent to spatial practices.
- Representations of space (conceived space) are a result of the knowledge society with its policy makers, architects, planners, developers or administration, as well as their concepts, maps, plans, models and designs. All these stakeholders have their own ideas and convictions as to what ageing means (or should mean). Such representations are laden with ideologies.
- Representational space (lived space) refers to passively, rather than actively (see above), experienced space – the way people subconsciously read and understand signs and symbols in space. These symbols help us to tell a road from a footpath or a playground from a park, but they also give us clues about where we can and cannot go, for example via signs of disorder that might symbolise crime in a certain area.

Applying such a lens to the relations between old-age, space and exclusion, results in a concept that prompts us to interpret every observation as an expression of a triadic relationship. However, it's not only space, but also age and exclusion that can be perceived, conceived, and lived. Like the triangulation of space, a triangulation of age and exclusion exists: modern neuroscience, for example, explains what it means to live with dementia (conceived age). Families feel insecure and believe that dementia villages offer optimum safety. Those who can afford it rent space there for their relatives; those who cannot afford it are left behind (perceived exclusion). Scholars label such neighbourhoods as 'geriatric ghettos' (conceived exclusion); older people read stories about their built environment in the newspapers and fear leaving their home (lived exclusion).

This interplay between different forms of perceiving, living and conceiving space, age and exclusion– depending on the power relations in society at a given time - results in narratives and paradigms used to analyse the older person in their environment and formulate recommendations for policy areas (such as the WHO "age-friendly cities" strategy). In this model space is considered to encompass an objective set of characteristics and a set of subjective elements, where it is imbued with meaning in the context of ageing and exclusion. As such we recognise the links between space and place in our interpretation, and accordingly use the terms interchangeably.

Figure 15.1 presents the ASE (Age, Space, and Exclusion) triangle derived from such a triadic thinking.

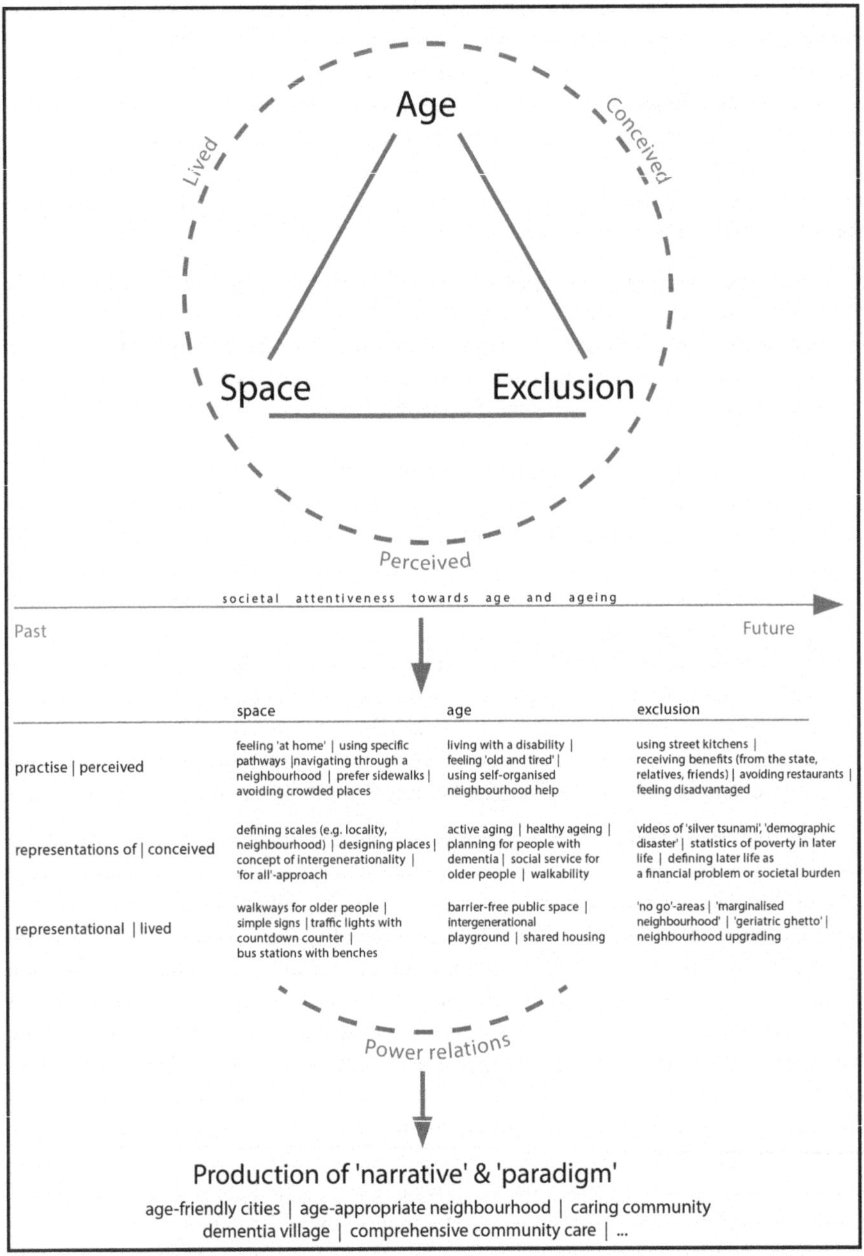

Fig. 15.1 How space, age and exclusion produces political narratives and paradigms – the “Age, Space and Exclusion ASE-Triangle”

After presenting our "Ageing, Space and Exclusion – ASE Triangle", the following section illustrates the interplay between space, age and exclusion using two examples: Greater Dublin (Ireland) and Pallouriotissa/Nicosia (Cyprus).

15.3 Ageing in Greater Dublin/Ireland: Experiences of Local Exclusion in Daily Life

Based on an on-going PhD project (Grove, n.d.) that explores whether older people's local environments support residents to 'age well', this case study uses a 'Qualitative GIS' approach, which integrates both qualitative and spatial data, and emphasises the importance of including *meaning* within mapping (Cope and Elwood 2009; Milton et al. 2015; Meijering and Weitkamp 2016). Twenty-four interviews and mapping exercises were carried out with 34 older people aged between 66 and 89 years old in a suburban and inner-city study area in Greater Dublin.[1] 'Go-along' interviews were also conducted with 20 of the participants. The results, presented here as an illustrative case, focus on an example of spatial exclusion from the project area, and the impact this is having on one of the participants. The ASE triangle model is applied to this example to think through how spatial practices, representational space, and representations of space all interact to produce different forms of spatial exclusion.

During interviews for this research, Anne (a pseudonym) shared that she was very distressed as a result of a new development happening in her local area.

There were several reasons for this distress. First, Anne was upset that she would lose her views of the mountains from her garden to the rear of her house as the development would create a significant obstruction. Anne highly valued these views which were a part of the characteristics of her home environment and which she had enjoyed for over 40 years. Second, Anne was concerned about safety as a result of the construction and completion of this new development. This related to both the building of a temporary alleyway to facilitate mobility through the neighbourhood during the development, and the intention to build a permanent lane at the back of her house.

For Anne, the imposed structures have created/will create potential spaces for antisocial behaviour hidden from external view and have further contributed to Anne not feeling safe in her neighbourhood. During her interview and go-along interview, she raised concerns about the behaviour of her neighbours, and how some of the newer residents did not seem to care about their local environment and would leave rubbish everywhere. She was also worried about people

[1] The Greater Dublin Area encompasses Dublin City and the six administrative counties (local authorities) of Fingal, Dun Laoghaire-Rathdown, South Dublin, Kildare, Meath and Wicklow.

jumping over the fence into her garden, affecting her sense of safety in her own home:

> 'Our lane was closed off, so that was ok. But these are leaving the lane as a walkthrough and... well, in the 80s we all had lanes behind the houses. But there was only unsociable... activity in them, so we fought and we got them all closed up. Now these [developers] are opening this up, and I was a young woman at that stage, now I'm 70 and they're bringing this on us.' (Main Interview)

Third, and linked to the construction of the temporary alleyway and her perceived lack of safety, Anne spoke about difficulties in maintaining social participation and connections with her trusted neighbours and friends in the area. A valued part of Anne's routine is to visit her friend's house. The usual route she takes is shown in Fig. 15.2 below (dotted green line), but the new alleyway has been created with tall fencing which makes it very dark, and there is a 'blind corner' where you can't see who is on the other side. Although it remains the most direct route, Anne no longer feels safe walking through it, and so in her mind it might as well not be there because she would not use it, and instead she is forced to walk a much longer route. From her perspective, she is more physically disconnected from her friend than she was before and describes this as an 'awful inconvenience':

> 'Oh I wouldn't go through that lane… oh my God… you see the way it's blocked off there, it's all black. Well then when you go up that lane it's completely black. Now, it's only going to be, I think, a temporary thing while they're building. But, the thing about it is, it's an awful inconvenience…' (Main Interview).

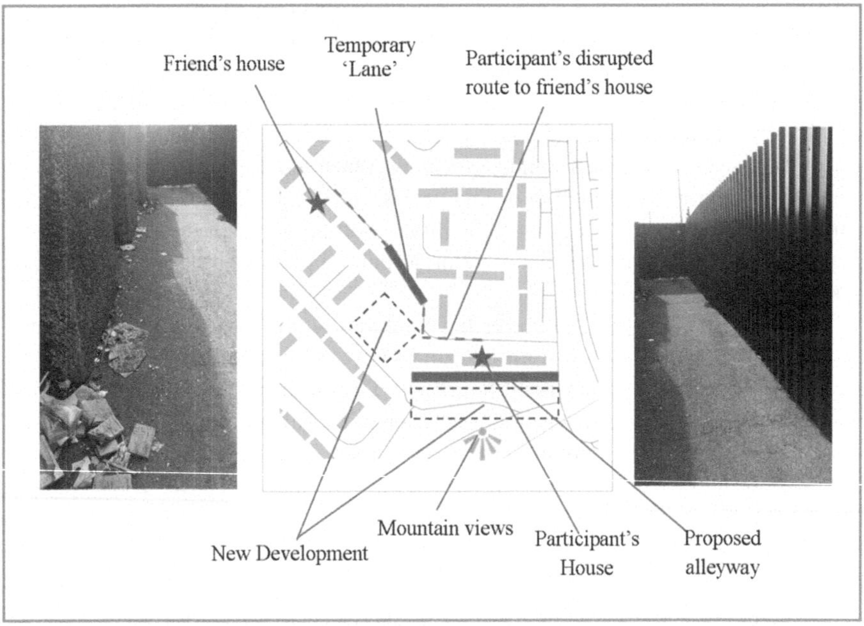

Fig. 15.2 Annotated map of participant's local environment (photographs taken by researcher during 'go-along' interview)

Turning now to triadic thinking: with regard to *spatial practices*, Anne's routes and routines have been disrupted by the temporary alleyway. To get to her friend's house, she previously had to walk a very short distance through a green space (less than 5 min), but now she has to 'go all around' the estate and walk over 10 min. This example reinforces that in order to better understand accessibility and forms of spatial exclusion for older people, there is a need to not just consider objective or physical distances to and from a place, but to also include more subjective components which may influence older adult behaviour. This may include perceived barriers about what a reasonable distance may be for an individual based on existing capabilities or habits, or perceptions of safety whilst navigating their local environment.

Closely connected to spatial practices, the notion of *representational space* leads to situations of *social exclusion*. Anne associated both the lane and the litter present in the lane with anti-social behaviour. The fact that there was no litter before the lane and now there is, introduces both the fear and confirmation of anti-social behaviour to this participant, which in turn creates an unwillingness to walk along the lane:

> 'And look at that, there's rubbish. That was never here. They're after creating more problems. Big change that I can see. Litter... It's too dangerous, you know.' (Go-along interview).

The fear around this lane also represents wider fears that the participant has about some of her neighbours, and about who might move into the new housing and whether she will be safe: 'Who's going to get them [the new houses]? They can get over your back wall. Depending on who it is.' (Go-along interview).

Finally, this example highlights that these considerations have perhaps not been taken into account during the planning phase, and illustrates the impact of a lack of consultation with residents, particularly older residents, concerning how to minimise disruption during this development. There are *representations of space* that show this site as a future development area or suburban infill development. In this instance it is represented as a map on a planning application for this development. This is the dominant representation, but perspectives of older people, and their subjective experiences and fears are absent from this traditional form of mapping.

By understanding older people's spatial practices and the meaning that they place on various signs and visual cues in the built environment, we can highlight everyday forms of spatial exclusion. These may also differ or contrast with policymakers' and professionals' experiences or understanding of the same place.

Within the broader study, many other narratives referred to other spatial and civic exclusion processes. For example, another participant was unable to walk through a green space shortcut to her community centre due to health and security challenges, and limited public transport and local shopping options meant that daily errands such as buying groceries and going to the doctor had become a challenge. Table 15.1 illustrates the three dimensions of older people's experiences of place-related exclusion identified in this case.

Table 15.1 Dominant patterns between age, space and exclusion in Greater Dublin

	Age	Space	Exclusion
Practices	- How people 'practise' and experience ageing varies (heterogeneity of older adults).	- Routines, daily activities. - Dependent on age (and mobility and health), and can in turn create either inclusion or exclusion when ageing in place. - Physical barriers/ enablers.	Physical practices of exclusion – *e.g.* lack of public transport, or no community centre.
Representations of (Of which policy is one form, but older adult representations are also needed). Some are more dominant than others.	- Dominant forms. - Types of 'ageing well' (successful, healthy, happy, active, positive). - 'Harder to reach' older adult subgroups not as well represented.	- Policymakers maps are dominant representations of space. - Qualitative GIS + go-along interviews help to make subjugated perspectives and experiences of place more visible.	- Raising awareness of forms of exclusion and inclusion. - Some older people can be so excluded they are not even represented; specific research methodologies can be a tool to resist this.
Representational	- Subjective experiences of ageing.	- Subjective/Meaningful (more place). - Influenced by what is important to individual – can also lead to more perceived barriers/enablers.	- Subjective aspects of exclusion (perceived exclusion), *e.g.* rubbish.

15.4 Ageing in the *Pallouriotissa* Suburbs, Nicosia/Cyprus: Suburbs as Both a Problem and Solution to Spatial Exclusion

This case study is based on the first results of research carried out by Frederick University (Ioannou 2018) that outlined the spatiality of ageing in the suburban context of Cyprus, in particular in the *Pallouriotissa* district that has undergone continuous suburban expansion during the last 80 years. Field data was derived from semi-structured interviews with 20 older people aged between 65 and 80 years old, car drivers and homeowners of Cypriot origin, which is the predominant group among the ageing population of Cyprus. Interviews were structured around the World Health Organisation (WHO 2015) age-friendly indicators most associated with the concepts of suburban development in Cyprus, specifically: walkability, accessibility of public spaces, and accessibility of public transport. Additionally, field observation provided a comparative assessment of human presence and quality of space and infrastructures. The aim of the approach was to investigate age-friendliness in terms of how the particular neighbourhood settings affect everyday lives.

The ASE triangle model is applied to this example to think through how *representations of space* influence perceptions of feeling old (perceived age) in place, and how these perceptions change during the different urban design epochs of Nicosia. This brings awareness that the ASE triangle is embedded in time and influenced by societal attentiveness towards age and ageing (see Fig. 15.1 'past and future' line).

The *Pallouriotissa* urban district is a very diverse place, with an old quarter dating to the Ottoman period and residential areas encompassing almost a century of suburban history in Nicosia through four distinct subareas (Fig. 15.3):

1. *initial old quarter* (Ottoman period); mixed use, irregular, narrow streets, compact fabric;
2. *early suburbia* (1940s-1970s); mixed use, medium/low density, shaped suburban fabric;
3. *postcolonial suburbia* (1980s-1990s); medium/low density, shaped suburban fabric;
4. *late suburbia* (2000s-2010s); very low density, incomplete suburban fabric.

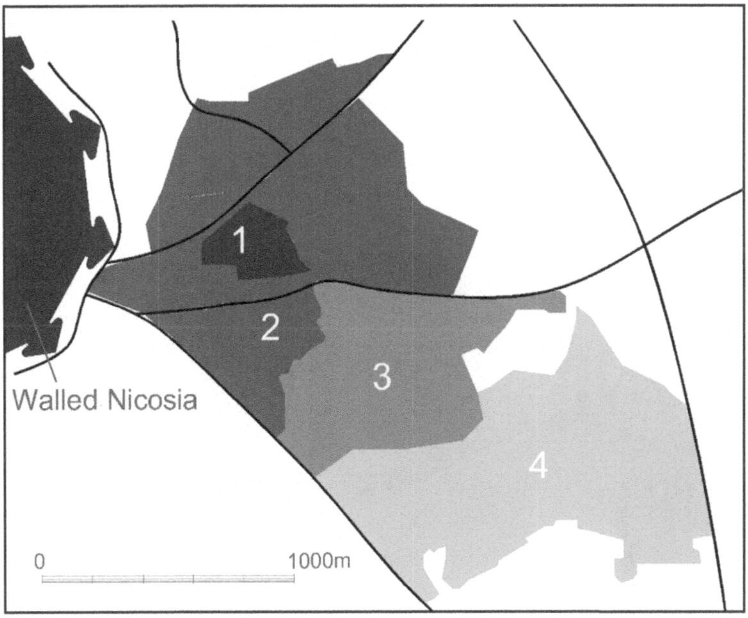

Fig. 15.3 Pallouriotissa urban district: Subareas 1–4

All four subareas are geographically and spatially shaped by the daily movements of their various resident groups, but mainly by the ageing group that spends most of its time at home.

The *initial old quarter* was perceived as a run-down area by the study participants due to the condition of the buildings, despite their architectural value as heritage structures. Place attachment is high, since most of the interviewees were born and grew up there. Place appropriation is also high, since they spend time gathering in places, such as their church or their old traditional cafes. But the general satisfaction with their place of living is low because of the complex traffic flows and the low levels of care invested in the public spaces, which together do not allow older people to benefit from the compact neighbourhood structure (Fig. 15.4).

> 'This place is like an old village in the city, though is very hard and dangerous to move.' (Interview)

The interviewees appreciated *early suburbia* because it combines its green and suburban character, which is a positive stereotype, with centrality and proximity to amenities. Place attachment is high, since most of the interviewees moved there during their youth. Place appropriation is high since they live close to relatives and old friends. There is a high satisfaction with their place of living in general.

> 'I bought this plot just when I migrated from my village during 1960s. It's green and quiet, My daughter has built the upper floor.' (Interview)

The *postcolonial suburbia* was also appreciated by the interviewees due to its suburban character. Place attachment is high, since most of the interviewees moved there during their youth or early adulthood. Place appropriation is high since they live close to relatives and old friends. Their overall satisfaction with their place is again high.

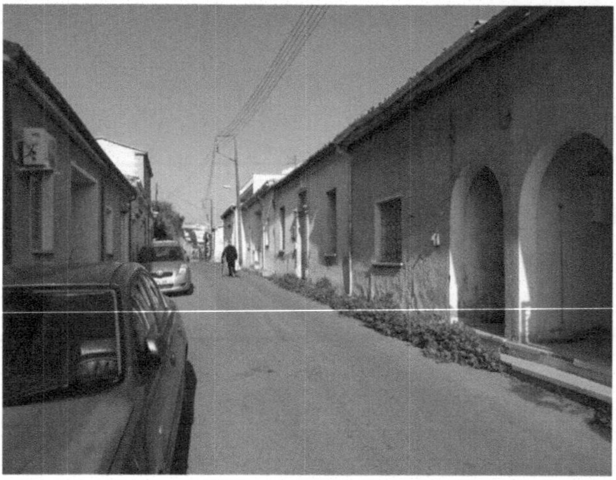

"This place is like an old village in the city, though is very hard and dangerous to move." (Interview)

Fig. 15.4 Pallouriotissa initial old quarter street view

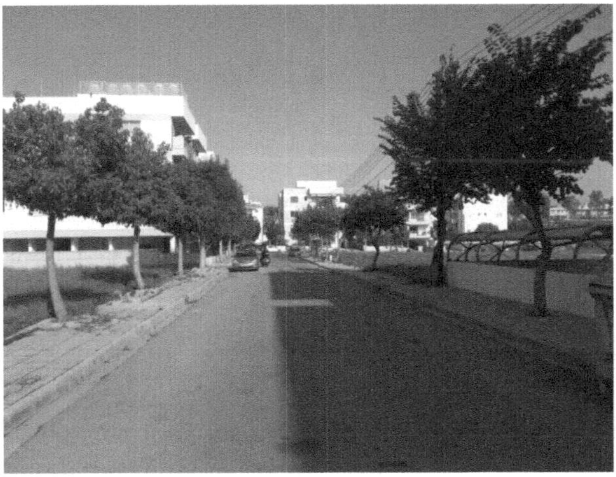

"Open sky, plenty of parking places, and quieter than our previous place." (Interview)

Fig. 15.5 Late suburbia street view

Late suburbia (Fig. 15.5) was appreciated by the interviewees due to its new buildings and quietness. Place attachment is low, since most of the interviewees moved there during their middle or late age. Place appropriation is low since they are effectively newcomers. Despite this fact, their overall satisfaction with their place is high: 'Open sky, plenty of parking places, and quieter than our previous place.' (Interview)

After gathering the interview data and observations in *Pallouriotissa/Nicosia* and analysing it using Fig. 15.1, Table 15.2 presents the three dimensions of older people's spatial experiences. In this case, however, and because of the age-friendly focus of the original study, we have structured the presentation according to the WHO indicators.

Regarding the *Age* aspects, the case study isolated the active and healthy ageing group (conceived age, see Fig. 15.1), setting as determining factors the attributes of *space* and *exclusion* in the urban environment. Residential mobility seems to be low in all cases, except *late suburbia*, but the perspective of ageing in place is high for all areas due to the supportive framework at the national level. The interviewees in the suburban sub-areas did not perceive exclusion as a visible threat. Exclusion may exist if they face any kind of disability, since the urban fabric is not adequately equipped for these cases.

On the other hand, in the initial quarter/compact neighbourhood, residents felt excluded by its differentiated fabric, both for the practical reasons previously mentioned, but also due to the perception of their place by others. Place seems to both define and be defined by age and exclusion constraints. Perception of place proves to be highly important. The *initial old quarter area* retained a number of virtues, like scale, proximity to amenities, character and compactness, which in the end are not much appreciated.

Table 15.2 Dominant patterns of age, space, and exclusion in Pallouriotissa/Nicosia structured by WHO indicators

	Initial old quarter	Early suburbia	Postcolonial suburbia	Late suburbia
AGE				
Population (No.)	291	2682	1608	2204
> 65 (% of total)	30	20	19	7
SPACE				
Indicator: walkability	- Limited space for pedestrians. Limited benches. - Low attractiveness of routes. - Narrow and interrupted footpaths. - Walking for both leisure and service. - Partly car dependent.	- Some space for pedestrians. No benches. - Medium attractiveness of routes - traffic. - Narrow and interrupted footpaths. - Walking for both leisure and service. - Car dependent.	- Some space for pedestrians. No benches. - Low attractiveness of routes - traffic. - Narrow and interrupted footpaths. - Walking mostly for leisure. - Car dependent.	- Adequate space for pedestrians. No benches. - High attractiveness of routes - no traffic. - Footpaths of adequate width – incomplete network. - Walking only for leisure. - Exclusively car dependent.
Indicator: infrastructures	- Green and shade: limited. - Streets and footpaths: cared for but narrow.	- Green and shade: adequate. - Streets and footpaths cared for.	- Green and shade: adequate. - Streets and footpaths cared for.	- Green and shade: limited. - Streets and footpaths: cared for and sufficient.
EXCLUSION				
Indicator: accessibility	Adequate foot access to retail, services and amenities.	Adequate foot access to retail, services and amenities.	Medium foot access to retail, services and amenities.	Difficult foot access to retail, services and amenities.
Indicator: human presence	Moderate	Moderate	Moderate	Low
Indicator: social contacts	Moderate to inadequate	Moderate	Moderate	Satisfactory

Late suburbia was lacking in the assessed dimensions but fell into the positive stereotype of newly built, low-density suburbia. Suburban subareas provide numerous and more amenable on-street parking places in close proximity to every dwelling. Older adults can use cars with limited traffic and parking stress. Parking difficulty was a very significant and frequent issue that prevents social contact and servicing. In the end, proximity did not equate to access.

Planning and urban design perceptions about 'age-friendly places' needed to become more informed about exclusion causes: how could the ASE triangle explain such exclusion processes? In the case study, where older adults of *Pallouriotissa* are car-dependent and active commuters, the attribute of accessibility and ease of car use was dominant. In many cases, it could define the range of older people's daily social contacts or even their level of happiness. Exclusion was perceived as the prevention of self-servicing or the loss of the lifestyle and commuting habits of the residents' early lives. On the other hand, older adults with disabilities could be excluded in the same way, regardless of the subarea they live in. Therefore, in the case of the initial old quarter area, *space* would not maintain its exclusive negative content, if *age* attributes were defined differently. Under this focus, *age* and *exclusion* may create a different perception or assessment of exactly the same place. Place assessment on the other hand has to consider the gravity of each indicator, especially those that vary for each user group. In this case in particular, the ease of car use is much more highly appreciated than all the other spatial aspects together.

15.5 Conclusion

There is no spaceless ageing and every placing of an (older) person has effects on their daily life. This chapter focuses on this interdependence, not simply limiting space to its physical dimensions. Such a concept is too narrow from our point of view and leads to a neglect of any spatial dimension beyond Euclidian definitions. In the case studies presented, space is also an emotional and social category. Places are actively visited, but the pathways planned for older people tend to be avoided by them. Objective reasons are never decisive in themselves.

In our analysis, we attempt to 'upgrade space' as a theory-led idea. Clearly, such a perspective has already been presented, for example in some of the seminal work within human geography (Rowles 1978). However, while Rowles continuously explored the "meaning of space" in an accurate and useful way for exploring new avenues in gerontology, his contribution rarely refers to critical (French/German) theory. Very interestingly, his perception of space, for older people at home, as a "surveillance zone" (Rowles 1981) does not refer to Foucault's panopticon; or, more recently, his interpretation of space as "habituation" of (little) changes in the meaning of place (Rowles 2000) neglects the "habitus" concept of Bourdieu. By referring to Lefebvre, our model clearly took the potential of such critical thinkers, *i.e.* the capacity to take into account the "meaning" of space as we age (as explored by Rowles), *and simultaneously* assumes contradictory conceptions of space. This is efficiently described within the first case study where the perception of space by Anne, due to the new development, is compared to the neglect of older people's perceptions during the planning phase of such development, in Greater Dublin.

In so doing, we clearly follow a similar avenue as the one suggested by Andrews and his colleagues (Andrews et al. 2013), *i.e.* contributing to a more complex and relational conception of space/place and age. While Andrews and his colleagues explores the crossings of "environmental gerontology" and of "geographical gerontology", they also acknowledge the general "spatial turn" in health and social sciences and the consequence of placing a higher importance on communities and the environment. Challenging the "static" vision of space and place in research, their model explores the potential of affects, following the human geography discipline. While affects are not central in our model, they nevertheless are part of the perceived space described in our two case studies. But most important, while Andrews and colleagues refer to public policies, they insist on the importance of global models of place and aging, like the WHO "age-friendly cities" strategy and indicators, to take better account of qualitative aspects of spatial life, like affects, to understand local variabilities. In our Cyprian example, the ASE Triangle directly helps to identify the limits of such indicators, where little attention is given to exclusion as a process. Therefore, in this case in the initial old quarter area, *space* would not maintain its exclusive negative content, if *age* attributes were defined differently. With such an example, we also admit that both our cases studies concern cities and their processes of suburbanization.

By arguing for a theoretically-based model inspired by critical thinkers, we hope to have contributed to a more complex and relational understanding of not only the "experience" of space, but of space and exclusion and the plurality of mechanisms that construct such experiences (*i.e.* "representation of space" and "space of representation"). We hope that international gerontology will benefit from our challenging model.

Editors' Postscript

Please note, like other contributions to this book, this chapter was written before the COVID-19 pandemic of 2020. The book's introductory chapter (Chap. 1) and conclusion (Chap. 34) consider some of the key ways in which the pandemic relates to issues concerning social exclusion and ageing.

References

Andrews, G. J., Evans, J., & Wiles, J. L. (2013). Re-spacing and re-placing gerontology: Relationality and affect. *Ageing & Society, 33*(8), 1339–1373.

Atkinson, A. (1998). Social exclusion, poverty and unemployment. In: A. Atkinson, & J. Hills, (Eds.), *Exclusion, employment and opportunity* (pp. 1–20). STICERD, *London School of Economics Discussion Papers Series CASE/4*.

Barnes, M., Blom, A., Cox, K., Lessof, C., Walker, A. (2006). *The social exclusion of older people: Evidence from the first wave of the English Longitudinal Study of Ageing (ELSA)*. London, Office of the Deputy Prime Minister, Social Exclusion Unit.

Casey, E. S. (2000/1987). *Remembering. A phenomenological study* (2nd ed.). Bloomington: Indiana University Press.

Chakravarty, S. R., & D'Ambrosio, C. (2006). The measurement of social exclusion. *Review of Income and Wealth, 52*(3), 377–398.

Cope, M., & Elwood, S. (2009). *Qualitative GIS: A mixed methods approach*. Thousand Oaks: Sage.

Drilling, M., & Schnur, O. (2019). Neighbourhood research from a geographical perspective. *DIE ERDE – Journal of the Geographical Society of Berlin, 150*(2), 48–60.

Grove, H., (n.d.) *Exploring the everyday experiences of older people in Greater Dublin: A qualitative GIS approach*. PhD thesis, Maynooth University, Maynooth.

Hodge, I., Dunn, J., Monk, S., & Fitzgerald, M. (2002). Barriers to participation in residual rural labour markets. *Work, Employment & Society, 16*(3), 457–476.

Ioannou, B. (2018). Concepts of suburban development in Cyprus: the spatiality of ageing. In *Constructing an Urban Future. The spatiality and resilience of cities – infrastructures, communities and architectures*, March 18-19, 2018, Abu Dhabi University (UAE). http://architecturemps.com/wp-content/uploads/2019/01/AMPS-Proceedings-13-Constructing-an-Urban-Future.pdf

Lefebvre, H. (1991). *The social production of space*. Oxford: Blackwell.

Meijering, L., & Weitkamp, G. (2016). Numbers and narratives: Developing a mixed-methods approach to understand mobility in later life. *Social Science & Medicine, 168*, 200–206.

Milton, S., Pliakas, T., Hawkesworth, S., Nanchahal, K., Grundy, C., Amuzu, A., Casas, J. P., & Lock, K. (2015). A qualitative geographical information systems approach to explore how older people over 70 years interact with and define their neighbourhood environment. *Health & Place, 36*, 127–133.

Moulaert, T., Wanka, A., & Drilling, M. (2018). The social production of age, space and exclusion: Towards a more theory-driven understanding of spatial exclusion mechanisms in later life. *Sociální studia/Social Studies., 1*(2018), 9–23.

Rowles, G. D. (1978). *Prisoners of space? Exploring the geographical experience of older people*. Boulder: Westview Press.

Rowles, G. D. (1981). The surveillance zone as meaningful space for the aged. *The Gerontologist, 21*(3), 304–311.

Rowles, G. D. (2000). Habituation and being in place. *The Occupational Therapy Journal of Research, 20*(1_suppl), 52S–67S.

Silver, H. (1994). Social exclusion and social solidarity: Three paradigms. *International Labour Review, 133*(5-6), 531–578.

Urbaniak, A., & Walsh, K. (2019). The interrelationship between place and critical life transitions in later life social exclusion: A scoping review. *Health & Place, 60*, 102234.

Walsh, K., Scharf, T., & Keating, N. (2017). Social exclusion of older persons: A scoping review and conceptual framework. *European Journal of Ageing, 14*(1), 81–98.

Wanka, A., Moulaert, T., & Drilling, M. (2018). From environmental stress to spatial expulsion – Rethinking concepts of socio-spatial exclusion in later life. *International Journal of Ageing and Later Life, 12*(2), 25–51.

Warf, B. & Arias, S. (ed.) (2009). Introduction. In B. Warf, & S. Arias (Eds.), *The spatial turn. Interdisciplinary perspectives* (pp. 3–10). London: Routledge.

Wiles, J. (2005). Conceptualizing place in the care of older people: The contributions of geographical gerontology. *International Journal of Older People Nursing, 14*(8), 100–108.

World Health Organization. (2015). *Measuring the age friendliness of cities. A guide to using core indicators*. Geneva: WHO Library Cataloguing-in-Publication Data.

Chapter 16
The Relationship Between Place and Life-Course Transitions in Old-Age Social Exclusion: A Cross-Country Analysis

Anna Urbaniak, Anna Wanka, Kieran Walsh, and Frank Oswald

16.1 Introduction

The international literature recognises that places can provide a significant social, cultural and economic context for major transitions in older people's lives (Buffel et al. 2013). Beyond this, there is also recognition that such transitions are in themselves spatial as well as temporal in structure (Diewald 2016). Coupled with evidence that where someone lives can protect against or intensify exclusion in older-age (Walsh et al. 2019), the relationship older adults maintain with their residential environment is likely to play an important role in, and perhaps mediate, their experiences of major transitions and related outcomes. In the context of social exclusion of older people, and the need to advance knowledge of its multidimensional and relative nature, unpacking such a role is fundamental to understanding how disadvantage and advantage can accumulate across critical junctures of older people's lives.

A. Urbaniak (✉)
Irish Centre for Social Gerontology, Institute for Lifecourse and Society,
National University of Ireland Galway, Galway, Ireland

University of Vienna, Vienna, Austria
e-mail: anna.urbaniak@univie.ac.at

A. Wanka
University of Vienna, Vienna, Austria

Research Training Group 'Doing Transitions', Goethe University Frankfurt am Main,
Frankfurt am Main, Germany

K. Walsh
Irish Centre for Social Gerontology, Institute for Lifecourse and Society,
National University of Ireland Galway, Galway, Ireland

F. Oswald
Goethe University Frankfurt am Main, Frankfurt am Main, Germany

K. Walsh et al. (eds.), *Social Exclusion in Later Life*, International Perspectives
on Aging 28, https://doi.org/10.1007/978-3-030-51406-8_16

However, there is often a failure to think about normative transitions in older-age in spatial terms (Cutchin 2003). Furthermore, while transitions can sometimes underlie models of environmental adjustment and relocation (Golant 2011), theoretical formulations of person-environment interactions rarely explicitly interrogate their meaning for later life exclusionary and inclusionary experiences in place. These deficits sit amidst broader knowledge gaps concerning how older-age transitions, as a set of processes and events, might construct multifaceted disadvantage (Grenier 2012). As a first step in responding to these circumstances, this chapter aims to explore the role of older adult place relationships in the inclusions and exclusions that may arise from two types of transitions considered as normative in older-age.

Our analysis focuses on bereavement and retirement. Bereavement is a life event that becomes a part of nearly everyone's later life experience (Stroebe et al. 2007). Retirement can be defined as an individual's exit from the workforce at the end of their careers (Wang and Shi 2014). Both transitions can be viewed as critical processes of change that may not only impact on aspects of social connectivity in older age (Cavalli et al. 2007), but may also result in objective changes in position and power within a community, and a subjective re-positioning of self. The older adult place relationship can be understood as derived from subjective and symbolic elements (*e.g.* roles and attachments) that cross-cut spatial/geographic, embedded service infrastructure, and social and cultural dimensions of place (Andrews et al. 2013). We draw on the definition of multidimensional exclusion, and its six domains, outlined earlier by Walsh et al. (this volume), to inform our analysis.

First, we provide an overview of existing work on the relationship between life-course transitions, exclusion in later life and the older adult place relationship. Second, we draw on the concept of person-environment exchange processes, in this case spatial agency and belonging, as a potential conceptual tool to deconstruct this interrelationship. Third, we present case studies from Germany, Ireland and Poland, focusing on individual experiences of retirement and bereavement. We do not aim at a cultural comparison, but the identification of similarities in the role of place across jurisdictions. Finally, we draw conclusions from overall analysis with a view to informing future conceptual understandings of place and exclusion across the life course.

16.2 Transitions, Exclusion and Place

Research shows that life-course transitions are crucial periods of risk in which social inequalities and exclusion can be (re-)produced, contributing to an accumulation of disadvantage across the life course (Dannefer 2003; also see Ogg and Myck, and Van Regenmortel et al. this volume). The domains of social exclusion discussed vary by transition. Even though contemporary life-course approaches emphasise the embeddedness, contextuality, and relationality of transitions across people, time, and place (Wanka 2019), it is the social and temporal and not the spatial dimensions of these transitions that is the focus of most research. One exception is the field of relocation and (forced) migration in later life (De Jong Gierveld et al. 2015). Consequently, we know little about how places are involved and may mediate the relationship between life-course transitions and social exclusion.

Research suggests that different dimensions of place (*e.g.* infrastructure, services, neighbourhood networks), and particularly the relationship older adults maintain to their residential environment, can play a crucial role in buffering and intensifying social exclusion (Walsh et al. 2019). Several conceptual frameworks recognise the agency of communities in constructing and/or protecting against exclusion (Jehoel-Gijsbers and Vrooman 2008), while others highlight how environmental change can exclude some older residents across different domains (Scharf and Bartlam 2008). In empirical work, relationships with neighbours are often discussed as resources to prevent social exclusion (Marquet and Miralles-Guasch 2015), while risks might be exaggerated through service retrenchment, lack of social services, community deprivation and transport in rural settings (Warburton et al. 2014), and redevelopment and relocation processes, the built environment, clustered deprivation as well as crime and safety in urban environments (Scharf et al. 2002; see also Drilling et al. this section for illustrative cases of the impact of redevelopment and issues around perceived safety). In their review of the interrelationships between place, exclusion and life transitions, Urbaniak and Walsh (2019) demonstrate that mediating mechanisms of place can stem from subjective and symbolic elements, social and cultural aspects, embedded service infrastructure, and environmental change. Potential circularity in the relations between the place-relationship, social exclusion and transitions are summarised in Fig. 16.1 (adapted from Walsh 2018). Here, multidimensional exclusion in general, and that arising directly from life-course transitions, may be mediated by an older adult's place relationship. Conversely, these transitions may also alter or disrupt an older person's relationship with place and, vice versa, an older person's relationship with place may alter or disrupt transitions. Ultimately, however, studies that explicitly consider life-course transitions in place as crucial turning points for the (re-)production of social exclusion remain rare.

16.3 Older Adults' Place Relationships: The Role of Agency and Belonging

Here, we focus on processes of agency and belonging as two key aspects of older adults' place relationships (Wahl and Oswald 2010), and how they may provide insights into the interrelationship between place, social exclusion and life transitions.

Following Bandura (2006), agency refers to the process of becoming a change agent in one's own life by means of intentional and proactive behaviours imposed on the physical-social environment. Agency is defined as the general capacity of self-regulation embedded in environmental determinants. The focus of agency lies

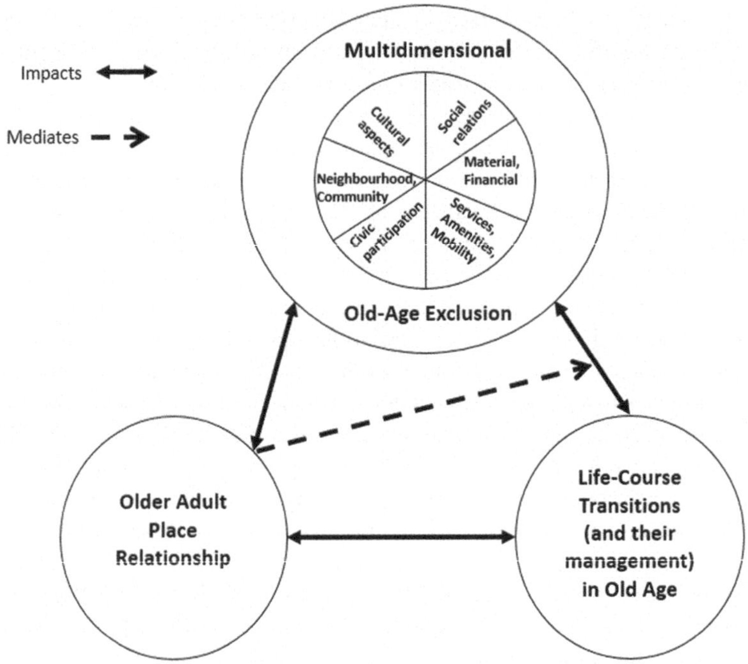

Fig. 16.1 Potential associations between older adults' place relationship, exclusion and transitions
Adapted from: Walsh 2018, p. 261

in actively making use of the objective physical-social environment, including acts of using, compensating, adapting, retrofitting, creating, and sustaining places. In contrast, belonging incorporates all non-goal-oriented cognitive and emotional aspects that make a space a place, the subjective and emotional evaluations and interpretations of places, as well as processes of attachment to places over time (Oswald and Wahl 2019). That is, belonging reflects the experiential connection of attachment and bonding with the physical environment (*e.g.* home as a refuge, personally meaningful objects), the social environment (*e.g.* family members, community of people) and their intersection (Rowles 1983). Whereas spatial agency is assumed to decrease from middle to late adulthood, place attachment and belonging is considered to increase.

However, within environmental gerontology, there have been calls for a more fine-graded situational perspective of spatial agency and belonging in older adults' everyday lives (Chaudhury and Oswald 2019). Such a situational perspective can inform understandings of how spatial agency and belonging evolve dynamically across the life course, change during the course of life-course transitions, and potentially impact on multiple domains of social exclusion. Across the life course, phases of increased agentic behaviour may alternate with phases of decreased agency. The same is possible for belonging.

With reference to Fig. 16.1, agency and belonging can be considered to play a key role within an older person's relationship with place operating across subjective and symbolic elements, and spatial/geographic, embedded service infrastructure, and social and cultural dimensions of place. Thus, a capacity for agency and belonging may mediate exclusion arising from transitions, or may in themselves be altered by those transitions. Table 16.1 summarises potential risks of such life-course transitions, and the mediating role spatial agency and belonging can play.

To explore how such risks and mediators of life-course transitions play out in individual life stories, we turn to empirical cases.

Table 16.1 The mediating role of agency and belonging processes in the face of critical life transitions and their effect on social exclusion in later life

Domains of social exclusion	Potential risks/ negative effects of transition	Mediating role of spatial agency	Mediating role of belonging
Social relations	Withdrawal from social networks	Making new or tightening existing relationships with neighbours (this might in turn increase one's sense of belonging)	Sense of belonging to the local community might psychologically comfort and compensate for the experienced losses
	R: Loss of working colleagues		
	B: Loss of significant other		
Material and financial resources	Decrease in material and financial resources	Relocation to a more affordable area or downsizing to make up for/cope with a reduced financial resources (this might in turn decrease one's sense of belonging)	Sense of belonging to the local community might psychologically compensate for lack of material and financial resources
	R: Decrease in employment income		
	B: Loss of spousal income		
Civic participation	Withdrawal from civic activities	Actively engaging in local volunteering (this might in turn increase one's sense of belonging)	Sense of belonging to a local community might prevent withdrawal from (local) civic activities
	R: Loss of role as an active union member		
	B: Loss of connection to clubs and parties		
Socio-cultural aspects	Loss of social roles and identity	Actively making use of local opportunities to develop new roles (this might in turn increase one's sense of belonging)	Sense of belonging might strengthen/create a local identity that compensates for identity loss
	R: Loss of professional role and identity		
	B: Loss of the role of a child/ spouse; loss of couple identity		

(continued)

Table 16.1 (continued)

Domains of social exclusion	Potential risks/ negative effects of transition	Mediating role of spatial agency	Mediating role of belonging
Services, amenities and mobility	Loss of mobility, decreased access to services and amenities	Actively supporting existing and/or creating new services within one's community	Sense of belonging might psychologically compensate shortcomings in local service infrastructure and diminish needs for mobility
	R: Loss of access to services granted by a former employer		
	B: Loss of mobility after the death of primary driver		

Note: potential risks/negative effects of transition: R – retirement transition; B – bereavement transition

16.4 Illustrative Cases

In this section, we present four empirical cases. In the first two cases of Harald and Krystyna, we focus on the mutual relationship between life-course transitions, spatial agency and sense of belonging. Since the transitions have been experienced fairly recently in each case, we cannot yet draw conclusions about the long-term effects of exclusionary impacts of transitions. With the subsequent cases of Jan and Patricia, we hence investigate further the interrelationships between transitions, older adults' place relationships and social exclusion.

The presented cases stem from three projects: "Interrelationship between life-course ruptures and place in old-age social exclusion – PLACED-Lives" (Ireland), "Social construction of retirement" (Poland), and "Doing Retiring" (Germany). Data collection in all projects focused on the experiences of older people in each of their areas and their experiences of different transitions in older-age. All projects follow a qualitative methodological approach and use a combination of narrative and problem-centred interviews for data collection. For the purpose of our analysis, first interviews, field notes and memos from the original studies were organised and thematically analysed (Braun and Clarke 2006) in order to capture the role of place in the bereavement and retirement transitions. Then, based on a group discussion, four illustrative cases were chosen to render visible in different ways the relationship between place, life-course transitions and social exclusion.

Case 1: Bereavement, Spatial Agency and Belonging

Harald's story illustrates how spatial agency and belonging can intensify when experiencing bereavement, and how this enhanced relationship to his residential environment helped him cope with his father's death.

Harald is 63 years old, married and has three adult children. He lives with his wife in a suburban town in Germany, and has hardly ever engaged in the life of his community. When his father died, Harald inherited his father's house and has since spent his days sorting out, looking through memories, and making plans for the future. In this process, however, he has become more locally involved. He got in touch with many local charities and people and this engenders a renewed attachment to his hometown.

When friends and acquaintances started long-distance travel in retirement, Harald realised that his preference was to spend time in his neighbourhood. For the future he wants his daughter and two grandchildren to move into the basement of his father's former home:

> 'The house, and the sorting out – it reminds me that I have a past here; and when my children and grandchildren move here, too, also a future.'

Case 2: Retirement, Spatial Agency and Belonging

Krystyna's story illustrates how retiring can negatively impact one's sense of belonging, but at the same time help to increase spatial agency.

Krystyna is 61 years old, single, has no children and lives alone in a medium-sized town in the south of Poland. She worked as a CEO in a large international company, but was forced to retire at age 55 years. Krystyna's experience of retirement has been characterised by feelings of exclusion from her employment and a loss of the role she had invested so much in:

> 'Financially, I'm really better off... but... it's about my dignity. I gave everything to this company [...] and am I now supposed to be a retiree who does nothing?'

Due to Krystyna's focus on her career she neglected to spend time embedding herself in her neighbourhood. Because of this, she has not developed a strong sense of belonging and has not relied on her community to support her in making her transition into retirement. Instead, Krystyna is looking to build relations with new places and people. This is evident in her purchase of a new apartment in a metropolitan city. While she wants to enjoy living there, at the same time she is not yet ready to move in permanently. As a result, she finds herself *betwixt and between* her hometown and the metropolitan city: "I feel that I'm somehow torn between here and there."

Case 3: The Mediating Role of Agency and Belonging in the Retirement Transition

Jan's story illustrates how retiring can intensify social exclusion, and how spatial agency can contribute to buffering these negative outcomes – at least in some domains of social exclusion.

Jan is 54 years old, married and has no children. He lives in a village with his wife and care-dependent mother-in-law. He has worked in various jobs and has regularly changed his place of residence. Therefore, he has not developed a strong sense of belonging to any place. In his early 50s, Jan became unemployed, was diagnosed with depression, and now receives a small disability pension. Losing touch with his former colleagues, Jan feels lonely and anxious. He has not been able to make any contacts or engage in the neighbourhood, and misses feeling like he belongs to a community:

> 'I was getting more and more anxious. Nobody calls, nobody knows what I'm doing, nobody cares, no friends, no employer. The employer at least had a social responsibility. When you are retired, you get your pension benefits, but apart from that, you get nothing. Who's supposed to care?'

At some point, however, Jan got in touch with an initiative in charge of organising intergenerational co-housing facilities. Finally, he and his wife moved into one of their housing projects. In this new home he has found a new sense of community both within the co-housing initiative and across the surrounding neighbourhood. Jan has now started to engage in various civic activities:

> 'And that's the reason for co-housing, because all of us want to grow old together, in one house, one community. Car-sharing, growing food together, saving money, saving CO2. And we are a gain for the neighbourhood, too – that's why we receive public funding. And we'll build benches and put them in front of the supermarket for old people to rest, and our theme nights are open to the public [...].'

While the transition to retirement made Jan feel lonely and socially excluded, the neighbourhood initiative helped him to find a community and build sustainable relationships with his neighbours.

Case 4: The Mediating Role of Agency and Belonging in the Bereavement Transition

Patricia's case illustrates how bereavement, place and social exclusion are intertwined in long-term effects of exclusionary impacts of a transition.

Patricia is 80 years old, widowed and has four children. She lives alone in a city in Ireland where she worked as a civil servant before she retired. Patricia's husband died unexpectedly when she was 59 years old. Before bereavement, she was primarily involved with her family and, while she had limited social contacts within the local community, she highlights the role of her neighbours during the transition into widowhood and talks specifically about the reciprocity of relationships:

> 'So these neighbours now they did come in for an hour and just check on me during the day and offer to drive me shopping or whatever as well because they knew that I didn't drive, in fact it's the other way around now because he [neighbour's husband] has passed away and I drive her because she never drove.'

Patricia indicates that the death of her husband was a particular turning point for her relationship with her community, where she is now embedded in networks of reciprocity and support. Over the years, this has expanded to civic activities she is engaged in and depends also on an experiential dimension in relation to her new roles within the community:

> 'Yeah I mean I'm proud of the life I've made for myself in [name of the city] and the fact that I have got so involved in my retirement [active retirement group] [...] I just feel I'm making a contribution that way you know.'

16.5 Discussion

We analysed four cases representing different stages and different settings of two types of life-course transition: bereavement and retirement. The aim was not to compare across cultures, but to highlight potential similarities in the insights that we can gather in applying a place lens to life-course transitions. The results show that bereavement and retirement impact across different domains of social exclusion and that their impacts might be mediated by spatial agency and belonging, as constituting forces within an older person's relationship with place.

Harald's and Patricia's cases illustrate the relationships between bereavement, place, and social exclusion. Harald's story demonstrates how, during the early stages of bereavement, older adults might become more agentic and develop a more intense sense of belonging to their neighbourhood. The increased involvement with his community, which might be perceived as exercising agency in place (Wahl and Oswald 2010), helped Harald to cope with his loss, knowing that, things once belonging to his parents can be used by others in the community. This newfound place-attachment might not only help in coping with transitions, but also potentially buffer exclusionary outcomes of future transitions. Patricia's story demonstrates not only the capacity of community to offer support against social exclusion that might arise from bereavement, but also the potential of individual agency in drawing on different dimensions of person-environment exchange processes (relational aspects of community, social connectivity and sense of belonging) and ultimately reinforcing the person-place relationship as a means to combat possible disadvantage in the exclusion domains of social relations, civic participation and socio-cultural aspects.

The cases of Harald and Patricia represent two different types of bereavement, yet they show similarities with regard to their interrelationships with place. Before experiencing bereavement, both were not particularly involved in their neighbourhoods. However, this changed in the course of the transition: both started to engage in local organisations, made new contacts, and acquired a renewed sense of home (Oswald and Wahl 2013). In both cases, agency (as openness and engagement in activities and social contacts in the neighbourhood) and belonging (as feeling at home and attached) to their neighbourhood increased. However, the timing *when* place would become relevant in the transition process differed: whereas Patricia's neighbours helped her cope with her grief from an early stage, Harald's spatial engagement occurred later in the process and was primarily mediated via the home and the objects he inherited.

We used the cases of Krystyna and Jan to illustrate relationships between retirement, place, and social exclusion. Krystyna's story highlights how during the liminal stage (Turner 1964) of the retirement transition, one's sense of belonging can diminish even if one's spatial agency increases. Krystyna's sense of belonging (Rubinstein 1989) to her hometown was mainly based upon professional connections that broke after retiring and her sense of belonging after transitioning decreased. At the same time, however, her agency increased, and she actively uses it to create new relationships to a new place. Jan's case highlights how transitions into retirement might result in exclusionary experiences across domains of social relations, material and financial resources and socio-cultural aspects. Through his spatial agency and sense of belonging, these effects are moderated as he tries to build up sustainable neighbourhood support networks among his co-housing neighbours, which could mediate his disadvantaged position through a newly established sense of belonging.

Both cases, albeit from the different cultural settings of Germany and Poland, represent similarities. They resonate with literature on the negative health and well-being impacts of involuntary exit from the labour market (Hershey and Henkens 2013). Both Krystyna and Jan lack a particular sense of belonging to their residential environment. Yet, place becomes relevant in their transitions, albeit in different ways. Whereas Krystyna acts out her liminal status by travelling and refusing to settle down, Jan longs for a sense of community and home, and relocates to an intergenerational housing facility to obtain it.

Whereas the four cases portray how place, and especially older adult's relationship to place, can mediate the relationship between life-course transitions and social exclusion, this mediating effect is not equally significant for all domains of social exclusion. In our cases, the buffering effect of the older adult's relationship to place was stronger for the domains of exclusion from social relationships, civic exclusion, and socio-cultural exclusion and less pronounced for the domains of economic exclusion and service exclusion. However, we can think of mediating effects on these domains, for example in neighbourhoods that undergo gentrification processes, where newly retired people decide to start their businesses.

Moreover, it is not only spatial agency and belonging that can mediate exclusionary processes, but vice versa. In all four cases, the possibilities to exert agency and gain a sense of belonging were facilitated by an accessible social and service infrastructure, involving clubs, voluntary organisations, or cultural initiatives. Patricia, for example, had many civic participation opportunities that she decided to pursue which allowed her to build a stronger sense of belonging that gave her a new identity, not only as a widow but as an active member of her local community. The same holds true for Jan, who could not have exerted agency in the way he did without the opportunity of an existing cohousing initiative. Krystyna and Jan relocated to access a better, more available and diverse infrastructure. Even though the cases show how spatial agency can buffer the exclusionary impacts of life-course transitions, to exert this kind of agency the respective infrastructure needs to be in place, or people need to have sufficient resources to relocate to another area – and this does not hold true for all environments and all people [see Cholat and Daconto, this volume].

16.6 Conclusion

The aim of this chapter was to explore the role of the older-adult place relationship in forms of inclusion and exclusion that may arise from two types of transitions in later life. Focusing on bereavement and retirement, we explored the complex and multidimensional exchanges between place, life-course transitions and social exclusion using four case studies from three countries. The intention was not to produce a cross-comparative cultural analysis of these relationships, but to identify potential broad commonalities in how these different factors might interrelate. Based upon these cases, we argued that there are a number of ways in which place can be involved with life-course transitions and the forms of exclusion that may sometimes arise. This includes the ways in which life-course transitions can impact on older people's relationship with place, how place can impact on the experiences of transitions themselves and how, in particular, the person-environment exchange processes of agency and belonging have the potential to hinder or magnify social exclusion that might result from life-course transitions. The presented cases are not suited to capturing the entire complexity of the interchanges between person and environments during life-course transitions, and in particular the degree of circularity in the dynamics between place, transitions and exclusion. However, the choice of cases demonstrates how spatial agency and a sense of belonging might mediate not only the way in which one experiences life-course transitions, but the way in which the transition may impact on different domains of social exclusion. Hence, certain levels of spatial agency and belonging can buffer the negative effects of life-course transitions on social exclusion, if they are enabled by respective local opportunities.

This chapter demonstrates why it is necessary to consider more actively the role of place, and the role older adults play in exerting agency in place, in processes of transition. It is exactly the interplay between locally existing opportunity structures and the way older adults make use of them and relate to them that can help buffer negative effects of life-course transitions on social exclusion in later life. Hence, simply stressing the role of individual agency is not sufficient – policy and practice instead need to enable older adults to exert spatial agency and develop a sense of belonging within a community, for example through supporting local initiatives for older adults.

This chapter has been exploratory in nature, and only in parts has hinted at macro and structural factors underlying the presented cases. Hence, we need to develop a more advanced and systematic understanding of the relationship between place, life-course transitions and social exclusion for further development of ageing policies that aim at combating social exclusion. Future research should systematically consider the ways in which national, cultural and structural contexts, different sorts of transitions, the diversity of people, neighbourhoods and communities might intersect with the role of place in exclusion arising from life-course transitions over time. This is necessary before we can conceptually map the dynamics of these complex forces with any certainty and explore their influence over the lived experience of older people in place. Nevertheless, our analysis has begun to unpack some of these dynamics and illustrates how we might begin the process of harnessing place to support older people at particular risk junctures in their lives.

Editors' Postscript

Please note, like other contributions to this book, this chapter was written before the COVID-19 pandemic of 2020. The book's introductory chapter (Chap. 1) and conclusion (Chap. 34) consider some of the key ways in which the pandemic relates to issues concerning social exclusion and ageing.

References

Andrews, G. J., Evans, J., & Wiles, J. L. (2013). Re-spacing and re-placing gerontology: Relationality and affect. *Ageing and Society, 33*(8), 1339–1373.

Bandura, A. (2006). Toward a psychology of human agency. *Perspectives on Psychological Science, 1*, 164–180.

Braun, V., & Clarke, V. (2006). Using thematic analysis in psychology. *Qualitative Research in Psychology, 3*(2), 77–101.

Buffel, T., Phillipson, C., & Scharf, T. (2013). Experiences of neighbourhood exclusion and inclusion among older people living in deprived inner-city areas in Belgium and England. *Ageing and Society, 33*(1), 89–109. https://doi.org/10.1017/S0144686X12000542.

Cavalli, S., Bickel, J. F., & Lalive d'Epinay, C. J. (2007). Exclusion in very old age: The impact of three critical life events. *International Journal of Ageing and Later Life, 2*, 9–31.

Chaudhury, H., & Oswald, F. (2019). Advancing understanding of person-environment interaction in later life: One step further. *Journal of Aging Studies, 51*, 100821. https://doi.org/10.1016/j.jaging.2019.100821.

Cutchin, M. P. (2003). The process of mediated aging-in-place: A theoretically and empirically based model. *Social Science & Medicine, 57*(6), 1077–1090.

Dannefer, D. (2003). Cumulative advantage/disadvantage and the life course: Cross-fertilizing age and social science theory. *The Journals of Gerontology Series B: Psychological Sciences and Social Sciences, 58*, 327–337.

De Jong Gierveld, J., Van der Pas, S., & Keating, N. (2015). Loneliness of older immigrant groups in Canada: Effects of ethnic-cultural background. *Journal of Cross-Cultural Gerontology, 30*, 251–268.

Diewald, M. (2016). Life course risks and welfare states' risk management. In M. J. Shanahan, J. T. Mortimer, & M. K. Johnson (Eds.), *Handbook of life course* (pp. 677–687). Cham: Springer.

Golant, S. M. (2011). The quest for residential normalcy by older adults: Relocation but one pathway. *Journal of Aging Studies, 25*, 193–205. https://doi.org/10.1016/j.jaging.2011.03.003.

Grenier, A. (2012). *Transitions and the lifecourse: Challenging the constructions of growing old.* Bristol: Policy Press.

Hershey, D. A., & Henkens, K. (2013). Impact of different types of retirement transitions on perceived satisfaction with life. *The Gerontologist, 54*(2), 232–244.

Jehoel-Gijsbers, G., & Vrooman, C. (2008). *Social exclusion of the elderly: A comparative study of EU member states.* http://aei.pitt.edu/9443/2/9443.pdf. Accessed 7 Jan 2020.

Marquet, O., & Miralles-Guasch, C. (2015). The Walkable city and the importance of the proximity environments for Barcelona's everyday mobility. *Cities, 42*, 258–266.

Oswald, F., & Wahl, H.W. (2013). Creating and sustaining homelike places in own home environments. In G. D. Rowles & M. Bernard (Eds.), *Environmental gerontology* (pp. 53–77). New York: Springer.

Oswald, F., & Wahl, H.W. (2019). Physical contexts and behavioral aging. In *Oxford research encyclopedia of psychology*. Oxford: Oxford University Press. https://doi.org/10.1093/acrefore/9780190236557.013.399.

Rowles, G. D. (1983). Geographical dimensions of social support in rural Appalachia. In G. D. Rowles & R. J. Ohta (Eds.), *Aging and milieu: Environmental perspectives on growing old* (pp. 111–130). New York: Academic.

Rubinstein, R. L. (1989). The home environments of older people: A description of the psychosocial processes linking person to place. *Journal of Gerontology: Social Sciences, 44*(2), 45–53. https://doi.org/10.1093/geronj/44.2.S45.

Scharf, T., & Bartlam, B. (2008). Ageing and social exclusion in rural communities. In N. Keating (Ed.), *Rural ageing: A good place to grow old?* (pp. 97–108). Bristol: Policy Press.

Scharf, T., Phillipson, C., Smith, A., & Kingston, P. (2002). *Growing older in socially deprived areas: Social exclusion in later life*. London: Help the Aged. https://www.ageuk.org.uk/documents/en-gb/for-professionals/communities-and-inclusion/id2255_a_growing_older_in_socially_deprived_areas_social_exclusion_in_later_life_2002_pro.pdf?dtrk=true. Accessed 7 Jan 2020.

Stroebe, M., Schut, H., & Stroebe, W. (2007). Health outcomes of bereavement. *The Lancet, 370*(9603), 1960–1973.

Turner, V. (1964). Betwixt and between: The liminal period in rites of passage. In J. Helm (Ed.), *Symposium on new approaches to the study of religion. Proceedings of the 1964 annual spring meeting of the American Ethnological Association* (pp. 4–20). Seattle: University of Washington Press.

Urbaniak, A., & Walsh, K. (2019). The interrelationship between place and critical life transitions in later life social exclusion: A scoping review. *Health & Place, 60*, 102234. https://doi.org/10.1016/j.healthplace.2019.102234.

Wahl, H.W., & Oswald, F. (2010). Environmental perspectives on aging. In D. Dannefer & C. Phillipson (Eds.), *International handbook of social gerontology* (pp. 111–124). London: Sage.

Walsh, K. (2018). Constructions of old-age social exclusion: In place and shaped by place. In M. Skinner, G. Andrews, & M. Cutchin (Eds.), *Geographical gerontology: Concepts and approaches* (pp. 252–266). London: Routledge.

Walsh, K., O'Shea, E., & Scharf, T. (2019). Rural old-age social exclusion: A conceptual framework on mediators of exclusion across the lifecourse. *Ageing and Society*, 1–27. https://doi.org/10.1017/S0144686X19000606.

Wang, M., & Shi, J. (2014). Psychological research on retirement. *Annual Review of Psychology, 65*, 209–233. https://doi.org/10.1146/annurev-psych-010213-115131.

Wanka, A. (2019). Change ahead—Emerging life-course transitions as practical accomplishments of growing old(er). *Frontiers in Sociology*. Online first: https://doi.org/10.3389/fsoc.2018.00045.

Warburton, J., Cowan, S., Winterton, R., et al. (2014). Building social inclusion for rural older people using information and communication technologies: Perspectives of rural practitioners. *Australian Social Work, 67*, 479–494.

Chapter 17
Ageing and Caring in Rural Environments: Cross-National Insights from Central Europe

Lucie Vidovićová, Monika Alisch, Susanne Kümpers, and Jolanta Perek-Białas

17.1 Introduction

In this chapter we discuss how difficulties in receiving undisrupted, good quality care can be understood as place-based social exclusion. We concentrate on the provision of broadly defined care services in rural areas, combining knowledge from three neighbouring European countries: Czechia, Germany and Poland [this and related topics have been addressed in section IV within Cholat and Dacanto, and Széman et al. this volume from the perspective of service exclusion]. Although these countries differ in size, degree of rurality, and in the ways older adult care services are organised, all three nations identify the social inclusion of older rural dwellers as a particular policy and practice concern.

Spatial exclusion can be located at the intersection of exclusion from social relationships, services, and the cultural and identity aspects of place in later life (Vidovićová and Tournier this section). Here, we understand place and space as an essential condition for the realisation of all social interactions, including the provision of care as a special type of both formal and informal interaction. As such, spatial factors can represent a significant set of mechanisms of social exclusion, leading to unintended and unwanted outcomes, such as reductions in mobility, community engagement and social participation (Buffel et al. 2013).

We adopt Walsh's (2018) approach and recognise embedded services, amenities and the built environment as encompassing exclusion from services embedded in

L. Vidovićová (✉)
Masaryk University, Brno, Czechia
e-mail: vidovicova@fss.muni.cz

M. Alisch · S. Kümpers
Fulda University of Applied Sciences, Fulda, Germany

J. Perek-Białas
Jagiellonian University, Kraków, Poland

K. Walsh et al. (eds.), *Social Exclusion in Later Life*, International Perspectives on Aging 28, https://doi.org/10.1007/978-3-030-51406-8_17

and delivered into place as a dimension of exclusionary processes. Recognising the multifaceted nature of social exclusion (Moffatt and Glasgow 2009) helps us to see how rural places per se are often perceived as marginal (Hooks et al. 2016), and how living (and caring) in rural areas is thus often understood as yet another minority status intersecting older-age (Vidovićová 2018). Evidence from various countries has demonstrated that professional services in rural areas are often less accessible, less specialised and more expensive than in urban settings (Kaye and Butler 2004; Goins et al. 2011), producing a form of spatial ageism or geographical injustice (Schlosberg 2007). However, how these processes operate in the contexts of Central European states has been rarely explored, and this chapter aims to address this gap.

For the cases studied here we employ a broad understanding of "care". Knijn and Kremer (1997, p. 330) suggest that "care includes the provision of daily social, psychological, emotional and physical attention for people". We will refer to care and support services as having various meanings, as this broad definition of care and caring activities include formalised and paid service provision as well as different forms of informal care activities. Thus, care will be understood as any activity, related to older people as primary recipients, undertaken with the goal of supporting their health and well-being and working against their exclusion.

Our approach combines country-level case studies (using aggregate statistical data) with a brief exploratory analysis of a European comparative survey (EU-SILC) to examine urban/rural differences in two arenas: first, we use the take-up of professional home care services as a proxy indicator of the availability of formal services (in the sense that they are provided, affordable, suited to, and actually needed by, older people); second, we compare data on retired people providing informal care or assistance in rural and urban areas, to examine the essential role of informal carers and more generally of volunteerism (Milligan and Conradson 2006) in rural settings.

17.2 Czechia, Germany and Poland – The Country Cases

With reference to Table 17.1, Czechia, Germany and Poland possess slightly different welfare regimes, socio-physical environments and cultures of expectation regarding care and support in later life (Mai et al. 2008), which in turn affect the ways care is provided to older adults within families and communities in rural areas. These three European countries are special cases within the EU, lying on the north-south and east-west divides evident in data on quality of life of rural dwellers (Eurofound 2019). Czechia and Poland have recently recovered from socialist experiments and still have much in common with other Eastern European countries. However, Poles and Czechs living in rural areas, according to the European Quality of Life Survey "EQLS" (Eurofound 2019), are not particularly deprived in terms of financial hardship and life satisfaction, which are problems often found in rural areas of Eastern and South European countries. As Table 17.1 shows, there was a dynamic change in at-risk-of poverty and exclusion rates between 2010 and 2018,

Table 17.1 Physical and population characteristics of Czechia, Germany and Poland (selection)

		CZ	DE	PL
Population (2019)	mio	10.69	83.10	38.38
Land area	km^2	78,668	357,386	321,679
Population density (2018)	pop/km^2	134	232	123
Sectoral contribution to gross value added (2019) % of value added OECD EU Average: Agriculture 1.6%; Industry 18.7%; Services 73.9%	Agriculture 1996	4.0	1.1	5.8
	Agriculture	2.1	0.9	2.3
	Industry	29.6	24.2	25.1
	Services	62.4	69.3	64.9
Employment rate (2016) (%)	Rural	71.3	77.4	62.5
	Town	71.6	75.3	63.1
	City	73.2	72.3	67.9
People at risk of poverty or social exclusion (%) [ilc_peps13]	2010 Rural	16.1	22.8	33.9
	2010 Urban	12.5	20.8	21.1
	2018 Rural	11.6	17.5	25.3
	2018 Urban	12.0	22.4	13.4
At-risk-of-poverty rate (%) [ilc_li43]	2010 Rural	10.2	18.8	23.5
	2010 Urban	8.2	16.2	11.0
	2018 Rural	9.2	15.8	21.2
	2018 Urban	9.5	18.4	9.6
Share of rural population (%) OECD	Rural	21.1	15.7	35.1
	Of which remote	–	2.2	6.4
Share of 65+ in total population (%)	1976	13.2	14.6	11.0
	1996	13.3	15.6	11.2
	2016	18.3	21.1	16.0
	2019	19.6	21.5	17.7
Share of 65+ in rural population (%) OECD 2019	Rural	20.3	22.6	17.0
	Rural and remote	(n.a.)	23.8	16.6
Share of 80+ in rural population (%) OECD 2019 (%) OECD	2019	4.3	6.8	4.3
Life expectancy at 65 (2015) – in years	Women	19.4	21.0	20.1
	Men	15.9	17.9	15.7
Healthy life expectancy at 65 (2015) – in years	Women	8.6	12.3	8.4
	Men	8.0	11.4	7.6
Living alone at 65+ (2015)	%	32.4	28.2	33.7

Sources: Eurostat; At risk poverty – EU-SILC, table [ilc_li43]; OECD 2010; OECD Regional Demography Database; https://stats.oecd.org/Index.aspx?DataSetCode=REGION_DEMOGR#; Agriculture, forestry, fishing, % of value added, 2005–2019; OECD National Accounts Statistics: National Accounts at a Glance (https://data.oecd.org/natincome/value-added-by-activity.htm)

which is important to note as previous research has shown that the national economy contexts actually make a difference in levels of urban vs. rural poverty (Hooks et al. 2016; Shucksmith and Brown 2016). We draw on Table 17.1 and other data to provide a brief contextual description of the three country cases.

Czechia is a midsize European country with more than ten million inhabitants, of which about one-fifth live in rural areas. There are few remote rural areas, especially in the context of international comparisons. The areas with the most challenges are found in so-called inner peripheries, *i.e.* peripheral regions located in the inner parts of the country, mainly along the borders of the administrative regions (*kraje*) (Musil and Müller 2008). While these include some rural parts, they are primarily the peripheral zones of metropolitan areas and regional centres, some of which are characterised by depopulation and difficulties in creating employment and in improving public transport and service access. This means that the problems usually documented in the rural literature are not exclusive to, or most prevalent in, rural Czech settings.

The population of rural areas are generally not declining, especially those with more than 500 inhabitants and outside the inner peripheries (Bernard and Šimon 2017). As a result, the ageing of the population is equally pronounced in big urban centres and small rural settlements. Older adult formal care services are governed by the principle of subsidiarity, with the regional and local governments having the main responsibility to provide services to citizens, including social care (Průša et al. 2015; Bareš and Víšek 2016). Regional governments also operate residential care and nursing homes. Finance is mostly provided to regional governments and/or care and service providers from the national budget. There is a cash benefit for frail people to cover the extra cost of services if needed, but long waiting lists for the required medical assessment for this benefit result in a high rate of non-take-up. Financing and quality are the most common issues in the political debates on care provision, since the regional availability of social services is considered medium to satisfactory, for both urban and rural regions (Průša et al. 2015).

There are also regional networks of charity and not-for-profit professional organisations active in providing various types of service (including care) to older people in rural areas. These networks are usually located in smaller regional centres, administrative districts of municipalities with extended competence ("*obce s rozšířenou působností*" (ORP)), serving older dwellers in surrounding villages (15–25 km). Non-professional care work is done almost exclusively by family members (Galčanová and Staveník 2020), community involvement in older adult support services has only a weak cultural tradition (see Table 17.2).

Germany has almost eight times the population of Czechia and is the most populous country in the EU with almost 83 million inhabitants. Germany also has the highest population density of the three nations, reflecting the fact that only 16% live in rural areas and only 2% of the population live in remote rural areas. While the agricultural sector is contracting, as with the other two countries (Destatis 2016), Germany is one of the few EU nations to actually have higher employment rates in rural places than in towns and cities.

Table 17.2 Czechia: Who helps rural dwellers 60+ with household chores and self-care?

	Help in the household (%)	Help with self-care (%)
Partner	48	6
Daughter	18	5
Son	10	3
Daughter-in-law	5	2
Son-in-law	1	–
Sibling	1	–
Care worker, other paid help	3	2
Friends, neighbours	3	–
Somebody else	3	1
Nobody	28	84

Source: Survey on ageing in rural areas 2016 (N = 1235; representative of people 60+ living in different types of rural settlement). Vidovićová (2018)

Germany has witnessed considerable depopulation in some areas, not limited but especially evident in the eastern rural districts where out-migration, especially by younger people, is most severe and is compounded by the general ageing of the population (Šimon and Mikešová 2013). These shifts within the structures and systems of local contexts peripheralise certain rural areas. Germany is the "oldest" of the three nations, with almost 22% of its population aged 65+, which rises to almost 24% in rural and remote areas.

Since 1996 Germany has had a system of long-term care insurance (divided into statutory and private components) to ensure services and care are provided to the ageing population. In contrast to German health insurance, the system is not meant to cover care needs completely, but to support families in managing the care of people living with disabilities and older people, similar to other conservative welfare states. Services are mainly provided by private enterprises, with a small proportion provided by non-profit organisations (Gerlinger and Röber 2009). Service development and delivery is mainly negotiated between care insurers, provider organisations and government agencies at the state level; regional and local actors (local authorities) have hardly any influence on service decisions, which remains an issue of political debate. Services provided do not cover personal care needs; this has led to significant pressure on families and the employment of a large number of migrant carers (estimates range to more than 400,000, *cf.* Rada 2016, p. 4), mostly from Eastern European countries, as live-in carers.

Poland is a large country of more than 320,000 square kilometres, nearly as big as Germany. However, population density is the lowest of the three nations, with the proportion of people living in rural areas (35%) twice that of Germany. Interestingly, the share of older people is actually a little lower than average in rural areas, which is another feature that sets Poland aside in the country comparison. Poland is also one of the two countries here affected by rural depopulation (Wojewódzka-Wiewiórska 2019).

Formal long-term care provision in Poland is considered to be largely residual (Perek-Białas and Racław 2014). Support in older-age is covered by the social security system (old-age and disability pension benefits), social assistance (care services and attendances), and health care (medical services, including long-term care). Local authorities ("*gmina*") are responsible for organising care services for home/residential care, day care (outpatient), and around-the-clock care. Social assistance centres determine the scope, measures, duration, and places where care is organised (Szczerbińska 2006). The policies which determine the quantity and quality of care services are drafted at the local level, with care allocations based on family and financial situations. By in large, the care needs of older people are mostly met by the immediate family, neighbours and relatives, and in some cases by directly employed migrant carers (Perek-Białas and Slany 2015; Kordasiewicz and Sadura 2017). Non-governmental care organisations for older people are rare in rural areas (Turek and Perek-Białas 2014). Such care arrangements are based on traditions and values still present in Polish society (Bojanowska 2008).

17.3 Comparing Czechia, Poland and Germany: An Urban/Rural Analytical Approach

As the previous paragraphs show, Czechia, Germany and Poland possess some differences and similarities in the care and support of older rural dwellers. In this section, we take advantage of data available from Eurostat and its revised three-category spatial classification. Cities (densely populated areas) equate to settings with at least 50% of the population living in urban centres; and rural areas (thinly populated areas) equate to areas with at least 50% of the population living in rural grid cells of 1 km^2. The third category of towns and suburbs has been omitted here.

17.3.1 The Use of Professional Home care Services

Often disregarding the homogeneity of rural places, it is generally agreed that "the spatial distribution of the population is a geographic feature of rural areas that makes service delivery difficult" (OECD 2010, p. 27). Therefore, while rural and urban citizens may have common needs and preferences, their location may lead to differences in service provision with rural communities often found to be underserved, in comparison with urban areas (Joseph and Cloutier-Fisher 2005). The data for Czechia, Germany, and Poland, however, suggest a more variable picture (Table 17.3).

If we disregard the five-percentage-point difference in the case of Poland, where urban dwellers report lower levels of subjective health than their rural counterparts, there are almost no differences in (subjective) health status between rural and urban

Table 17.3 People 65+ using professional home care services by household type and people 65+ in poor health by degree of urbanisation (%)

	Single household 65+				Two-adult household, at least one 65+				People 65+ in poor or very poor health (rural)	People (rural single household in poor health)
	all areas	urban	rural	r-u diff.	all areas	urban	rural	r-u diff.	%	%
Czechia	8.3	6.8	10.6	−3.8	4.7	3.7	6.1	−2.4	22	48
Germany	1.7	1.6	2.3	−0.7	3.0	2.5	2.7	−0.2	14	16
Poland	2.3	2.7	1.9	0.8	2.4	3.3	1.7	1.6	33	6
EU27	7.5	7.6	8.0	−0.4	5.1	5.0	5.0	0.0	18	44

Source: https://ec.europa.eu/eurostat/web/degree-of-urbanisation/data/database; table [ilc_ats13] (Data from 2016). Subjective health table [ilc_lvhl01] (data 2018). Own calculations
Note: r-u diff. = difference between rural and urban areas

dwellers in any of the three countries studied here. While subjective health status is only indicative of possible (prospective) need for care, it may provide us with an interesting comparison. On one hand a "healthier" country like Germany has a smaller proportion of people using professional home care services, which is what one would expect. On the other hand, people using home care services represent only about half of those who have serious health conditions in Czechia (48%) while in Germany and Poland this is 16% and 6% respectively. The share of home care users is greater in rural Czechia and Germany, but in Poland it is the urbanites who are more frequent users of services, and that holds for single-person households, as well as for couples.

To respond to the limited availability of different services – in Germany, for example – a growing number of rural communities have founded local aid associations to support disadvantaged older people. These self-organised agencies describe their work as "to help each other make life easier, to commit oneself to others, to volunteer to help and to gain from mutual help" (Rosenkranz and Görtler 2013, p. 12). They offer assistance in everyday activities, trying to complement or even compensate for the lack of public services. Local authorities strive to provide them with formal or organisational support. However, it has been shown that such self-organised help is fragile and depends on people who are active in the aid associations. Consequently, volunteers are often overwhelmed by the amount of work, increasing the risk of unsustainable provision (Alisch et al. 2018). In Poland, regional authorities decided to establish "Centers for Supporting Informal Carers" in order to collaborate with and promote voluntary agencies providing older adult services, as well as to support informal caregivers. However, despite the original plan to spread these centres across regions, most are located in urban areas. Thus, rural areas, which are more in need of such support, are left behind.

17.3.2 *Informal Care and Assistance*

Unsatisfactory, underperforming state-funded services often create a need to mobilise voluntary-sector organisations and volunteers to provide caring services. But the care provided by family and friends is not included in the usual measurement of voluntary sector activity (Skinner and Hanlon 2016). Yet, the person-hours spent by family and friends in acts of care represent a considerable share of the care services provided to older people [as is the case in Hungary and Russia, as outlined in Széman et al. this volume].

Here, we look specifically at older people's involvement in the provision of this type of care and support. As we have seen already in this chapter, partners are an especially important source of this type of help. Providing that there is a strong age homogamy in marriages we may assume that the partners of those being cared for are themselves older. This greater age of the carer hypothesis holds also in the case of adult children (60+) taking care of their very old parents (80+).

There are at least two reasons to expect that the level of informal care will be higher in rural regions than in urban areas: closer social relationships in rural areas, including family co-residence, and less availability of formal care and services, which then need to be supplemented by informal help. Figure 17.1 supports this expectation and provides an overview of the involvement of retirees in providing informal care or assistance as recorded by the EU-SILC database.

While, on average, there seems to be little difference between rural and urban areas in the EU27, we can see quite a notable variation in our three nation cases. The differences are both across countries and across rural/urban settings. Comparatively

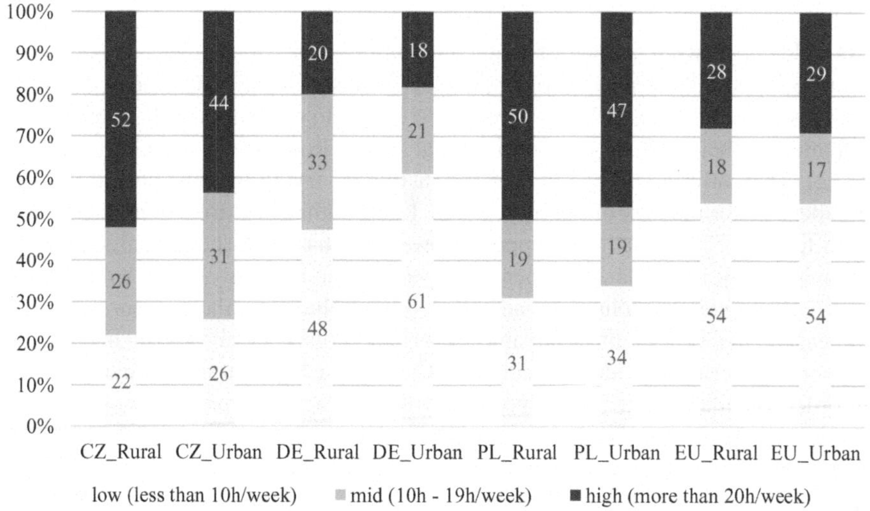

Fig. 17.1 Retirees providing informal care or assistance by degree of urbanisation and intensity of care measured as hours per week (in %)

Source: Ad hoc module EU-SILC 2016; table [ilc_ats18]; https://ec.europa.eu/eurostat/web/degree-of-urbanisation/data/database

speaking, older people in rural Czechia have the greatest involvement in providing care, followed by Polish rural older adults (inter-country comparison). Although a smaller proportion, German rural carers are still considerably more involved than German urbanites. An additional dynamic can be brought to light by applying a gender perspective. Despite the EU averages for rural and urban women being the same, women in cities provided less of the most intensive care (20 h+/week) than their rural counterparts in all three countries.

A qualitative research project in the Małopolska region found that informal caregivers were often left with minimal or no support, and without adequate information about other caring options. These results from Poland (Stypińska and Perek-Białas 2014) and elsewhere, direct our attention to the multidimensional risk of social exclusion for caregivers in rural areas (Racław 2012), including but not limited to financial hardship, lost status and relationships, isolation and constrained involvement in social and community activities (Keating and Eales 2017).

17.4 Discussion

As Walsh (2018, p. 254) summarises, there are two approaches to how place interacts with the processes of exclusion: first, the characteristics of place, and the factors that shape those characteristics, shape the exclusionary experiences of place (place as a domain of exclusion); and second, place functions as a fundamental determinant of exclusionary experiences in old-age, both in relation to place and to various other aspects of life in older-age (place as a mediator of exclusion). The provision of care to an ageing population is an interesting example of how different dimensions can inform the inclusion-exclusion continuum.

In the previous paragraphs we presented three case studies on the Czech Republic, Germany and Poland, the main goal of which was to try to evaluate possible interconnections between social exclusion from services and community/spatial exclusion. Care constitutes the principal element in welfare provision and the welfare state institutional network and also highlights the importance of care activities for the social integration of those working in and receiving care (Geissler and Pfau-Effinger 2005). The embeddedness of (delivering) care activities in a particular place seems to be at least two-fold: service/care delivery is: (a) a special kind of social interaction that is hindered or supported by the appropriates of the place; and (b) enabled and/or hindered by the policies which usually originate at the level of the nation and move down the spatially categorised levels of government, policy making and practice delivery. Both of these features seem to be specifically challenged in rural areas.

> 'Very few national governments explicitly guarantee that public services should be uniformly available across their territory; there remains a growing perception […] that spatial equality of access should be part of the statutory rights of citizens.' (OECD 2010, p. 24)

Many of the services seniors consume are considered to be core entitlements, so it is difficult or even impossible to restrict availability; just maintaining the traditional service infrastructure of these areas, ignoring the service implications of depopulation, may in the future not be enough to address the increasing demand for care in ageing populations. The low number of the working-age population entering the care profession and the need to recognise that the wages for these carers might be under threat are another two factors that may add to an increase in the overall costs, which are already high in rural settings. Asthana et al. (2003) specifies the following characteristics of rural areas that impact the costs of service delivery: economies of scale; additional travel costs, high levels of unproductive time; additional communication costs; and poorer access to training, consultancy and other support services to local providers.

While voluntary and grass-roots organisations are often relied upon to cover blind spots, our case studies show that this strategy may be threatened by prevailing cultures and customs. Shucksmith and Brown (2016) collected examples from various countries of how governmental strategies to address rural vulnerability had fed on narratives of community self-help to pass responsibility to local citizens, which involved both rescaling responsibility and shifting it from the state to the market and civil society. Skinner and Hanlon (2016, p. 4) make a similar point when they identify a gap "within prevailing discourses on ageing that emphasise the involvement of voluntary sector organisations and their volunteers (*i.e.* the "voluntary turn"), but do not take into account the crucial differences place makes to explain the uneven landscapes of volunteerism".

The situation of non-existent (Czechia), unstable (Germany), or dysfunctional (Poland) self-organised groups has been also described by Cloutier-Fisher and Joseph (2000) in Canada. The authors see this situation as one of the steps in more general processes of exclusion embedded in vulnerable places, resulting in significant service gaps, including deficiencies in sheltered housing, transport and mobility services, respite care, palliative care and mental health services. If attempts are made to address such gaps, there is a tendency to leave out the voluntary sector, both financially, and in terms of providing coordination and support. This reinforces:

> 'the reliance on voluntary-sector agencies and local governments for the provision of an important sub-set of community support services, and thereby perpetuates the systemic bias against rural communities exemplified by small over-burdened volunteer networks and limited tax bases.' (Joseph and Cloutier-Fisher 2005, p. 136)

Our case studies show that, regardless of the size of the country or its proportion of remote or depopulating areas, there can be similar discourses on care in rural areas. But the data, sometimes counter-intuitively, show that there is a lot of variation. For example, a lot of informal caring is provided both in the family-oriented Polish countryside and in Czechia, a country with a midsize rural population and comparatively common use of professional home care services, indicating a promising belt-and-braces approach to securing care provision. This pattern confirms spatiality as a useful, if not crucial, lens for evaluating social exclusion from services. The country level contexts may give additional information on the heterogenous results obtained at the community level and underline the importance of a culturally sensitive approach. The processes of policy making would greatly benefit from recognising these interconnections between different levels of places and spaces and how they exercise influence over social exclusion outcomes in terms of service and care delivery and use. That may also include the rehabilitation of rural areas as those "on average worse off".

17.5 Conclusion

The analysis presented in this chapter is exploratory and as such faces many limitations. We were limited by the comparability of available data and with this data originally collected for a different purpose. Further, we decided to use the often rightly criticised urban/rural duality in our analytical approach, and to leave out the middle category of towns, as this category deals with yet another set of issues related to its sometimes "hybrid" character. By limiting ourselves to these two distinct categories we recognise we have lost depth and explanatory power, but we hope we have gained a simplicity, and clarity in our exploration. While emphasising the "importance of place in determining the experience of rural ageing" (Joseph and Cloutier-Fisher 2005, p. 146), we should not ignore the intertwining double heterogeneity of rural contexts and their, often increasingly, heterogeneous older populations (Scharf et al. 2016; Skinner and Winterton 2018). The scope of this study and datasets available didn't allow us to tackle these important intersections in any great breadth or depth, but instead illustrate the extensive set of questions that are left to be addressed in future work.

Editors' Postscript

Please note, like other contributions to this book, this chapter was written before the COVID-19 pandemic of 2020. The book's introductory chapter (Chap. 1) and conclusion (Chap. 34) consider some of the key ways in which the pandemic relates to issues concerning social exclusion and ageing.

Acknowledgements The study presented here was supported by national grants:

Czechia: Ageing in rural environments: unanswered questions in social gerontology (GACR grant No. 16-20873S)

Germany: The "BUSLAR – Citizens' aid associations and social cooperatives as partners for public services and care. Model development for supplementary assistance for older people in rural areas" funded by the Federal Ministry of Education and Research (0FK, 3FH004SB4, 2014-2017) and "Age4Health" a subproject of the research consortium PartKommPlus – German Research Consortium for Healthy Communities, funded by the Federal Ministry of Education and Research 2015 – 2017 and 2018 – 2020 (01EL 1423G).

Poland: "Opienkunowie rodzinni osób starszych – problem, potrzeby, wyzwania dle polityki społcznej" financed by the Regional Center of Social Policy, Małopolska, Kraków (2015) and the project "Sytuacja opiekunów rodzinnych w kontekście sprawowania opieki nad osobami w wieku 60+ z terenu województwa łódzkiego" by "ARC Rynek i Opinia" financed by the Regional Center of Social Policy in Łódź (2017).The cooperation of the authors has been made possible by the COST ROSEnet Action CA15122.

References

Alisch, M., Ritter, M., Boos-Krüger, A., Schönberger, C., Glaser, R., Rubin, Y., & Solf-Leipold, B. (2018) *„Irgendwann brauch' ich dann auch Hilfe ...!" – Selbstorganisation, Engagement und Mitverantwortung älterer Menschen in ländlichen Räumen. Beiträge zur Sozialraumforschung, Band 17*. Opladen/Berlin/Toronto: Barbara Budrich Verlag.

Asthana, S., Gibson, A., Moon, G., & Brigham, P. (2003). Allocating resources for health and social care: The significance of rurality. *Health and Social Care in Community, 11*(6), 486–493. https://doi.org/10.1046/j.1365-2524.2003.00454.x.

Bareš, P., & Víšek, P. (2016). Dostupnost služeb sociální péče ve správních obvodech obcí s rozšířenou působností v Jihočeském kraji. *Fórum sociální politiky, 10*, 1.

Bernard, J., & Šimon, M. (2017). Vnitřní periferie v Česku: Multidimenzionalita sociálního vyloučeníve venkovských oblastech. *Sociologický časopis/Czech Sociological Review, 53*(1), 3–28.

Bojanowska, E. (2008). Opieka nad ludźmi starszymi. In P. Szukalski (Ed.), *To idzie starość Warszawa*. Instytut Spraw Publicznych.

Buffel, T., Phillipson, C., & Scharf, T. (2013). Experiences of neighbourhood exclusion and inclusion among older people living in deprived inner-city areas in Belgium and England. *Ageing & Society, 33*, 89–109.

Cloutier-Fisher, D., & Joseph, A. (2000). Long-term care restructuring in Rural Ontario: Retrieving community service user and provider narratives. *Social Science and Medicine, 50*(7–8), 1037–1045.

DESTATIS Older People in Germany and the EU. (2016). https://www.destatis.de/EN/Themes/Society-Environment/Population/Current-Population/Publications/Downloads-Current-Population/brochure-older-people-eu-0010021169004.pdf?__blob=publicationFile

EUROFOUND. (2019). *Is rural Europe being left behind? EUROFOUND European quality of life survey*. Luxembourg: Publications Office of the European Union. https://www.eurofound.europa.eu/publications/policy-brief/2019/is-rural-europe-being-left-behind.

EUROSTAT. (2020). (database) https://ec.europa.eu/eurostat/data/database

EU-SILC. (2016). Ad hoc module; table [ilc_ats18]; https://ec.europa.eu/eurostat/web/degree-of-urbanisation/data/database

Galčanová, L., & Staveník, A. (2020). Ageing in the changing countryside: The experience of rural Czechs. *Sociologia Ruralis, 60*(2), 329–356. https://doi.org/10.1111/soru.12292.

Geissler, B., & Pfau-Effinger, B. (2005). Change in European care arrangements. In B. Geissler & B. Pfau-Effinger (Eds.), *Care and social integration in European societies* (pp. 3–20). Bristol: Policy Press.

Gerlinger, T., & Röber, M. (2009). *Die Pflegeversicherung*. Bern: Huber.

Goins, R. T., Spencer, S. M., & Byrd, J. C. (2011). Research on rural caregiving. In R. C. Talley, K. Chwalisz, & K. C. Buckwalter (Eds.), *Rural caregiving in the United States. Research, practice, policy* (pp. 103–132). Berlin: Springer.

Hooks, G., Lobao, L., & Tickamyer, A. (2016). Spatial inequality and rural areas. In M. Shucksmith & D. L. Brown (Eds.), *Routledge international handbook of rural studies* (pp. 553–571). Routledge.

Joseph, A., & Cloutier-Fisher, D. (2005). Ageing in rural communities. In G. Andrews & D. Phillips (Eds.), *Ageing and place: Perspectives, policy, practice* (pp. 133–146). Oxon: Routledge.

Kaye, L. W., & Butler, S. (2004). *Gerontological social work in small towns and rural communities*. New York: Routledge.

Keating, N., & Eales, J. (2017). Social consequences of family care of adults: A scoping review. *International Journal of Care and Caring, 1*, 153–173. https://doi.org/10.1332/239788217X14937990731749.

Knijn, T., & Kremer, M. (1997). Gender and the caring dimension of welfare states: Toward inclusive citizenship. *Social Politics: International Studies in Gender, State & Society, 4*(3), 328–361. https://doi.org/10.1093/oxfordjournals.sp.a034270.

Kordasiewicz, A., & Sadura, P. (2017). Clash of public administration paradigms in delegation of education and elderly care services in a post-socialist state (Poland). *Public Management Review, 19*(6), 785–801.

Mai, R., Naderi, R., & Schimany, P. (2008). Who should take care for them? In C. Höhn, D. Avramov, & I. Kotowska (Eds.), *People, population change and policies. Lessons from the population policy acceptance study – Volume 2: Demographic knowledge, gender, ageing* (pp. 45–63). Dordrecht: Springer.

Milligan, C., & Conradson, D. (Eds.). (2006). *Landscapes of voluntarism: New spaces of health, welfare and governance*. Bristol: Policy Press.

Moffatt, S., & Glasgow, N. (2009). How useful is the concept of social exclusion when applied to rural older people in the United Kingdom and the United States? *Regional Studies, 43*(10), 1291–1303. https://doi.org/10.1080/00343400903002697.

Musil, J., & Müller, J. (2008). Vnitřní periferie v České republice jako mechanismus sociální exkluze Sociologický časopis. *Czech Sociological Review, 44*(2), 321–348.

OECD. (2010). *Strategies to improve rural service delivery*. https://www.oecd-ilibrary.org/urban-rural-and-regional-development/strategies-to-improve-rural-service-delivery_9789264083967-en. Data access Mar 2020.

OECD (database). Regional demography: Demographic indicators by rural/urban typology, Country level. https://stats.oecd.org/Index.aspx?DataSetCode=REGION_DEMOGR#. Data access Mar 2020.

Perek-Białas, J., & Racław, M. (2014). Transformation of elderly care in Poland. In M. Leon (Ed.), *The transformation of care in European societies* (pp. 256–275). London: Palgrave Macmillan.

Perek-Białas, J., & Slany, K. (2015). The elderly care regime and migration regime after the EU accession: The case of Poland. In U. Karl & S. Torres (Eds.), *Ageing in contexts of migration* (pp. 27–38). Routledge.

Průša, L., Bareš, P., Holub, M., & Šlapák, M. (2015). *Vybrané aspekty péče o seniory z hlediska sociálního začleňování* [Selected aspects of care for the elderly in terms of social inclusion]. Praha: VÚPSV, v.v.i.

Racław, M. (2012). Opiekunowie nieformalni. Krótkookresowa funkcjonalność nieopłaconej pracy. In J. Hrynkiewicz (Ed.), *O sytuacji ludzi w starszym wieku*. Warszawa: RRL.

Rada, A. (2016). *Pflegekräftemigration aus den neuen EU-Mitgliedstaaten nach Deutschland*. Frankfurt/Main: Institut für Sozialarbeit und Sozialpädagogik e. V.

Rosenkranz, D., & Görtler, E. (2013). *Wegweiser zur Gründung und Gestaltung von „Seniorengenossenschaften". Neue Formen verbindli-cher Unterstützung im Alter. Hrsg. vom Bayerisches Staatsministerium für Arbeit und Soziales, Familie und Frauen*. München.

Scharf, T., Walsh, K., & O'Shea, E. (2016). Ageing in rural places. In M. Shucksmith & D. L. Brown (Eds.), *Routledge international handbook of rural studies* (pp. 50–61). Routledge.

Schlosberg, D. (2007). *Defining environmental justice. Theories, movements, and Nature*. Oxford: Oxford University Press.

Shucksmith, M., & Brown, D. L. (Eds.). (2016). *Routledge international handbook of rural studies*. Routledge.

Šimon, M., & Mikešová, R. (2013). *"Demographic change in Central Europe. A socio – economic background analysis"*. Sociologický ústav AV ČR, v.v.i. (research report).

Skinner, M., & Hanlon, N. (2016). *Ageing resource communities: New frontiers of rural population change, community development and voluntarism* (Hardback) (1st ed.). Routledge.

Skinner, M. W., & Winterton, R. (2018). Interrogating the contested spaces of rural aging: Implications for research, policy, and practice. *The Gerontologist, 58*(1), 15–25. https://doi.org/10.1093/geront/gnx094.

Stypinska, J., & Perek-Białas, J. (2014). Working carers in Poland-successful strategies of reconciliation of work and care of an older adult. *Anthropol Notebooks, 20*(1), 87–104.

Szczerbińska, K. (Ed.). (2006). *Dostępność opieki zdrowotnej i pomocy społecznej dla osób starszych w Polsce*. Kraków: Wydawnictwo Uniwersytetu Jagiellońskiego.

Turek, K., & Perek-Białas, J. (2014). Older volunteers in Poland: The heritage of a socialist regime. In A. Principi, P. Jensen, & G. Lamura (Eds.), *Active ageing: Voluntary work by older people in Europe* (p. 173).

Vidovićová, L. (2018). Age-friendly rural areas. The challenges of measurement and evaluation in Czech older adults. *Sociální studia/Social studies*. https://journals.muni.cz/socialni_studia/article/view/11218.

Walsh, K. (2018). Constructions of old-age social exclusion: In place and shaped by place. In M. Skinner, G. Andrews, & M. Cutchin (Eds.), *Geographical gerontology: Concepts and approaches* (pp. 252–266). London: Routledge.

Wojewódzka-Wiewiórska, A. (2019). Depopulation in rural areas in Poland – Socio-economic local perspective. *Research for Rural Development, 2*, 126–132. https://doi.org/10.22616/rrd.25.2019.059126-132.

Section VI
Civic Exclusion

Chapter 18
Introduction: Framing Civic Exclusion

Sandra Torres

18.1 Introduction

The topic of old-age social exclusion has received increased attention as studies that measure the prevalence of this multidimensional phenomenon have shown its spread across countries; see Ogg (2005) who focuses on Europe, Hrast et al. (2013) who considers Central and Eastern Europe, and Macleod et al. (2019) who measure exclusion in the UK. The three chapters that belong to this section pay specific attention to two of the domains which Walsh et al. (2017) refer to as civic participation and socio-cultural aspects in their framework on exclusion in later life. In this book, we refer to them as civic exclusion [see Walsh et al. this volume]. It is worth noting that this domain has received the least scholarly attention so far within the literature (Van Regenmortel et al. 2016; Walsh et al. 2017), even though there is clear evidence that civic engagement and socio-cultural aspects of exclusion can have an impact on self-rated health (Poortinga 2006). Thus, the purpose of the chapter is to offer an abridged introduction to the topic of civic exclusion in later life in order to offer context to the three chapters in this section.

18.2 Civic Exclusion and the Life Course

First, to the part of this domain that deals with exclusion from civic participation. In the old-age exclusion conceptual framework formulated by Walsh et al. (2017), the domain of civic exclusion is about what the lack of participation in generic civic activities, volunteering and community involvement, voting and the political sphere can mean for older people's ability to exercise their citizenship rights to the fullest.

S. Torres (✉)
Department of Sociology, Uppsala University, Uppsala, Sweden
e-mail: sandra.torres@soc.uu.se

K. Walsh et al. (eds.), *Social Exclusion in Later Life*, International Perspectives on Aging 28, https://doi.org/10.1007/978-3-030-51406-8_18

Grenier and Guberman (2009) call this domain "socio-political exclusion". They define this type of exclusion as being about "barriers to civic and political participation resulting from a lack of involvement in decision-making, collective power, and limited clout of agency" (ibid: 118). Macleod et al. (2019) – who rely on another framework for the study of exclusion in later life – call this domain civic participation but define the scope of it in a much broader sense than Walsh et al. (2017) do. Macleod et al. (2019) propose namely that this domain "encompasses cultural, educational, and political engagement, factors that enable a person to connect with and contribute to their society, and be involved in its decision making" (ibid: 82).

Serrat et al. (2020) have recently published a scoping review of 50-years of research into older people's civic participation that shows that most of this research focuses on either social (particularly volunteering), or political participation. This means that citizenship and generic civic activities are the dimensions of civic exclusion that remain relatively unexplored. In their review, they identify the critical gaps that need to be addressed as well, and the ways in which these gaps affect not only the conceptualisation of old-age civic exclusion, but also the ways in which contextual aspects are addressed. Relatively little research has taken a life-course approach to the study of civic exclusion, and the ways in which diverse and potentially marginalised groups of older people experience civic exclusion remains a topic in dire need of scholarly attention. With regard to the latter, Torres and Serrat (2019) have argued that the lacuna of research on older migrants' civic participation means that the role that migratory life-courses play in civic participation in older-age remains unexplored. In the latest measurement of the prevalence of civic exclusion amongst older people in the UK, Macleod et al. (2019) have shown that those who are "non-white were more excluded /…/ and that those born outside of the UK score higher" (ibid: 97), which is why a diversity-informed agenda for the study of civic exclusion in later life is needed.

We turn our focus now to the second part of this domain, socio-cultural aspects of exclusion. According to Walsh et al. (2017), the socio-cultural domain brings attention to the symbolic and discursive sphere (and the ways in which public discourses and imagery promote the exclusion of older people from wider society), ageism and age discrimination (which is about how these discourses get translated into exclusionary practices), and identity exclusion (which they define as a "reduction to one-dimensional identities") (Walsh et al. 2017, p. 90). Canadian scholars have, as already mentioned, their own framework, but they have two domains rather than just one to refer to the socio-cultural aspects alluded to here. They differentiate namely between the domain they call symbolic (which is about the negative representations mentioned earlier), and the one they call identity (which they define as "dismissal or diminishment of the distinctive and multiple identities of the person or group through reduction to one identity such as age", (Grenier and Guberman 2009, p. 118). In the framework used by Macleod et al. (2019), the socio-cultural domain is called "discrimination" instead, which they define as the domain that "includes symbolic exclusion: negative representation or prejudicial treatment for a particular characteristic or group membership, and identity exclusion: disregard of one's whole identity by only recognising a single characteristic/ identity" (Macleod et al.

2019, p. 82). Irrespective of which framework one relies on, the socio-cultural aspect of exclusion is about the ways in which societal discourses lead not only to the exclusion of older people, but also to neglecting the complex identities they have, and the variety of circumstances, experiences and needs with which these are associated. Studies focusing on these forms of exclusion not only consider the positionality of ageing within societal values systems and structures, but also often its intersection with the construction of other social locations, such as gender, ethnicity and migration status, disability and health conditions.

18.3 Outline of This Section

Like other contributions to this book, these chapters were written before the COVID-19 pandemic of 2020. However, the relevance and importance of the themes, and the forms of exclusion, documented within this section is only heightened by the barriers and discourses that emerged to impact civic engagement and socio-cultural aspects of ageing during the virus outbreak.

The chapter by Serrat et al. in this section exposes the angles of investigation that deserve scholarly attention if exclusion from civic engagement in later life is to be studied in a useful manner. This chapter also maps out what a future agenda for this research field could look like while arguing for the need to take into account that civic exclusion plays an important part of what old-age social exclusion entails. They propose that there are four areas that future research should address: the multidimensionality of civic engagement; the diversity of the older population; the dynamics and experiences of engagement across the life course; and the culturally-embedded processes that characterise civic engagement. In arguing that these are the areas that deserve scholarly attention at this point in time, Serrat and colleagues offer us a roadmap for future research on this topic.

The chapter by Gallistl brings attention to exclusion from cultural activities in later life and exposes how consumption patterns relating to cultural activities change as we grow older, and how we sometimes position these activities in relation to cultural identities stratified by socio-economic status. Gallistl's contribution gives us insight into how socio-economic determinants, as well as changes over the life course, affect someone's engagement in cultural activities, and why policies to advance cultural participation need to more actively consider ageing and later life. In doing so, this chapter offers ample empirical evidence for some of the arguments that Walsh et al. (2017) have made. They have namely argued that "old-age exclusion /…/ (varies) in form and degree across the older adult life course", and that "its complexity, impact and prevalence are amplified by old-age vulnerabilities, accumulated disadvantage for some groups, and constrained opportunities to ameliorate exclusion" (ibid: 93). Thus, through its use of quantitative data on older Austrians' cultural consumption patterns, this chapter shows the intrinsic interconnectedness of the domains of social exclusion since both material and financial resources, as well as access to services, amenities and mobility affect older people's participation in cultural activities.

The last chapter in this section (by Gallassi and Harrysson) is also a contribution that exposes the interconnectedness of domains, but does so from the perspective of identity. The chapter by Gallassi and Harrysson is a prime example of how the horizons that have informed policy formulation (which is influenced by, and can formulate, societal discourses) can inadvertently lead to the neglect of older people's multiple identities. In their chapter, they discuss older migrants' truncated labour participation, and the effects this has on their retirement. They argue that it is Swedish policies lack of mobility know-how that complicates these older people's pension access. Thus, by showing how policy formulation can reduce the needs of older people to just one dimension, this chapter makes a contribution to our understanding of socio-cultural exclusion that is concerned with identity, which Walsh et al. (2017) have argued is also about the "mechanisms in relation to social security individualization, globalization, social stratification" (ibid: 90–91). With its focus on older migrants this chapter clearly shows also why I have for years argued that the peculiarities of the migratory life-course are not always taken into account when non-migrant life-courses are regarded as the norm (Warnes et al. 2004; Torres 2012).

This introductory chapter has contextualised what the contributions of the following three chapters are. This has been done by alluding to the fact that the scholarly debate on civic exclusion (incorporating both civic participation and socio-cultural aspects of exclusion) is in its infancy but the contributions made in this section advance the ways in which we make sense of how mechanisms associated with this type of exclusion operate. The call by Serrat and colleagues for more research on civic exclusion, that uses the agenda for future research they delineate in their chapter, urges scholars of ageing to pay more attention to civic participation in older-age, and the ways in which a lack of civic participation affects the social exclusion that older people can experience later in life. The contributions by Gallistl on cultural exclusion, and by Gallassi and Harrysson on older migrants' retirement, offer policy makers suggestions for areas that require further attention. Taken together, these contributions expand our imagination on old-age social exclusion by bringing attention to how civic forms of exclusion are constructed, why attention to this domain is necessary, and how social exclusion, in relation to civic participation and socio-cultural aspects, works in later life.

References

Grenier, A. M., & Guberman, N. (2009). Creating and sustaining disadvantage: The relevance of a social exclusion framework. *Health and Social Care in the Community, 17*(2), 116–124.

Hrast, M. F., Mrak, A. K., & Rakar, T. (2013). Social exclusion of elderly in Central and Eastern Europe. *International Journal of Social Economics, 40*(11), 971–989.

Macleod, C., Ross, A., Sacker, A., Netuveli, G., & Windle, G. (2019). Re-thinking social exclusion in later life: A case for a new framework for measurement. *Ageing & Society, 39*, 74–111.

Ogg, J. (2005). Social exclusion and insecurity among older Europeans: The influence of welfare regimes. *Ageing & Society, 25*, 69–90.
Poortinga, W. (2006). Social capital: An individual or collective resource for health? *Social Science & Medicine, 62*(2), 292–302.
Serrat, R., Scharf, T., Villar, F., & Gomez, C. (2020, February). Fifty years of research into older people's civic participation: Recent trends, future directions. *The Gerontologist, 60*(1), e38–e51. https://doi.org/10.1093/geront/gnz021.
Torres, S. (2012). International migration: Patterns and implications for exclusion in old age. In T. Scharf & N. C. Keating (Eds.), *From exclusion to inclusion in old age: A global challenge* (pp. 33–49). Bristol: The Policy Press.
Torres, S., & Serrat, R. (2019, September). Older migrants' civic participation: A topic in need of attention. *Journal of Aging Studies, 50*. https://doi.org/10.1016/j.jaging.2019.100790.
Van Regenmortel, S., De Donder, L., Dury, S., Smetcoren, A. S., De Witte, N., & Verté, D. (2016). Social exclusion in later life: A systematic review of the literature. *Journal of Population Ageing, 9*, 315–344.
Walsh, K., Scharf, T., & Keating, N. (2017). Social exclusion of older persons: A scoping review and conceptual framework. *European Journal of Aging, 14*, 81. https://doi.org/10.1007/s10433-016-0398-8.
Warnes, A. M., Friedrich, K., Kellaher, L., & Torres, S. (2004). The diversity and welfare of older migrants in Europe. *Ageing and Society, 24*(3), 307–326.

Chapter 19
Reconceptualising Exclusion from Civic Engagement in Later Life: Towards a New Research Agenda

Rodrigo Serrat, Thomas Scharf, and Feliciano Villar

19.1 Introduction

Social exclusion in later life remains a major challenge for ageing societies. Despite widespread acceptance of the multidimensional nature of exclusion in later life, research and policy debates have tended to focus on exclusion from material resources or social relations, often overlooking other recognised dimensions of social exclusion. In this context, and as outlined by Torres when introducing this section (Chap. 18), exclusion from civic engagement has been by far the least studied dimension of social exclusion in later life (Walsh et al. 2017). Older people's civic engagement has been highlighted as a key feature in policy debates around participatory democracy (Barnes et al. 2011) as well as in initiatives aimed at promoting active and successful ways of ageing (United Nations 2002; WHO 2002) or implementing age-friendly communities (Buffel et al. 2012). While research on the topic has grown steadily since the 1960s, many areas remain in need of improvement (Serrat et al. 2019). In this chapter, we argue that research and policy initiatives that are aimed at reducing exclusion around older people's civic engagement should consider four interrelated and often disregarded aspects. First, we need to embrace the multidimensionality of the concept of civic engagement, which includes a range of qualitatively different activities. Second, it is necessary to account for the diversity of the older population, since this shapes who is, in practice, able to engage civically and in which ways individuals are able to participate. Third, attention should be paid to the dynamics and experiences of engagement across the life course, in order to understand better the causes and consequences of civic

R. Serrat (✉) · F. Villar
Department of Cognition, Development and Educational Psychology, University of Barcelona, Barcelona, Spain
e-mail: rserrat@ub.edu

T. Scharf
Population Health Sciences Institute, Newcastle University, Newcastle upon Tyne, UK

K. Walsh et al. (eds.), *Social Exclusion in Later Life*, International Perspectives on Aging 28, https://doi.org/10.1007/978-3-030-51406-8_19

engagement trajectories as people age. Fourth, we need to consider exclusion from civic engagement as a culturally-embedded process that is shaped by the particular socio-political context in which engagement occurs. Before reviewing these four aspects, we explore how civic engagement has been conceptualised and comment on the scope and nature of the evidence available. To develop these points, we draw on the findings of a recent scoping review on older people's civic engagement (Serrat et al. 2019), which allows us to show the four key gaps that future studies should address.

19.2 Conceptualising Civic Engagement

Civic engagement is an inherently multidimensional concept that embraces a broad repertoire of activities (Hustinx and Denk 2009). While civic engagement was initially restricted to the act of voting in elections, in recent decades the number of activities considered as civic has expanded rapidly (van Deth 2001). Understandings of civic activities now typically include contacting political representatives, participating in political organisations, being involved in protest activities or social movement organisations, volunteering, or engaging in charitable work. This rapid expansion has transformed civic engagement into an umbrella concept that encompasses a highly diverse range of activities, which may blur its definition and limits. Consequently, its utility both as a tool for exploring and comparing civic activities across empirical studies and as a social policy framework to promote older people's active involvement in community life may be challenged (Theocharis 2015). To avoid such imprecision, there have been numerous attempts to provide systematic criteria to define and organise the diversity of civic activities (*e.g.* Adler and Goggin 2005; Ekman and Amnå 2012).

Civic activities can be classified according to their objective and format. Consideration of the activity's objective allows us to distinguish between volunteering and political engagement. While volunteering includes activities aimed at helping others or producing common good, political engagement combines activities that are explicitly aimed at influencing decision-making processes on political issues. While most scholars generally agree upon this differentiation, volunteering has sometimes been labelled as social or community engagement (*e.g.* Ekman and Amnå 2012; Barrett and Brunton-Smith 2014). However, the specific activities that should be included under these two forms of civic engagement remains open to debate, suggesting the need to consider a further axis of classification.

Consideration of the activity's format permits a differentiation between formal or informal volunteering, and between institutionalised or non-institutionalised forms of political engagement. As noted by Jones and Heley (2016):

> '… formal volunteering encompasses those activities conducted under the auspices of formal organisations and programmes. Informal volunteering refers to engaging in activities without the umbrella of a prescribed organisation, and includes undertakings that benefit family and friends.' (p. 182)

In the case of political engagement, that distinction echoes the traditional dichotomy between conventional forms of engagement, such as working on campaigns, contacting political representatives or participating in political organisations or forums, and non-conventional activities, such as signing petitions, boycotting or participating in protest activities or new social movements (Offe 1985). While the former refers to activities channelled by recognised regulated political agents and procedures, the latter encompasses less formal, bottom-up forms of political engagement. So, exclusion from civic engagement refers to older people's inability to engage in informal and formal activities aimed at seeking improved benefits for others, the community, or wider society, or impacting on collective decision-making processes.

19.3 Assessing the Scope and Nature of Research on Older People's Civic Engagement

A recent scoping review of research on older people's civic engagement identified not only a substantial growth in publications relating to this topic since the 1960s, and especially since the late 1990s, but also highlighted some key features of the 429 English-language papers that met the review's inclusion criteria (Serrat et al. 2019).[1] The overwhelming majority of papers included in the review (83%) focused on collective forms of social engagement, primarily volunteering. Such papers considered, for example, older people's engagement in a broad array of volunteering organisations, including health, educational, social, religious, entrepreneurial, and community organisations. Far fewer papers addressed collective forms of political engagement (13%; mainly engagement in political organisations or forums or in social movements) or considered individual forms of political engagement (11%; primarily with a focus on voting behaviours) or of social engagement (6%; mainly exploring informal helping behaviours outside the family). More than half of the papers included in the review drew on US samples (55%), with studies conducted in other western nations such as Australia (7%), the United Kingdom (4%), Canada (4%), The Netherlands (3%) and Spain (3%) lagging well behind. Only a handful of papers considered civic engagement of older people in non-western nations.

In relation to the process of civic engagement, most papers considered by Serrat et al. (2019) in their scoping review focused on antecedents of engagement (61%).

[1] Searches were conducted in four databases (Psycinfo, Sociological Abstracts, Web of Science, and Scopus) using the following keywords: (Ageing OR Aging OR Aged OR Old age OR older people OR older persons OR older adults OR seniors OR senior citizens OR elder* OR later life OR third age) AND (all the combinations between civic OR civil OR citizen* OR political OR social OR community AND participation OR engagement OR involvement, OR volunteering). Searches were limited to empirical, review, or conceptual/theoretical papers written in English. We did not use any year of publication limit. Searches were carried out in April 2017 and updated in May 2018.

This was especially the case in terms of papers considering individual forms of political engagement (100%; exploring, for example, the association of such engagement with human and social capital variables (*e.g.* Nygård and Jakobsson 2013), political attitudes or public policy changes) and collective forms of political engagement (85%; assessing, for example, the association of engagement with such aspects as human and social capital, motivations, political attitudes, political generation, or personality variables). While just under two-fifths of papers (37%) addressed outcomes of civic engagement, this proportion varied significantly across the different types of civic activity. Studies addressing older people's experiences of engagement were far less frequent (14%), with most of these considering collective forms of social engagement. Finally, it is important to note that, with some exceptions (*e.g.* Postle et al. 2005; Tang et al. 2009), most papers did not use social exclusion as a frame of reference to analyse older people's civic engagement.

19.4 Developing a New Research Agenda on Older People's Civic Engagement

Although research into older people's civic engagement has significantly increased in recent decades (Serrat et al. 2019) as have studies on social exclusion in later life (Walsh et al. 2017), the two strands of literature have hardly overlapped. Drawing on the scoping review concerning engagement in civic activities in later life (Serrat et al. 2019), we propose that there are four key dimensions that future research should address in order to understand older people's exclusion from these activities: the multidimensionality of civic engagement; the diversity of the older population; the dynamics and experiences of engagement across the life course; and the culturally-embedded process that characterises civic engagement. These four areas underpin a conceptual framework aimed at guiding future studies and policy initiatives aimed at reducing exclusion from civic engagement in later life (Fig. 19.1).

19.4.1 Multidimensionality of Exclusion from Civic Engagement

To move research on older people's civic engagement forward implies broadening the concept's meaning. As suggested by Greenfield (2010), definitions have important practice and social policy consequences, as they "… serve to identify not only the *what is*, but also the *what could be* and the *what should be*" (p. 6). Gerontological research has tended to equate civic engagement with volunteering, overlooking the many other ways in which older people engage. Although this trend may reflect the growing interest in older people as active contributors to ageing societies (United Nations 2002; WHO 2002), it also risks embedding cultural expectations regarding what it is to be a *good old person* and a *good old citizen* (Martinson and Halpern

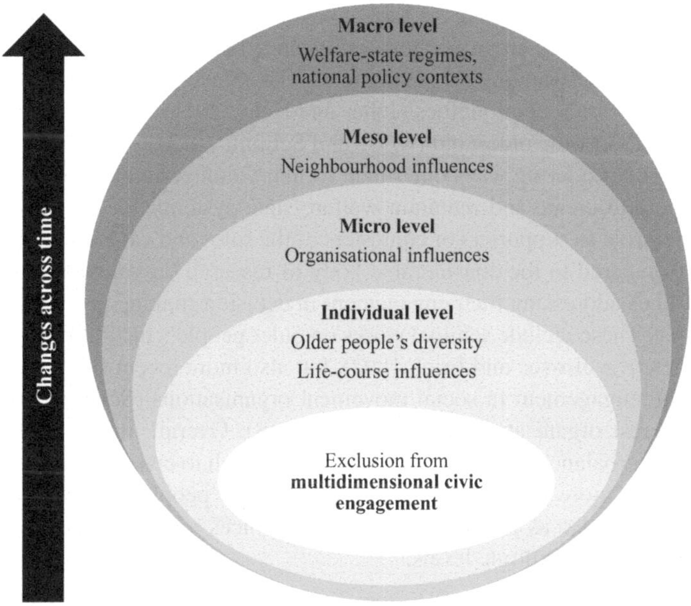

Fig. 19.1 Proposed conceptual framework for studying exclusion from civic engagement in later life

2011), naturalising formal volunteering as the "right" way to contribute. This approach may lead to the stigmatisation of people who are unable or unwilling to formally volunteer, and also to the invisibility of those who engage through other channels (Martinez et al. 2011). Such circumstances also illustrate how processes and cultures associated with dominant discourses of voluntarism may function to exclude older people who engage civically in different ways. Consequently, studies on exclusion from civic engagement in later life may benefit from paying greater attention to informal helping behaviours inside and outside the family, and to political engagement.

It is the relative invisibility of these informal helping behaviours in the ageing literature that is paradoxical, given the fact that caregiving to family members and helping non-kin are far more common among older people than formal volunteering (*e.g.* Kruse and Schmitt 2015). Critical gerontologists have highlighted that this responds to a gendered construction of what should and what should not be considered civic engagement (*e.g.* Martinson and Halpern 2011; Nesteruk and Price 2011). This also connects with other forms of social exclusion in later life, such as identity and symbolic exclusion, as valuing some contributions and labelling them as "civic" over others could lead to the depreciation and marginalisation of those who engage in different ways. As noted by Herd and Meyer (2002), if the concept includes activities seeking improved benefits for others, the community, or wider society "…what could possibly fit these definitional requirements better than care work?" (p. 674). Although researching informal helping behaviours may be more challenging than studying formal volunteering, given that they are less easy to quantify, more likely to occur in a private sphere, and less likely to be recognised as civic activities by those who perform them, they are of greatest significance for creating and maintaining the social glue, especially among people at greater risk of exclusion in later life, such as people ageing in rural communities (Jones and Heley 2016), older migrants (Torres and Serrat 2019), or the oldest old (Kruse and Schmitt 2015).

As well as considering ways other than formal volunteering in which older people contribute to create and maintain welfare-state systems, we need to take into account their role as supporters or contesters of the rules and values governing these systems. Compared to the considerable body of research on volunteering by older people, studies addressing their engagement in decision-making processes are relatively scarce. These include seminal works on older people's institutionalised political activities (*e.g.* Jirovec and Erich 1992), but also more recent studies addressing older adults' engagement in social movement organisations (Schwarz 2019) or in seniors' interest organisations (Serrat et al. 2018). Overall, this line of research helps to counterbalance a prevailing apolitical approach to civic engagement in later life, allowing a more nuanced picture in which older people are not only seen as social actors but also as political agents whose voices must be heard in decision-making processes at multiple levels.

19.4.2 Diversity of the Older Population

Broadening the scope of civic engagement also offers scope to acknowledge the growing diversity of the older population, and therefore the many forms in which older adults engage outside formal volunteering. This not only provides the basis to recognise and value equally all older people's contributions, but also foregrounds the power imbalances that govern later life. Consequently, a second strategic direction for research into civic engagement in later life places the spotlight on older people's diversity. Although social gerontology discourse has increasingly emphasised the importance of considering this diversity, it has been scarcely explored in empirical studies (Stone et al. 2017), and particularly in those addressing civic engagement in later life (Serrat et al. 2019). This is partially due to the omission or underrepresentation in household surveys of some people most at risk of social exclusion (Levitas et al. 2007). Diversity shapes aspects such as who takes part (Petriwskyj et al. 2017) and who benefits from engagement (Morrow-Howell et al. 2009), or in which ways older people participate (Nesteruk and Price 2011). Research and policy initiatives aimed at reducing older people's exclusion from civic engagement may consider the particular challenges that potentially marginalised groups of older people may confront to their full inclusion in civic activities, including older migrants (Torres and Serrat 2019), older people living in long-term care institutions (Villar et al. in this volume), the oldest old (Kruse and Schmitt 2015), or older people experiencing health problems or disabilities (Principi et al. 2016).

Research into older people's exclusion from civic engagement may particularly benefit from simultaneously taking into account multiple dimensions of diversity. Intersectionality theory highlights that people occupying particular social positions experience the non-additive effects of multiple forms of inequality. As argued by Calasanti and Kielcot (2012), age may be considered as a system of inequality as "... membership in age categories shape self-concepts and interactions in ways that have material consequences and thus influence life chances" (p. 271). Consideration of diversity in studies on civic engagement must therefore take into account how age interacts with other systems of inequalities, such as gender, disability, living situation, or migrant status, to shape older people's inclusion or exclusion from civic engagement.

Acknowledging older people's diversity has a direct impact on practice and social policy initiatives, raising questions about issues of representation and representativeness. Barnes and Newman (2003), among others, warn about the risks of using a single identity category (such as "older people") to determine how public actors are defined. This raises questions about how diverse groups of older people can be taken into account in decision-making processes, and also regarding which voices represent (and which do not) those who effectively gain a seat at the table (Petriwskyj et al. 2014). As argued by Barnes et al. (2011):

> '...the question of whether participants can be considered legitimate representatives of older people requires consideration of the basis on which they might be able to 'speak for' older people who are not directly involved, and whether they can and should be accountable to them.' (p. 263)

Against this background, diversity should be prioritised both in future research aimed at understanding civic engagement and in social policy initiatives seeking to encouraging greater engagement of older people and to reduce opportunities for exclusion from civic activities in later life.

19.4.3 Exclusion from Civic Engagement as a Culturally-Embedded Process

Exclusion from civic engagement in later life should be understood as a culturally-embedded process, as it is decisively influenced by where and when engagement occurs. However, this contextual aspect of civic engagement has been underexplored in previous research (Serrat et al. 2019). In order to move research on older people's civic engagement, and their exclusion from that engagement, forward, we should consider at least three possible levels in which exclusion from civic engagement may occur: micro (related to organisational influences), meso (connected to neighbourhood and communities influences), and macro (referring to the influence of welfare-state regimes and national policy contexts).

At the micro level, an emerging body of studies has shown that organisations play a key role in aspects such as recruiting and retaining older people (Devaney et al. 2015) or even the benefits they obtain from their engagement (Hong and Morrow-Howell 2013). Importantly, exclusionary processes are also in place within organisations. This means that some older people may be excluded from civic engagement altogether, while others gain a seat at the table but experience that their contributions are not as valued as those of others. According to Young (2000), when organisations are inaccessible to older people because of individuals' physical or cognitive needs, their socio-economic status or their literacy level, then external exclusion takes place. When those who access organisations do not participate in the ways expected, and their opinions are considered less important, internal exclusion occurs. Notwithstanding recent efforts to incorporate an institutional approach into the study of older people's civic engagement (Hong et al. 2009), there is clearly a need for more research addressing these organisational influences.

At the meso level, it is important to consider how neighbourhood and community aspects shape older people's opportunities and constraints for civic engagement [see Tournier and Vidovićová, this volume], as well as the way in which micro organisations are often embedded in particular neighbourhood and community contexts. Recent studies on urban settings show that older people's engagement in formal volunteering is associated with objective municipality characteristics as well as with people's perceptions of social and physical features of their neighbourhood, including connectedness, satisfaction, security, and availability of services and amenities (Dury et al. 2016; Gonzales et al. 2016; see also Urbaniak et al. this volume). Moreover, studies in rural communities highlight the many civic contributions of older people living in these settings, both at formal and informal levels, but also the particular constraints and limitations that rural elders must face to engage civically (Skinner and Hanlon 2015; Jones and Heley 2016; Warburton and Winterton 2017). However, there is clearly a need for more studies analysing the role of spatial aspects on exclusion from civic engagement in later life.

Finally, at the macro level, civic engagement is decisively influenced by the particular socio-political context in which engagement occurs (Goerres 2009). Until fairly recently, most literature on civic engagement in later life emanated from the United States. However, more recent studies focus on other world regions with quite different political and cultural contexts. These include findings from different countries of Europe (Principi et al. 2014) and Asia (Morrow-Howell and Mui 2012), and emerging comparisons across countries in different world regions (Serrat et al. 2018). This body of literature highlights the crucial importance of understanding the macro context when addressing older people's exclusion from civic engagement. It is particularly relevant to explore how different welfare state (Warburton and Jeppsson Grassman 2011) or policy (Castles and Obinger 2008) regimes shape seniors' possibilities for civic engagement. However, research from this perspective remains underdeveloped.

19.4.4 Dynamics and Experiences of Older People's Exclusion from Civic Engagement

Finally, civic engagement should be understood as a dynamic rather than static phenomenon, as people may be included or excluded from civic engagement at different points of the life course. Yet most existing research focuses exclusively on later life circumstances, and therefore fails to explain how civic engagement begins and develops across the life course (Serrat et al. 2019). Moreover, people may experience changes that reach beyond simply moving in and out of engagement. For example, the ways in which individuals engage or their level of commitment may change over time. However, biographical aspects of civic engagement in later life has been scarcely explored in previous research (Serrat and Villar 2019).

When addressing dynamic aspects of civic engagement, it is useful to distinguish between age-graded influences (*i.e.* changes associated with particular developmental trajectories), history-graded influences (*i.e.* historical events and changes that affect specific cohorts of older people), and non-normative influences (*i.e.* positive and negative events that the individual cannot anticipate) (Baltes 1987; Heckhausen 1999). Regarding history-graded influences, for instance, many western nations are currently experiencing the ageing of the 1968 "generation", people largely in their late teens and early twenties who engaged in non-conventional forms of political protest in the late 1960s. People belonging to this birth cohort may well be engaged in different types of civic activity compared to previous or later cohorts, a point argued by Bruns et al. (2007) in relation to the situation in Germany.

As well as dynamics of civic engagement, experiences of engagement have been largely overlooked in research (Serrat et al. 2019). Studies on the experiences of engagement are aimed at overcoming the idea of civic engagement as a "black box" which older people enter if they have the resources, motivations, and opportunities (antecedents), and which they exit with increased levels of health and well-being (outcomes). Thus, this line of research is aimed at taking a closer look at the experiences and processes occurring inside the "black box" of civic engagement. Most of this research addresses issues of retention, that is, longer permanence within activities and organisations (Tang et al. 2009; Devaney et al. 2015), with a smaller number of studies exploring the informal learning processes occurring through engagement in civic activities and organisations (Piercy et al. 2011; Chen 2016). However, there are still significant opportunities for further studies addressing older people's negative and positive experiences of civic engagement and their role in issues such as retention, satisfaction, or benefits accruing from the activity.

19.5 Conclusion

In this chapter, we have sought to make a contribution to conceptual understandings of social exclusion in later life by focusing our attention on the exclusion from civic engagement as the least studied dimension of older people's social exclusion. Drawing on a state-of-the-art review of evidence concerning older people's engagement in civic activities, we make the case that future research should address four key dimensions of older people's exclusion from civic engagement: the multidimensionality of civic engagement; the diversity of the older population; the dynamics and experiences of engagement across the life course; and the culturally-embedded process that characterises civic engagement. In exploring these dimensions of exclusion from civic engagement, there is clearly further merit in considering the ways in which this particular form of social exclusion interacts with other forms of disadvantage, thereby exacerbating experiences of exclusion in later life for individuals or groups of older adults.

Editors' Postscript

Please note, like other contributions to this book, this chapter was written before the COVID-19 pandemic of 2020. The book's introductory chapter (Chap. 1) and conclusion (Chap. 34) consider some of the key ways in which the pandemic relates to issues concerning social exclusion and ageing.

Acknowledgement This work was supported by Spain's Ministry of Economy and Competitiveness, Reference PSI2016-77864-R. Rodrigo Serrat is a Serra Húnter Tenure-Track Lecturer.

References

Adler, R. P., & Goggin, J. (2005). What do we mean by "civic engagement"? *Journal of Transformative Education, 3*(3), 236–253. https://doi.org/10.1177/1541344605276792.

Baltes, P. B. (1987). Theoretical propositions of life-span developmental psychology: On the dynamics between growth and decline. *Developmental Psychology, 23*(5), 611–626. https://doi.org/10.1037/0012-1649.23.5.611.

Barnes, M., & Newman, J. (2003). Constituting "the public" in public participation. *Public Administration, 81*(2), 379–399. https://doi.org/10.1111/1467-9299.00352/full.

Barnes, M., Harrison, E., & Murray, L. (2011). Ageing activists: Who gets involved in older people's forums? *Ageing and Society, 32*(2), 261–280. https://doi.org/10.1017/S0144686X11000328.

Barrett, M., & Brunton-Smith, I. (2014). Political and civic engagement and participation: Towards an integrative perspective. *Journal of Civil Society, 10*(1), 5–28. https://doi.org/10.1080/17448689.2013.871911.

Bruns, P., Bruns, W., & Böhme, R. (2007). *Die Altersrevolution: wie wir in Zukunft alt werden*. Berlin: Aufbau-Verlag.

Buffel, T., Phillipson, C., & Scharf, T. (2012). Ageing in urban environments: Developing "age-friendly" cities. *Critical Social Policy, 32*(4), 597–617. https://doi.org/10.1177/0261018311430457.

Calasanti, T., & Kielcot, K. (2012). Intersectionality and aging families. In R. Blieszner & V. Bedford (Eds.), *Handbook of families and aging* (pp. 398–434). Santa Barbara: Praeger.

Castles, F. G., & Obinger, H. (2008). Worlds, families, regimes: Country clusters in European and OECD area public policy. *West European Politics, 31*(1–2), 321–344. https://doi.org/10.1080/01402380701835140.

Chen, L. K. (2016). Not just helping: What and how older men learn when they volunteer. *Educational Gerontology, 42*(3), 175–185. https://doi.org/10.1080/03601277.2015.1085786.

Devaney, C., Kearns, N., Fives, A., Canavan, J., Lyons, R., & Eaton, P. (2015). Recruiting and retaining older adult volunteers: Implications for practice. *Journal of Nonprofit & Public Sector Marketing, 27*(4), 331–350. https://doi.org/10.1080/10495142.2015.1015373.

Dury, S., Willems, J., De Witte, N., De Donder, L., Buffel, T., & Verté, D. (2016). Municipality and neighborhood influences on volunteering in later life. *Journal of Applied Gerontology, 35*(6), 601–626. https://doi.org/10.1177/0733464814533818.

Ekman, J., & Amnå, E. (2012). Political participation and civic engagement: Towards a new typology. *Human Affairs, 22*(3), 283–300. https://doi.org/10.2478/s13374-012-0024-1.

Goerres, A. (2009). *The political participation of older people in Europe: The greying of our democracies*. Basingstoke: Palgrave Macmillan.

Gonzales, E., Shen, H. W., Wang, Y., Martinez, L. S., & Norstrand, J. (2016). Race and place: Exploring the intersection of inequity and volunteerism among older black and white adults. *Journal of Gerontological Social Work, 59*(5), 381–400. https://doi.org/10.1080/01634372.2016.1224787.

Greenfield, E. A. (2010). Identifying the boundaries and horizons of the concept of civic engagement for the field of aging. In L. Carstensen, G. O'Neill, & S. Wilson (Eds.), *Civic engagement in an older America* (pp. 4–12). Washington, DC: The Gerontological Society of America.

Heckhausen, J. (1999). *Developmental regulation in adulthood: Age-normative and sociostructural constraints as adaptative challenges*. Cambridge: Cambridge University Press. https://doi.org/10.1017/CBO9780511527852.

Herd, P., & Meyer, M. H. (2002). Care work invisible civic engagement. *Gender and Society, 16*(5), 665–688. https://doi.org/10.1177/089124302236991.

Hong, S., & Morrow-Howell, N. (2013). Increasing older adults' benefits from institutional capacity of volunteer programs. *Social Work Research, 37*(2), 99–108. https://doi.org/10.1093/swr/svs028.

Hong, S., Morrow-Howell, N., Tang, F., & Hinterlong, J. (2009). Engaging older adults in volunteering: Conceptualizing and measuring institutional capacity. *Nonprofit and Voluntary Sector Quarterly, 38*(2), 200–219.

Hustinx, L., & Denk, T. (2009). The "black box" problem in the study of participation. *Journal of Civil Society, 5*(3), 209–226. https://doi.org/10.1080/17448680903351693.

Jirovec, R., & Erich, J. (1992). The dynamics of political participation among the urban elderly. *Journal of Applied Gerontology, 11*(2), 216–227. https://doi.org/10.1177/073346489201100207.

Jones, L., & Heley, J. (2016). Practices of participation and voluntarism among older people in rural Wales: Choice, obligation and constraints to active ageing. *Sociologia Ruralis, 56*(2), 176–196. https://doi.org/10.1111/soru.12073.

Kruse, A., & Schmitt, E. (2015). Shared responsibility and civic engagement in very old age. *Research in Human Development, 12*(1–2), 133–148. https://doi.org/10.1080/15427609.2015.1010353.

Levitas, R., Pantazis, C., Fahmy, E., Gordon, D., Lloyd, E., & Patsios, D. (2007). *The multidimensional analysis of social exclusion*. London. https://doi.org/10.1177/1744987110370529.

Martinez, I., Crooks, D., Kim, K., & Tanner, E. (2011). Invisible civic engagement among older adults: Valuing the contributions of informal volunteering. *Journal of Cross-Cultural Gerontology, 26*(1), 23–37. https://doi.org/10.1007/s10823-011-9137-y.

Martinson, M., & Halpern, J. (2011). Ethical implications of the promotion of elder volunteerism: A critical perspective. *Journal of Aging Studies, 25*(4), 427–435. https://doi.org/10.1016/j.jaging.2011.04.003.

Morrow-Howell, N., & Mui, A. (2012). *Productive engagement in later life: A global perspective*. New York: Routledge.

Morrow-Howell, N., Hong, S. I., & Tang, F. (2009). Who benefits from volunteering? Variations in perceived benefits. *The Gerontologist, 49*(1), 91–102. https://doi.org/10.1093/geront/gnp007.

Nesteruk, O., & Price, C. (2011). Retired women and volunteering: The good, the bad, and the unrecognized. *Journal of Women & Aging, 23*(2), 99–112. https://doi.org/10.1080/08952841.2011.561138.

Nygård, M., & Jakobsson, G. (2013). Senior citizens and political participation: Evidence from a Finnish regional study. *Ageing & Society, 33*(1), 159–180. https://doi.org/10.1017/S0144686X11001139.

Offe, C. (1985). New social movements: Challenging the boundaries of institutional politics. *Social Research, 52*(4), 817–868.

Petriwskyj, A., Warburton, J., Everingham, J., & Cuthill, M. (2014). Seniors' motivations for participation in local governance: Evidence from an Australian study. *Local Government Studies, 40*(2), 240–263. https://doi.org/10.1080/03003930.2013.790812.

Petriwskyj, A., Serrat, R., Warburton, J., Everingham, J., & Cuthill, M. (2017). Barriers to older people's participation in local governance: The impact of diversity. *Educational Gerontology, 43*(5), 259–275. https://doi.org/10.1080/03601277.2017.1293391.

Piercy, K. W., Cheek, C., & Teemant, B. (2011). Challenges and psychosocial growth for older volunteers giving intensive humanitarian service. *The Gerontologist, 51*(4), 550–560. https://doi.org/10.1093/geront/gnr013.

Postle, K., Wright, P., & Beresford, P. (2005). Older people's participation in political activity making their voices heard: A potential support role for welfare professionals in countering ageism and social exclusion. *Practice, 17*(3), 173–189. https://doi.org/10.1080/09503150500285123.

Principi, A., Jensen, P., & Lamura, G. (2014). *Active ageing: Voluntary work by older people in Europe*. Bristol: The Policy Press.

Principi, A., Galenkamp, H., Papa, R., Socci, M., Suanet, B., Schmidt, A., et al. (2016). Do predictors of volunteering in older age differ by health status? *European Journal of Ageing, 13*(2), 91–102. https://doi.org/10.1007/s10433-016-0377-0.

Schwarz, C. H. (2019). Collective memory and intergenerational transmission in social movements: The "grandparents' movement" iaioflautas, the indignados protests, and the Spanish transition. *Memory Studies*. https://doi.org/10.1177/1750698019856058.

Serrat, R., & Villar, F. (2019). Lifecourse transitions and participation in political organisations in older Spanish men and women. *Ageing & Society, 40*, 2174–2190. https://doi.org/10.1017/S0144686X19000618.

Serrat, R., Warburton, J., Petriwskyj, A., & Villar, F. (2018). Political participation and social exclusion in later life: What politically active seniors can teach us about barriers to inclusion and retention. *International Journal of Ageing and Later Life, 12*, 53–58. https://doi.org/10.3384/ijal.1652-8670.18395.

Serrat, R., Scharf, T., Villar, F., & Gómez, C. (2019). Fifty-five years of research into older people's civic participation: Recent trends, future directions. *The Gerontologist, 60*, e38–e51. https://doi.org/10.1093/geront/gnz021.

Skinner, M., & Hanlon, N. (2015). *Ageing resource communities: New frontiers of rural population change, community development and voluntarism*. London: Routledge.

Stone, M. E., Lin, J., Dannefer, D., & Kelley Moore, J. A. (2017). The continued eclipse of heterogeneity in gerontological research. *The Journals of Gerontology Series B: Psychological Sciences and Social Sciences, 72*(1), 162–167. https://doi.org/10.1093/geronb/gbv068.

Tang, F., Morrow-Howell, N., & Hong, S. (2009). Inclusion of diverse older populations in volunteering: The importance of institutional facilitation. *Nonprofit and Voluntary Sector Quarterly, 38*(5), 810–827. https://doi.org/10.1177/0899764008320195.

Theocharis, Y. (2015). The conceptualization of digitally networked participation. *Social Media + Society, 1*(2), 1–14. https://doi.org/10.1177/2056305115610140.

Torres, S., & Serrat, R. (2019). Older migrants' civic participation: A topic in need of attention. *Journal of Aging Studies, 50*. https://doi.org/10.1016/j.jaging.2019.100790.

United Nations. (2002). *Madrid international plan of action on ageing*. Madrid.

van Deth, J. W. (2001). Studying political participation: Towards a theory of everything? *European Consortium for Political Research*, 1–19.

Walsh, K., Scharf, T., & Keating, N. (2017). Social exclusion of older persons: A scoping review and conceptual framework. *European Journal of Ageing, 14*(1), 81–98. https://doi.org/10.1007/s10433-016-0398-8.

Warburton, J., & Jeppsson Grassman, E. (2011). Variations in older people's social and productive ageing activities across different social welfare regimes. *International Journal of Social Welfare, 20*(2), 180–191. https://doi.org/10.1111/j.1468-2397.2009.00691.x.

Warburton, J., & Winterton, R. (2017). A far greater sense of community: The impact of volunteer behaviour on the wellness of rural older Australians. *Health and Place, 48*, 132–138. https://doi.org/10.1016/j.healthplace.2017.10.005.

WHO. (2002). *Active ageing: A policy framework*. Geneva.

Young, I. M. (2000). *Inclusion and democracy*. New York: Oxford University Press.

Chapter 20
Cultural Exclusion in Old-Age: A Social Exclusion Perspective on Cultural Practice in Later Life

Vera Gallistl

20.1 Introduction

Expanding the cultural participation of socially marginalised groups is a major concern of cultural policies around the world (Morrone 2006). However, cultural exclusion in later life is conceptually under-developed and empirically under-explored. Even though cultural activity in later life has received attention in gerontology since the 1980s (Fisher and Specht 2000) and has been revived as a research topic in the last 10 years (Bernard and Rickett 2016), it is hardly analysed outside of therapeutic interventions (Fraser et al. 2015) and even less so as an aspect of exclusion in later life. Despite the positive impacts of cultural participation, for example, participatory arts (Tymoszuk et al. 2019), writing (Sabeti 2014), music (Perkins and Williamon 2014), singing (Coulton et al. 2015), and visiting museums (Thomson et al. 2018) having been extensively analysed, its barriers in access as well as the impacts of exclusion on cultural participation are scarcely evident in gerontological research. This results in a lack of knowledge concerning the mechanisms through which cultural exclusion is produced and which policy instruments support the cultural inclusion of older adults.

This chapter explores exclusion from cultural participation in later life, as an example of civic exclusion, by taking three steps: first, a theoretical framework of cultural exclusion in later life is developed, which draws on social-gerontological theories of social exclusion as well as a sociology of the arts and culture; second, the phenomenon of cultural exclusion is explored with representative survey data on cultural activity of the older Austrian population (60 years and over); third, results are discussed in light of the proposed concept of old-age cultural exclusion.

V. Gallistl (✉)
Department of Sociology, University of Vienna, Vienna, Austria
e-mail: vera.maria.gallistl@univie.ac.at

K. Walsh et al. (eds.), *Social Exclusion in Later Life*, International Perspectives on Aging 28, https://doi.org/10.1007/978-3-030-51406-8_20

20.2 An Exclusion Perspective on Cultural Practice in Old-Age

Culture has been a well-studied topic in gerontology, however, from very different perspectives. Intervention studies have shown that involving older adults in creative activities has significant positive outcomes for well-being, health, and self-image (for reviews, see Fraser et al. 2015; Bernard and Rickett 2016). Studies with representative survey data have highlighted that even though adults aged 65 years and over attend more cultural events compared to the general population (Toepoel 2011) and 45-54 year olds are the most culturally active group (van Eijck 2005), participation declines in most European countries after the age of 65 years. This indicates an inverted U-shaped relationship between age and cultural participation (Falk and Katz-Gerro 2015). By contrast, research in cultural gerontology (see, *e.g.* Twigg and Martin 2015) has highlighted the role of culture in the construction of age and ageing in late-modern societies. This variety of approaches directs our attention to the heterogeneity of understandings of culture in gerontological research and the often-complicated relationship between cultural practice and social exclusion.

For the sake of this article, we can identify two notions of culture in gerontology. First, culture can be understood as the ubiquitous symbolic nature of human existence (Reckwitz 2008/2010), making culture an inherent part of our everyday lives. From this perspective, we can argue that all people are involved in culture in their everyday lives and might understand practices of consumption (for example, ways of dressing, travelling or eating), practices of everyday life (for example, ways of reading or arranging our furniture) or shared values and beliefs (for example ways of framing age and ageing) as a part of *cultural practice* in a society. Culture is an inherent part of our society, which "can be seen as discursively constituted as a web of signs, so that the central focus of analysis becomes the interpretation and deconstruction of these" (Twigg and Martin 2015, p. 353).

Second, culture can be understood as a field of social differentiation within a society, dedicated to the production of aesthetic knowledge through arts and cultural institutions (Reckwitz 2008/2010) in which some social groups participate, and others do not. *Cultural participation*, hence, describes taking part in specific activities related to arts institutions. This understanding allows us to question hierarchies in cultural practice (Bourdieu 1979/2013): While going to renowned theatres might be highly valued as a cultural activity, watching rock-concerts on TV might be valued differently. Participation in specific, "highbrow" forms of culture is therefore involved in the depiction of high social status and we can differentiate between "highbrow" (legitimate) and "lowbrow" (less legitimate) forms of culture.

How do these approaches inform understandings of old-age cultural exclusion? Drawing on conceptual frameworks of social exclusion in older-age (Walsh et al. 2017), this chapter puts forward the notion of cultural exclusion in later life to describe the separation of older individuals and groups from highly appreciated forms of culture in a society. This definition encompasses two aspects: First, it emphasizes the manifold ways in which older individuals might experience barriers and challenges in accessing "highbrow" forms of culture, through *e.g.* physical and emotional distance or declining mobility in later life, decreasing their chances of *cultural participation* as a result. Second, it acknowledges the ubiquitous nature of *cultural practice* and asks through which processes certain forms of cultural practice are appreciated and addressed as forms of cultural participation, while others are not.

To develop a concept of cultural exclusion in later life, we must, hence, not only ask which age groups participate in culture and which ones do not, we must also ask how our understandings of culture are influenced by social power structures. Studies on arts participation in later life often find that the majority of older adults report no arts participation (Tymoszuk et al. 2019), which reflects not only decreasing participation by older adults, but also the limits of measurements used. Problematic in these understandings of cultural participation is that they are often not sensitive to changes and vulnerabilities over the life course – especially in old-age, cultural participation is not always an active behaviour (Morrone 2006), and might include consuming media, listening to music, or inventing stories while talking to friends and family, which are often not covered in traditional surveys. It might also include the consumption of easier and more accessible "lowbrow" cultural activities than in other life stages. Studies on late-life cultural participation, hence, are often somewhat at risk of reproducing an oversimplified image of older adults as frail, inactive, and excluded through the idea that cultural activity is only possible through health, activity, and independence. What comes to count as participation in later life requires acknowledging cultural practice that happens at home, or in less visible ways. Conceptualising cultural exclusion, hence, means to draw a comprehensive picture of the maybe less obvious ways in which older adults participate culturally.

One more nuanced framework to understand the dimensions of cultural participation was introduced by Morrone (2006), who defines cultural participation as a threefold construct. It comprises, first, cultural activities that happen outside of the home ("*culture de sortie*"—"going-out culture"). This dimension includes activities that are usually understood and measured as cultural practice, for example going to theatres, museums, and galleries. Second, Morrone (2006) understands cultural activities that happen at home as part of cultural participation (*"culture d'appartement"—"home-bound culture"*), such as media consumption, reading, or listening to music. Third, he acknowledges amateur creative activities as a part of cultural participation; as part of an "identity culture" ("*culture identitaire*").

Further, an understanding of cultural exclusion in later life needs to take the differentiation between "highbrow" and "lowbrow" forms of culture into account and ask in which forms of culture older adults participate in. Although often contested, the notion of "highbrow" culture has signified the aesthetic refinement of the well-educated since the beginning of the nineteenth century (Hanquinet and Savage 2015), while the term "lowbrow" taste was used to describe the culture of the socio-economic less well off, for example through their preference for folklore music, art, and dance. From that perspective, high social socio-economic status was connected to the appreciation of "highbrow" forms of culture, while lower socio-economic status led to "lowbrow" cultural activity and taste (Bourdieu 1979/2013).

This dichotomy has, however, been significantly contested in the last 20 years, especially through the concept of the *omnivore*, which offers a more nuanced understanding of social inequalities in cultural consumption and taste (Sullivan and Katz-Gerro 2006). Introduced by Peterson and colleagues in the 1990s, it follows the hypothesis that "[c]ontemporary elites no longer use highbrow taste to demonstrate their cultural distinction, but are better characterized as inclusive 'omnivores', happy to consume both high and low culture." (Peterson and Kern 1996). Groups higher in social status can thus be characterised by a broad interest in cultural goods from all levels (Radošinská 2018). This might include both patterns of cultural voraciousness (meaning that consumers have a large appetite for all forms of cultural consumption) and taste eclecticism (meaning that they intentionally cut across boundaries between highbrow and lowbrow culture as a means of distinction) (Chan and Goldthorpe 2007). Studies on hipsters (Busman 2019) and modern cosmopolitanism (Cicchelli and Octobre 2018) show that the concept of the omnivore can be applied in different contexts to explain dominant forms of cultural participation.

Applied to the study of old-age, two different hypotheses might apply. First, considering the strong influence of activity theory (Havighurst 1961) in gerontology, it might be that it is the general level of activity that is of special value in later life, rather than a specific taste orientation. This leads to the hypothesis that older adults with high status tend towards cultural omnivorousness, interested in consuming any kind of culture that demonstrates activity. On the other hand, Peterson (1992) suggests that in a generational shift in cultural practice, dominant taste might become more subcultural as an effect of the ageing of new social groups (for example baby boomers or ageing hippies). This leads to the hypothesis that subcultures and narrow cultural tastes (especially those oriented towards pop and rock 'n' roll taste) are highest in status in older-age.

Applying Morrone's (2006) framework and combining it with Schulze's patterns of taste (2014), the present study examines patterns of cultural participation of older adults and their relationship with socio-economic status by answering the following three research questions:

First, what types of cultural participation can be observed among older adults and how does cultural participation change in later life? Second, what is the association between different forms of cultural participation in later life (high-brow and low-brow) and socio-economic status? Third, to what extent is high socio-economic status in later life related to cultural omnivorousness?

20.3 Materials and Methods

20.3.1 Data Collection and Sample

This study was conducted within the context of "Cultures of Ageing" project, a 3-year project that addresses the diverse sites of older adults' cultural participation. This paper is based on a representative survey of older adults in Austria aged 60 years and over. Data was collected via CATI (Computer-assisted telephone interview), to reach a random sample of 1531 community dwelling older adults. Participants ranged from 60 to 98 years, with a mean of 71.9 years (SD = 8.3). Females account for around half of the sample (55.3%), and 29% finished only primary and 8.6% completed tertiary education. The majority of the sample (89.8%) were unemployed, unable to work, or retired and 10.8% were employed or self-employed. Data was weighted to ensure representation of the average older population in Austria. Data collection was conducted exclusively in German.

20.3.2 Measurement

The investigation was based on a specific part of the data that explored participants' cultural participation. Participants were asked about a total of 24 activities and asked how frequently they had engaged in these activities in the 12 months (for all activities included see Table 20.1). The analysis also included variables concerning the respondents' socio-demographic background (*e.g.* sex, education, place of residence, subjective health, size of household, age, income). Low socio-economic status was measured as having low education, social class and income as three most commonly used measures of social stratification in later life (Grundy and Holt 2001). Analysis also included a short version of Schulze's (2014) scheme of aesthetic preferences, to measure taste preferences in three schemes: (1) High culture scheme (highbrow taste); (2) Trivial scheme (folk taste); (3) Excitement scheme (pop taste).

20.3.3 Data Analysis

Data was analysed using SPSS V. 24 software. The first step involved a factor analysis of the data describing the frequency of participating in different cultural activities using principal components extraction and varimax rotation with Kaiser Normalisation. The accepted factors had an eigenvalue of at least 1.0 and reported factor loadings were at least 0.4. Factor labels resulted from the authors' interpretation of common characteristics of the activities in each factor. The identified factors were then subjected to a two-step cluster analysis, classifying groups of older adults

Table 20.1 Factors and factor loadings for exploratory factor analysis of three dimensions of cultural activities

Dimension (KMO)	Factor (Eigenvalue)	Activities included in the factor	Factor loading	Variance explained
Culture d'Appartement (0.578)	Reading and music (2.063)	Listening to music	0.623	17.194
		Reading books	0.823	
		Reading newspapers and magazines	0.556	
		Using a computer	0.427	
	Radio (1.737)	Listing to radio shows	0.819	14.475
		Listening to radio (music)	0.798	
	Relaxation (1.410)	Gardening	0.611	11.750
		Praying and meditating	0.741	
	TV (1.082)	Watching TV	0.856	9.013
	Games (1.009)	Playing chess or other games	0.903	8.405
		Doing crosswords or Sudoku	0.451	
Culture de Sortie (0.816)	Highbrow culture (3.751)	Concerts	0.735	31.256
		Theatre, ballet, opera	0.799	
		Dance performances, musicals	0.622	
		Comedy shows	0.557	
		Museum, galleries, exhibitions	0.802	
		Historical sights	0.702	
		Public libraries	0.552	
	Local culture (1.643)	Local events	0.809	13.694
		Services, church	0.530	
		Eating at home with 10+ people	0.641	
	Entertainment culture (1.341)	Cinema	0.705	11.171
		Sport events	0.643	

Note: Data was weighted. N = 1.518. Pairwise case deletion. Principal component extraction and varimax rotation with Kaiser normalisation. Factors included based on an eigenvalue of at least 1. Only loadings of at least 0.4 are presented. The five factors explained 61% of variance (culture d'appartement) and 57% of variance (culture de sortie). Creative activities (writing, making music, crafting, creative cooking, creative sports, painting and drawing, acting, taking photos or movies, dancing) were measured as binary variables and therefore summed for index construction

with similar cultural activity patterns as clusters. The identified clusters were named by the author based on the interpretation of each clusters' involvement in cultural activities. The next step involved analysing differences in these lifestyles according to socio-economic background and taste using cross-tabulations and chi-square tests as well as one-way analysis of variance (ANOVA) and Bonferroni post hoc tests. Unless otherwise stated, all reported findings were significant at or above the 0.05 level.

20.4 Results

20.4.1 The Structure of Cultural Participation in Later Life

Factor analysis on the frequency of participation in 24 cultural activities revealed eight activity factors (Table 20.1): three in the *culture de sortie* (going-out culture) and five for activities in the *culture d'appartement* (home-bound culture). For *culture identitaire* (identity culture), an index was constructed based on the variables in the dataset.

Factor analysis for the *culture de sortie* activities revealed the importance of space as well as taste as a part of going-out culture. First, the *highbrow culture* factor included all cultural activities that usually require leaving the neighbourhood or community and are usually seen as highbrow cultural activity, such as visiting the theatre, museums, galleries, exhibitions, or historical sites. Second, the *local culture* factor included all cultural activities that can usually be done close to the home. It included activities connected to a local or community culture, like going to the church, visiting local events, or inviting more than ten persons for a meal. Third *entertainment culture* included all variables that were connected to a lighter cultural experience, such as going to the cinema or visiting sports events.

Factor analysis for the *culture d'appartement* showed that some cultural activities engaged in at home were oriented towards the medium, while others were oriented towards the aim of the activities. The largest factor, *reading and music,* involved all variables that were connected to consuming media in either a visual or auditory form. Most importantly, this factor included reading books, listening to music, or reading newspapers and magazines. The second-largest factor, *radio,* included both variables that described consumption of the radio as a cultural format (radio shows and radio music). The third-largest factor, *relaxation,* included cultural activities at home that were oriented towards self-reflection as well as relaxation (gardening and praying/meditating). Finally, *television* (TV) and *games* factors were clearly associated with specific activities, watching TV (TV), and playing chess, crosswords, Sudoku, or other games (games).

Analysing the age patterns for different activity factors reveals that while there are some groups of activities in which participation declines with age, this is not the case for all observed factors. Three factors (*highbrow culture, entertainment culture, reading, and music)* show clear patterns of decreased participation in higher age groups (changes larger than 0.5). Four factors (*creative activities, local culture, TV,* and *games*) point to continuity between age groups (changes smaller or equal to 0.5). Two activity factors (*radio, relaxation)* even increase with age (changes smaller than 0.0 and negative values). This points to patterns of age-related change in cultural activities rather than a simple decrease (Fig. 20.1).

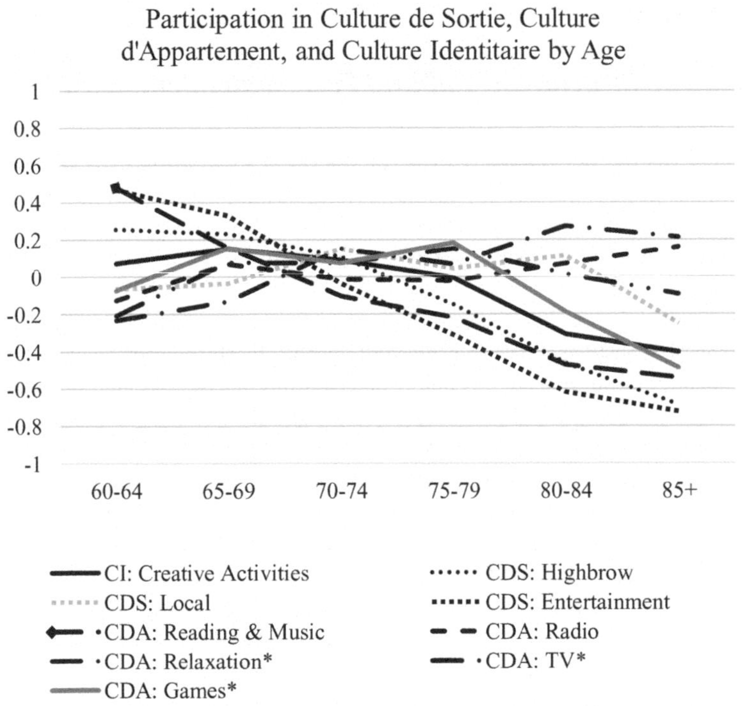

Fig. 20.1 Factors of cultural participation by age of respondents

Note: Data were weighted. N = 1518. Significance was tested using one-way ANOVA with Bonferroni post hoc tests. Standardised means (z-score). Significance tested with one-way ANOVA with Bonferroni post-hoc test. All associations significant ($p < 0.05$)

20.4.2 Clusters of Cultural Participation

Cluster analysis of the eight factors of cultural activities produced an optimal three-cluster solution for Austria's older population (Table 20.2). The identified clusters showed significant differences in their cultural activities as well as taste orientation and general appreciation of culture and the arts.

The first cluster, which accounted for about one-fifth of the total sample (19.9%) was named '*Omnivores*', based on the cluster's tendency to consume a wide variety of cultural products—from highbrow cultural activities (for example museums, theatre) to lowbrow cultural activities (for example religious services, sports, games). Involvement in creative activities, highbrow, and local cultural activities, as well as listening to the radio, meditating, and gardening were most prevalent in this group. This group also displayed a high overall tendency towards highbrow taste. In line with this, this cluster of respondents was also most likely to state that the culture and the arts were very important to them.

The second and largest cluster (53.7%) was labelled '*Univore–TV*', as this cluster showed a strong selectivity in its cultural consumption, and strongly

Table 20.2 Clusters of cultural participation

Variable	Omnivore	Univore – TV	Univore – Entertainment
Participation factor[a]			
CI: Creative activities	1.23	−0.38	−0.15
CDS: Highbrow	0.86	−0.57	0.50
CDS: Local	0.97	−0.12	−0.49
CDS: Entertainment	0.42	−0.49	0.68
CDA: Reading & Music	−0.02	−0.39	0.80
CDA: Radio	0.49	0.01	−0.38
CDA: Relaxation	0.78	0.10	−0.80
CDA: TV	−0.06	0.16	−0.29
CDA: Games	0.60	−0.05	−0.35
Cultural scheme (taste)[a]			
High culture (highbrow)	0.41	−0.23	0.15
Trivial (folk)	0.10	0.28	−0.65
Excitement (pop)	0.08	−0.26	0.48
Appreciation of culture and the arts[b]	81.8	45.4	69.5
Weighted N	302	815	399
Percentage of sample	19.9	53.7	26.3

Note: Data were weighted. Weighted N = 1518. Significance was tested using one-way ANOVA with Bonferroni post-hoc tests. [a]Standardised means (z-score). [b]How important are the arts and culture to you? Summed percentage for 'very important' and 'rather important'

characterised by a high level of watching TV. Furthermore, this cluster was also characterised by a specific taste orientation: Analyses of Schulze's aesthetic schemes showed that this cluster was most likely to be oriented towards trivial and folk taste, which emphasises a high appreciation of folk music and films with a regional background and love stories. Likewise, this cluster also showed the lowest subjective appreciation of highbrow culture and the arts in general.

The third cluster (26.3%) was labelled *'Univore–Entertainment'*. Like *Univore–TV*, this cluster was characterised by involvement in specific cultural activities. In this case, however, selectivity was associated with going to the cinema and sports events (*entertainment culture*), as well as reading books, or listening to music through traditional media or a computer (*reading and music*). Hence, this cluster was also characterised by a preference for going-out culture, which again was connected to a specific taste orientation. This cluster was most likely to react positively to the excitement scheme (pop taste).

The three clusters showed significant ($p < 0.01$) differences according to age. *Univores-TV* showed to be the oldest of the three clusters. For men and women, older participants were more likely to belong to the '*Univore–TV*' cluster, with 86% of the male and 92% of the female population belonging to that cluster. On the other hand, analysis revealed that the *'Univore-Entertainment'* cluster was the youngest clusters for both men and women (Fig. 20.2).

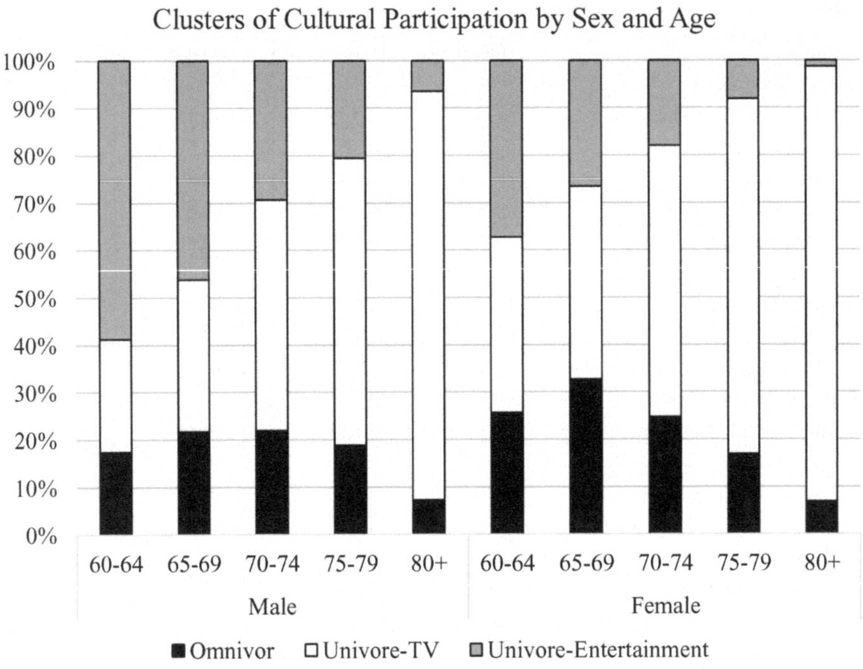

Fig. 20.2 Clusters of cultural participation by sex and age

Note: Data were weighted. N = 1518. Significance was tested using chi-square statistics. All associations significant ($p < 0.05$)

20.4.3 Socio-economic Differentiation in Cultural Practice

Nine socio-economic variables were associated significantly with clusters of cultural participation (Table 20.3). Generally, the *Omnivores* had a socio-economic status that was average to the sample, with deviations towards a high socio-economic status (*Univore–Entertainment*) and lower socio-economic status (*Univore–TV*) in both directions.

Univores-TV showed a higher tendency to be female (61.2%), have low levels of education (with 42.1% only having compulsory education), and to live in rural areas with less than 5000 inhabitants (46%). As they were the oldest cluster (73.2 years on average), they also showed a tendency towards poor subjective health (with 61.7% feeling that their health is average, bad, or very bad), being retired (85.5%), or unable to work (10.6%). In line with their lower level of education, they also showed the lowest average household income of €1350 per month. This was reflected the pattern that they were both more likely to have never been employed (10%) or to hold elementary occupations (11.3%). This cluster was also most likely to live alone (39.3%).

In contrast, *Univores-Entertainment* were more likely to be male (60.2%), higher educated (23.6% academics), and live in rural areas with more than 10,000 inhabitants (43.8%). Corresponding to their high levels of education, they showed the

Table 20.3 Background characteristics of participation clusters

Variable	Omnivore	Univore – TV	Univore – Entertainment
Sex			
Female	59.9	61.2	39.8
Male	40.1	38.8	60.2
Education			
Compulsory education (Primary)	23.8	42.1	6.3
Lower than academic (Secondary)	68.0	56.6	70.2
Academic (Tertiary)	8.3	1.3	23.6
Place of residence (No. of inhabitants)			
< 5,000	45.7	46.0	28.7
5,000 – 10,000	34.1	32.8	27.5
> 10,000	20.2	21.2	43.8
Health			
(Very) Good	69.2	38.3	77.8
Average, (Very) Bad	30.8	61.7	22.3
Size of household			
1 Person	20.9	39.3	24.5
> 1 Person	79.1	60.7	75.5
Work status			
Retired	85.4	85.5	73.2
Employed or self-employed	10.3	3.9	25.3
Other[a]	4.3	10.6	1.5
ISCO[b]			
Managers and professionals	12.2	3.0	26.3
Technicians and associate professionals	8.3	4.7	13.7
Support workers	73.6	71.0	58.7
Elementary occupations	2.3	11.3	0.5
Never employed	3.6	10.0	0.8
Age (mean)	69.2 [68.5, 69.9]	75.3 [74.7, 75.9]	66.9 [66.4, 67.5]
Income (median)	1750	1350	1833

Note: Data represent % of the sample and were weighted. N = 1518. Chi-squared statistics were significant ($p < 0.05$) for all attribute category cross-tabulations. Income and age were tested using one-way ANOVA and were significant ($p < 0.01$). (a) (b) (c) (d) mark significant ($p < 0.05$) differences between groups according to Bonferroni post-hoc tests.[a] Unemployed, disabled, working in household, other [b] ISCO-08 in correspondence with ISCED-97, armed forces occupations excluded due to low case numbers

highest mean household income (an average of € 1833 per month) and had the highest probability of being either managers or professionals (26.3%) or technicians and associated professionals (13.7%). Given that they were the youngest cluster (66.9 years on average), they were also the cluster with the highest ongoing labour market participation (25.3% being employed or self-employed), and the best health (77.8% reported good or very good health).

Given that the first two clusters showed either a tendency towards a higher or lower socio-economic status in general, the *Omnivores* tended toward the sample average for most variables (income, education). This cluster was characterised by their higher probability of living in areas with 5000—10,000 inhabitants (34.1%) and living in a household with more than one person (79.1%). They also showed a higher tendency to be support workers (73.6%).

20.5 Discussion

The central contribution of this study is to put forward the notion of cultural exclusion in later life and to explore this concept based on representative survey data. Drawing on conceptual frameworks of social exclusion in older-age (Walsh et al. 2017), this chapter puts forward the notion of cultural exclusion in later life to describe the separation of older individuals and groups from highly appreciated forms of culture in a society. This topic has been explored with empirical data along three research questions. First, what types of cultural participation can be observed among older adults and how does cultural participation change in later life? Second, what is the association between different forms of cultural participation in later life (high-brow and low-brow) and socio-economic status? Third, to what extent is high socio-economic status in later life related to cultural omnivorousness?

First, data shows that cultural participation shifts, rather than declines, in later life, as this study identified patterns of decline in participation for some cultural activities, however, not for all. This was especially true for activities that are most favourably appreciated for their high artistic quality (for example highbrow cultural activities, but also interests related to cinema to some extent). Participation in highbrow as well as entertainment culture was clearly lower in higher age groups. Further, data showed that the older study participants were more likely to participate in cultural activities that occur predominantly in or close to their own home. As many other studies in gerontology have shown, this emphasises later life as a phase where disengagement from public space (Wanka 2017) and more of a focus on private spaces can be more prevalent, and highlights how spaces operate as opportunity structures for cultural participation (Brook 2016) [also see Tournier and Vidovićová, this volume]. The data therefore shows that cultural participation in later life does not only shift from more "high-brow" to more "low-brow" cultural activities, it also shifts from public to private spaces.

Second, this study suggests that lower rates of participation in cultural activities in later life might not (only) be a function of declining health, but also a function of marginalisation of specific taste orientations. While those groups with high culture taste were more likely to be culturally engaged, it was those with trivial (folk) taste that showed the lowest participation. These findings situate the changes in late-life cultural practice not only within the context of health and mobility, but also in the context of taste. Future research might critically explore how far the taste orientation of older adults is represented in the art world and the sort of consequences this representation has for their participation. Future research might also unpack the extent to which the classification of certain forms of culture as "high culture" is *per se* exclusionist (Crowther 2003) and marginalises the taste orientations of specific age groups.

Third, regarding the omnivore thesis and socio-economic status, this study suggests that the older omnivores are characterised by their participation in different kinds of (highbrow and lowbrow) cultural activities; however, this group was socio-economically within the average population of the sample. By contrast, the *Univores-TV* showed the lowest and the *Univores-Entertainment* showed the highest socio-economic status. The results therefore show how dominant forms of cultural participation in later life do not follow the patterns of the omnivores. Rather, the highest social groups showed preferences usually associated with young audiences (for example, sci-fi, pop- and rock'n'roll taste). Dominant cultural participation and taste in later life, therefore, might not be omnivorous, but—in times of a consumeristic third age and anti-ageing cultures (Gilleard and Higgs 2000) — "young".

Further, this study argues that cultural policies need to take diverse groups of older adults into account when supporting the inclusion of socially marginalised older people in arts and culture. In order to build more age-inclusive cultures across Europe, policy should address the diversity of older adults' cultural participation and provide support in bringing marginalised practices into public spaces. Enabling cultural participation in inclusive societies (UNESCO 2006 (see Morrone 2006) means to understand older adults as a heterogeneous arts and culture target group. Results suggest that both questions of accessibility (for example, building accessible cultural institutions), as well as symbolic representation in the program (for example, targeting not only towards "highbrow", but also "folk" tastes) might support cultural inclusion of older adults.

20.6 Conclusion

This chapter identifies cultural practice in later life as an important area of study for critical gerontology. Future research in gerontology needs to problematise older adults' exclusion from cultural practice as a matter of spatial and taste marginalisation. Participation in culture and the arts is not merely a topic to be watched from the side-lines but is a field of study that shows which social groups are both structurally and symbolically marginalised in late-modern societies. It also shows that as the study of ageing becomes increasingly interested in culture (Twigg and Martin 2015), social inequalities might not only be a matter of access and barriers, but of cultural and symbolic representation in the cultural field.

The study had several limitations, including the cross-sectional nature of the data, which does not allow for analysing causalities, and the lack of data concerning support structures needed to enable higher rates of cultural participation. Most importantly, this means that the analysis presented here can only highlight associations. Moreover, the data presented in this study did not differentiate between various forms of cultural consumption (for example, reading Goethe or a sci-fi novel) as well as the social embeddedness of cultural activities (for example, going to the theatre alone or in groups) and did not assess the extent to which people felt excluded from cultural participation or the degree to which exclusionary mechanisms actually drove different rates of participation – outside of social stratification variables. Finally, this study was limited to the context of Austria. While this means that results may be relevant to western European countries, which have a similarly structured cultural sector, the case might be different in non-European contexts.

Editors' Postscript

Please note, like other contributions to this book, this chapter was written before the COVID-19 pandemic of 2020. The book's introductory chapter (Chap. 1) and conclusion (Chap. 34) consider some of the key ways in which the pandemic relates to issues concerning social exclusion and ageing.

References

Bernard, M., & Rickett, M. (2016). The cultural value of older people's experiences of theatermaking: A review. *The Gerontologist, 57*(2), e1–e26. https://doi.org/10.1093/geront/gnw093.

Bourdieu, P. (1979/2013). *Distinction: A social critique of the judgement of taste*. London: Routledge. (Original work published 1979).

Brook, O. (2016). Spatial equity and cultural participation: How access influences attendance at museums and galleries in London. *Cultural Trends, 25*(1), 21–34.

Busman, J. K. (2019). From hipster to hillbilly: Death, bluegrass, and gospel according to David Crowder. *Journal of the Society for American Music, 13*(3), 338–358.

Chan, T. W., & Goldthorpe, J. H. (2007). Social stratification and cultural consumption: Music in England. *European Sociological Review, 23*(1), 1–19. https://doi.org/10.1093/esr/jcl016.

Cicchelli, V., & Octobre, S. (2018). Omnivorism and aesthetico-cultural cosmopolitanism. In *Aesthetico-cultural cosmopolitanism and French youth* (pp. 109–134). Cham: Palgrave Macmillan.

Coulton, S., Clift, S., Skingley, A., & Rodriguez, J. (2015). Effectiveness and cost-effectiveness of community singing on mental health-related quality of life of older people: Randomised controlled trial. *The British Journal of Psychiatry, 207*(3), 250–255.

Crowther, P. (2003). Cultural exclusion, normativity, and the definition of art. *The Journal of Aesthetics and Art Criticism, 61*(2), 121–131.

Falk, M., & Katz-Gerro, T. (2015). Cultural participation in Europe: Can we identify common determinants? *Journal of Cultural Economics, 40*(2), 127–162. https://doi.org/10.1007/s10824-015-9242-9.

Fisher, B. J., & Specht, D. K. (2000). Successful aging and creativity in later life. *Journal of Aging Studies, 13*(4), 457–472.

Fraser, K. D., O'Rourke, H. M., Wiens, H., Lai, J., Howell, C., & Brett-MacLean, P. (2015). A scoping review of research on the arts, aging, and quality of life. *Gerontologist, 55*(4), 719–729. https://doi.org/10.1093/geront/gnv027.

Gilleard, C., & Higgs, P. (2000). *Cultures of ageing: Self, citizen and the body*. London: Routledge.

Grundy, E., & Holt, G. (2001). The socioeconomic status of older adults: How should we measure it in studies of health inequalities? *Journal of Epidemiology & Community Health, 55*(12), 895–904.

Hanquinet, L., & Savage, M. (Eds.). (2015). *Routledge international handbook of the sociology of art and culture*. London/New York: Routledge.

Havighurst, R. J. (1961). Successful aging. *The Gerontologist, 1*(1), 8–13. https://doi.org/10.1093/geront/1.1.8.

Morrone, A. (2006). *Guidelines for measuring cultural participation*. Montreal: UNESCO.

Perkins, R., & Williamon, A. (2014). Learning to make music in older adulthood: A mixed-methods exploration of impacts on wellbeing. *Psychology of Music, 42*(4), 550–567.

Peterson, R. A. (1992). Understanding audience segmentation: From elite and mass to omnivore and univore. *Poetics, 21*(4), 243–258.

Peterson, R. A., & Kern, R. M. (1996). Changing highbrow taste: From snob to omnivore. *American Sociological Review, 61*, 900–907.

Radošinská, J. (2018). Omnivore vs univore. *European Journal of Media, Art and Photography, 6*(2), 98–109.

Reckwitz, A. (2008/2010). *Unscharfe Grenzen*. Bielefeld: Transcript.

Sabeti, S. (2014). Creative ageing? Selfhood, temporality and the older adult learner. *International Journal of Lifelong Education, 34*(2), 211–229. https://doi.org/10.1080/02601370.2014.987710.

Schulze, G. (2014). Alltagsästhetische Schemata. *Zusammenstellung sozialwissenschaftlicher Items und Skalen*. https://doi.org/10.6102/zis60.

Sullivan, O., & Katz-Gerro, T. (2006). The omnivore thesis revisited: Voracious cultural consumers. *European Sociological Review, 23*(2), 123–137. https://doi.org/10.1093/esr/jcl024.

Thomson, L. J., Lockyer, B., Camic, P. M., & Chatterjee, H. J. (2018). Effects of a museum-based social prescription intervention on quantitative measures of psychological wellbeing in older adults. *Perspectives in Public Health, 138*(1), 28–38.

Toepoel, V. (2011). Cultural participation of older adults: Investigating the contribution of lowbrow and highbrow activities to social integration and satisfaction with life. *International Journal on Disability and Human Development, 10*(2), 123–129. https://doi.org/10.1515/ijdhd.2011.027.

Twigg, J., & Martin, W. (2015). The challenge of cultural gerontology. *The Gerontologist, 55*(3), 353–359.

Tymoszuk, U., Perkins, R., Spiro, N., Williamon, A., & Fancourt, D. (2019). Longitudinal associations between short-term, repeated, and sustained arts engagement and well-being outcomes in older adults. *The Journals of Gerontology: Series B*, gbz085. https://doi.org/10.1093/geronb/gbz085.

van Eijck, K. (2005). No more need for snobbism: Highbrow cultural participation in a taste democracy. *European Sociological Review, 21*(5), 513–528. https://doi.org/10.1093/esr/jci038.

Walsh, K., Scharf, T., & Keating, N. (2017). Social exclusion of older persons: A scoping review and conceptual framework. *European Journal of Ageing, 14*(1), 81–98.

Wanka, A. (2017). Disengagement as withdrawal from public space: Rethinking the relation between place attachment, place appropriation, and identity-building among older adults. *The Gerontologist, 58*(1), 130–139.

Chapter 21
Sidestepping Rights: An Analysis of the Intersection of Human Rights Obligations and Their Practical Implications for Older Migrants

Ada Lui Gallassi and Lars Harrysson

21.1 Introduction

In this chapter, ageing and migration is placed within the setting of international human rights law and its relevance to reducing civic forms of exclusion. International legal treaties are presented within a mobility perspective to assess whether the protection mechanisms of human and labour rights are in line with the international migration movements brought by globalization. With the example of Sweden as a host country, we analyse the principles of equality and non-discrimination as the pillars for the protection of human rights, in order to assess their capacity to support the right to work and the right to social security for ageing migrants. These rights are presented as possessing the characteristics of socio-rights, which can serve to circumvent mechanisms of civic exclusion, in this case socio-cultural processes connected to identity-based and discriminatory practices, and secure better socio-economic outcomes for older migrants. Finally, the consequences of the difficulties experienced by migrants in accessing the formal labour market are analysed to evaluate the need for further legislation and policy to support the rights of this group. As illustrated by Pickett and Wilkinson (2009), equal societies perform better in regards to inclusion, and as Therborn (2012) harshly notes, inequality provides a "killing field" for the cohesion of societies. Socio-economic status, as discussed in this chapter, represents a strong force in both social inclusion and social exclusion, and thus an important aspect of any person's sense of civic positionality in a society, or lack thereof. If, as our empirical example illustrates, systems that are introduced to provide income support serve instead to widen the income inequality gap, groups

A. Lui Gallassi (✉)
Örebro University, Örebro, Sweden
e-mail: ada.lui-gallassi@oru.se

L. Harrysson
Lund University, Lund, Sweden

K. Walsh et al. (eds.), *Social Exclusion in Later Life*, International Perspectives on Aging 28, https://doi.org/10.1007/978-3-030-51406-8_21

with low- or erratic-income histories, like many migrants in Sweden, are specifically vulnerable to the impacts of socio-cultural based processes that can undermine their civic and social positionality and status.

21.2 Principle of Equality and Non-Discrimination – Pillars for the Protection of Human Rights

International human rights law has created several mechanisms to combat human rights violations and to protect a vast number of basic fundamental rights. It intends to universally preserve and protect such rights (Lechner and Boli 2008) by transcending national borders. This is one of its' most important aspects, and means that the international setting of human rights law incorporates variations of culture and tradition in national legal systems and citizenship (Alston and Goodman 2013). In analogy with Hannah Arendt (Arendt 1979) and her argument on human rights and citizenship, international human rights law aims at providing individuals the 'right to have rights', where 'belonging to humanity' (Hamacher and Wetters 2004) is the one and sole relevant criteria to be entitled to rights.

The idea of a common world culture is conveyed through the intensified globalization that the world is currently experiencing (Friedman 2007), in which place of birth, origin, or residence should not interfere with one's fundamental rights (Nussbaum 2010). As a result, concepts of transnationalism and cultural pluralism, as well as cosmopolitanism versus localism, are central to a debate and understanding of the global migration phenomenon (Friedman 2007). Values such as human rights are essential to this global community (Held 1995).

The principles of equality and non-discrimination, enshrined as preamble articles to the various international human rights treaties, are central to the inclusive universality of human rights.[1]

When discussing the principle of equality, it is important to ask ourselves what we mean by the term. Our standpoint rests in Amartya Sen's way of linking equality to "our capability to achieve valuable functioning that make up our lives, and more generally, our freedom to promote objectives we have reasons to value." (Sen 1992, p. xi). What are the conditions for human rights law to encompass the idea that everyone should be treated equally before the law? In an attempt to answer this question there are two approaches to the principle of equality that we will take into consideration, namely formal equality and substantive equality. Formal equality establishes equal treatment to everyone in similar or equal cases. Substantive equality considers material differences and employs a difference in treatment between groups or individuals (*e.g.* positive discrimination) that, due to their status or

[1] These principles are not only included in all the core international human rights instruments, but also in several specialized human rights and labor rights conventions.

specific conditions, is required to achieve equal outcomes, de facto equality (Moeckli 2010; Sageant 2018).

For the purpose of achieving the core ideal of human rights, and because ageing migrants are a specific group, the two approaches tend to live parallel lives. Sen (1992) argues that the principles do have a tendency to be in conflict when politicised. In practice however, they often exist on different levels. The formal equality approach safeguards the "sameness" of people on an institutional level, while the substantive equality approach focuses on the aim and ideal to "try to correct the wrong" and in taking into account the reality of the position of ageing migrants on a concrete practical level. Sageant (2018) argues for the latter to be the more appropriate approach to utilise when considering the circumstances of older migrants. Thus, for the realization of de facto equality, it is in many occasions necessary to establish positive discrimination policies in order to equalize the conditions of the less favoured group or individual in a given society. For instance, this is employed in many countries in relation to employment practices through quota schemes that ensure representation of disadvantaged groups *e.g.* indigenous populations and other minority groups (Smith 2007).

Both approaches, formal and substantive equality, are likely to be powerful instruments in securing equality of treatment for older migrants, thereby reducing a core set of exclusionary outcomes.

The principle of non-discrimination is particularly relevant for groups in vulnerable positions. The empirical study referred to in this chapter clearly indicates how migrants in Sweden may end up in precarious economic situations as a result of lacking labour market integration. Possessing problematic working life trajectories can enhance exclusionary experiences in later life, illustrating a lack of "aligned biographies" (Bommes 2000). Then we look into the International Covenant on Economic, Social and Cultural Rights (ICESCR),[2] the articles regarding non-discrimination are viewed as a core principle to the treaty as a whole and specifically provides the inclusive focus behind the Covenant (see art. 2.2 ICESCR). Even though the principle of non-discrimination comes as a separate right and article in international human rights law, the goal behind it and the principle of equality is very similar in essence. Furthermore, the protection of members of minorities against discrimination and the goal to achieve the vital concept of equality are central concerns for most liberal nation-states (Alston and Goodman 2013, p. 526).

Two important aspects of discrimination concerning ageing migrants are highly relevant to civic forms of exclusion in many western nations; discrimination based on older-age and discrimination based on race/ethnicity and nationality. In combination, they lead to increasingly precarious living conditions for people belonging to both groups, not least to ageing migrants. In line with understandings of socio-cultural exclusion, these dimensions of discrimination can reduce older migrants to single identities, excluding them from expressing their intersectional and complex

[2] The International Covenant on Economic, Social and Cultural Rights (ICESCR) is considered a core legally binding instrument of international human rights law for socio-economic rights, which is the focus of this chapter.

selves, and excluding them from adequate representation of their personhood. Allowing these principles to be part of a policy judgement tool for evaluation of social protection models would help illuminate systematic tendencies towards increased exclusionary consequences. They would serve as warning signals when distributive effects of a system may strengthen inequality, thus expose people to social exclusion.

21.3 Work and Social Security as Benchmarks of Inclusion

The right to work and the right to social security (protection)[3] are part of the so-called social rights established by international human rights treaties.[4] They are crucial provisions to ensure basic democratic rights to promote socio-economic integration and to combat exclusion of ageing migrants in the host countries. As defined by Marshall, social rights are "the whole range from the rights to a modicum of economic welfare and security to the right to share to the full in the social heritage and to live the life of a civilized being according to the standards prevailing in society" (Marshall 2006, p. 30).

Regarding the right to work, apart from the basic idea that everyone should have the right to work or to engage in a productive activity, this right also underlines the importance of having "access to employment, freedom from forced labour, and security in employment" (Smith 2007, p. 280). In other words, this refers to the right to adequate employment, with a decent wage, under the minimum international labour standards. The right to work and its related rights are established in several international human rights and labour standards treaties, *i.e.* Universal Declaration of Human Rights (UDHR) and International Covenant on Civic and Political Rights (ICCPR) among others. Analysing this right for ageing migrants through the lenses of equality and non-discrimination means, "the realization of the right to work implies equal access to employment, equal opportunities for promotion, and equality in terms and conditions of work" (Smith 2007, p. 282). Following the goal of de facto equality, to overcome the disadvantages within the ageing migrant group, positive discrimination, or affirmative action measures should be taken into account to remedy any inequality of opportunity faced by this group. Of course, some restrictions or discrimination based on national origin for instance may still exist based on the type of work accessible to older migrants, such as limited opportunities to undertake public administration jobs with an increased security level.

Let us then move to our example, the Swedish case of social protection – the right to work and to a retirement income.

---

[3] It is important to note that from an international legal setting, social protection and social security rights are seen as synonyms and can have interchangeable meanings – see CESCR (2008, para. 4).

[4] See the International Covenant on Economic, Social and Cultural Rights (ICESCR).

21.4 Social Protection, Equality and Non-discrimination in Sweden

Sweden has signed several international human rights treaties that guarantees the right to equality and non-discrimination. Examples are the International Covenant on Civil and Political Rights and the International Covenant on Economic, Social and Cultural Rights, the International Convention on the Elimination of All Forms of Racial Discrimination (ICERD) and the Convention on the Elimination of All Forms of Discrimination against Women (CEDAW). Against this legal backdrop, let us explore the right to work and to have a retirement income, and the principles of equality and non-discrimination in addressing forms of civic exclusion that can impede the achievement of these rights. Our focus is on migrants and inclusionary and exclusionary patterns in relation to ageing.

> 'I have never during my 26 years in Sweden ... never met one single immigrant who has said that – I don't want to work in Sweden. /.../ the question rather is: How does the structures in society look, and what preconditions and opportunities are there for a person to be part of the labour market?' (Social worker, interview)

As claimed by international legal instruments, based on the principles of equality and non-discrimination, the right to work and the right to social security should be ensured equally for people legally within its jurisdiction, citizen or not. Even though Sweden has developed an inclusive policy towards migration and enacted the various anti-discrimination laws, the tendency towards marginalization of the migrant population in society, and the difficulties for the migrant group in gaining access to employment, particularly white-collar jobs, is an ongoing fact (Castles et al. 2014). According to Woolfson et al. (2014) even migrants holding a work permit in Sweden, either temporary or linked to an employer, encounter abuse by employers. This has detrimental impacts on labour ties and working conditions, creating new spaces for migrant precariousness. The vulnerabilities linked to such precarious working conditions and a lack of labour standards guaranteeing access to decent work and strong employment ties bring consequences such as instability, poor social protection, insecurity and socio-economic exclusion. It contradicts the right to work and the right to social security (Anderson 2013). This becomes particularly clear in a retirement perspective where a life-time-earnings-based system (see below) is prevalent, thus making latecomers' situation difficult. The ageing migrant's position, other things equal, relatively worsens as time goes by (Harrysson et al. 2016).

There is a strong relationship between the right to paid work and the right to social security, as the latter is considered a direct consequence of the right to work, being based on labour market participation and taxable income. This is particularly the case in relation to benefits linked to illness, disability, maternity, employment, injury, unemployment, old-age, or death of a family member (CESCR, General Comment 19, para. 2). A broader definition of social security rights also encompasses social assistance, moving from an individual right to a "collective all-embracing right" (Nussberger 2007). For the scope of this chapter, the right to social security solely refers to the individual right to social protection benefits after retirement due to old-age.

The importance of the right to social security lies in that while it provides a social safety net, it also has positive impacts on income equality and in combating poverty (Ben-Bassat and Dahan 2008, p. 108). This right is seen as one out of the five social rights that should be included in a Constitution, to ensure the 'right to live in dignity'. (ibid, p. 105). For the Universal Declaration of Human Rights, this right is considered a core guarantee for the right of everyone to an adequate standard of living (Art.25 UDHR). According to the International Labour Organization, "Social Security systems are one of the most powerful institutional expressions of social solidarity." (International Labour Office 2011, p. 71). Social protection benefits are essential mechanisms to eliminate socio-economic exclusion and marginalization in society. As outlined by Claudio Bolzman, "given the development and growth of the welfare state, social security has become the main means of protecting individuals from poverty and insecurity" (Bolzman 2012, p. 105). To those with migrant backgrounds, first generation Swedes, lacking "aligned biographies" (Bommes 2000), the inclusion in these systems is vital for integration, and clearly the opposite if actively excluded as victims of discriminatory systems and/or stigmatizing political discourses. We will next use an empirical example of the lived experience of this system, the manifestation of key exclusionary processes that are rooted in civic dimensions, and the consequences for socio-economic outcomes.

21.5 Retirement in Sweden: A Lived Experience

Retirement in Sweden, as in other western economies, relates to moving into a decommodified part of life, a time when we do not need to think of earning our living through paid work (Esping-Andersen 1990). However, retirement is strongly related to long-term dependence on paid work, as we live the consequences of our working life trajectory. A trajectory should illustrate how we prepare for our lives in later life. However, financial preparations, commonly discussed in terms of individual choices, are choices made in a context of specific system requirements. In the pension system these requirements regard both time spent in Sweden and incomes earned and taxed, as well as type of employment contracts in play. Many migrants do not meet them as they deviate from the expected life course in three central dimensions: education, employment and retirement (Harrysson et al. 2016). In these dimensions our life inclusion outcomes are dependent on national welfare institutions providing protection to us as their members.

The data collection for the study (Harrysson and Werner 2015), which this chapter draws on, was carried out in the southern Swedish city of Helsingborg. It was an action research inspired project in which migrants who arrived in Sweden in the 1990s and later reflected upon how they navigate and form strategies to handle the retirement and pension contexts. The study was based on individual and group interviews with migrants of mostly non-European origin, who arrived in Sweden while of working age. We also interviewed and had workshops with professionals in social work and social insurance as well as private insurance and banking. Some of the respondents were already retired, most were not. Data collection focused on general experiences of migration, work, family life, health and economy. The empirical data demonstrated significant complexity in the migration process and a diversity in retirement preparations that reflect biographies that do not conveniently fit into institutionalised expectations. These participants found themselves in a transitional position as job seekers, where they often had been for quite some time, and often as a group at risk of receiving low pensions in the future (Harrysson et al. 2016).

The Swedish public pension system, as referred to among pension researchers, is based on notional individual accounts (fictive savings) providing accrued pension rights on a lifetime income principle and assumes that a person is independent of their spouse in most respects. The income and premium pensions are fully portable and may be drawn from more or less anywhere in the world where there is a banking system. They are intended to cover about 60–70 per cent of final income for those also drawing a pension from an occupational benefit scheme, which is a part of collective agreements in the labour market in Sweden. However, as Harrysson et al. argues, the "generous" part of the system's design is not typically accessible to people with limited opportunities to build up pension rights, such as migrants arriving in Sweden in later life or those with only intermittent access to paid work in a workplace with a collective agreement. These latter groups are instead dependent on the other part of the public pension system that takes the form of paid supplements, *e.g.* guaranteed pension and maintenance support for pensioners. Such supplements are limited in their portability, thus forcing people to stay in Sweden to receive long-term payments. They are also restricted by factual residency. "This attribute of the Swedish pension system reflects a historically well-established duality of the Swedish welfare state. The advantage of a relatively generous social insurance in terms of income maintenance with less individualised social control /../, is balanced by a tradition of poverty relief with quite harsh restrictions on mobility /../." (Harrysson et al. 2016, p. 535).

The consequence of a labour market not absorbing newly arrived groups, and existing labour market policies not facilitating a more appropriate integration of migrants into paid labour, will be low pensions. Many older migrants participating in this research were well aware of this:

> 'The pension system is not made for foreigners, it is made for Swedes who work here, live here and die here.' (Focus group with migrants)

Pension levels very close to the relative poverty line, defined as older people that may not have enough resources to buy four necessary items, are reported by *Pensionsmyndigheten* to be the case for around 245,000 individuals (approx.12%) and this in large is explained by how the system is designed (Pensionsmyndigheten 2019a, b). The poverty measure used combines the levels of guaranteed pension and income maintenance support with housing subsidies. However, many older people pay low rent, and thus are not eligible for such rental subsidies. This is not exclusively a case for migrants, but all persons having had erratic working life trajectories may encounter the very same situation. The system's core is an income-related pension, which is strongly connected to lifetime earnings. This is in terms of an evenly distributed income over a working life. The public system does not generate pension rights on incomes above 538,700 SEK or below 20,008 SEK in 2020 (Pensionsmyndigheten, 2020). Thus, a short time in the labour market and an uneven income distribution (below the threshold in some years and above in other years) is not favoured by the system. The introduction of an income maintenance support scheme with an intention of freeing people from means testing procedures of social assistance, has not altered its historical foundation in poverty relief and locking in effects (Harrysson et al. 2016).

> 'If I, for example, have worked in the health care here in Sweden, then I have only worn down my body. I don't earn any pension. Maybe I should have been a housewife instead, then I would have received 6000 crowns anyway! It would have been better if I had these thoughts today, then I wouldn't have worked a day and still have the right to the 6000.' (Focus group with migrant women)

In sum, the pension system does not discriminate in its design on anything but income, but shows some awkward negative consequences for people not fitting the model citizen upon which the system is designed. At the same time, the system is positively discriminating some particular life situations as to withstand unwelcome effects on pension equality. Time off work due to childbearing, military services and higher education provide some pension credits. Further, as the social insurance schemes concerning unemployment, sickness, occupational injury and parental leave are income-compensating systems, pension credits are counted as equal to wage incomes. Since these insurances all have eligibility rules, capped entitlements and defined durations, their strength as social protection mechanisms for older migrants can be questioned (Harrysson and Werner, 2015).

> 'Pension!, but that is nothing but social assistance by another name.' (Man (not ironically) telling us that his job is to search for jobs)

> '… you are Einstein, Aristotle and Plato, but you don't get a job! Bueno, full stop.' (Focus group with women)

The system's strong focus on lifetime income has also shown a disadvantage to women in those generations planning within the former system, which focused on the best 15 of 30 years of wage earnings as eligibility criteria for an adequate pension level. Staying at home to care for children or working part time does not pay off in the new system's eligibility rules in the same way. However, for some migrant women, the system, as individualized as it is, has provided them with a personal income that they never before had access to as they were dependent on their husbands' incomes (Harrysson and Werner, 2015).

21.5.1 Living Unequal Outcomes

First generation migrants do not fit the standard case of a Swedish retirement planner. Despite that, the system is intended to treat all entrants the same. The effects of a life-income-based savings system causes large variations in subsistence opportunities among groups of legally residing people in Sweden. Seen in a perspective of subsistence, which is what people mostly think of when pensions are discussed (Harrysson and Werner 2015), it often opposes a pure insurance argument.

However, we would argue that the system in itself is not discriminatory towards migrants as such, but rather positively discriminating groups with shorter time in Sweden. This is because the system is in effect compensating for a lack of eligibility in terms of required years of contribution (40 years of contributions required for full guarantee pension) through an income maintenance system.

Harrysson and Werner argue that those that are really hit by the system's way of working are people with erratic income patterns over life, earning only a guaranteed pension after a full working life in Sweden. This situation fuels a populist argument against migrants' rights to income maintenance, regardless of the very low levels of support provided. In this regard, such arguments do not help foster a better understanding of the precarious position that many migrants find themselves in due to major difficulties in entering the labour market in the first place, and due to typically having to work in sectors paying less and with worse working conditions.

In a worst-case scenario people are forced to work in the black market not earning any public pension rights at all. Combined with this we find the issue of migrants being less informed of what is expected and what is required to build pension rights. In some respects people live in a "vacuum" judging their situation from a standpoint founded in their former home country's cultural setting and system, and in myths, arguably wrong, about how the Swedish system works (Harrysson and Werner 2015). But still, people were adamant about the need for not giving up:

> Participant 1: 'Sure, it is the question, but what other solutions are there? Life goes on and you can become bitter, but you can't stay bitter because then your whole life "marshy", what do you then make of it, what solutions are there? Family ties for example – family, the collective. How do you do to make life go on? These are things you think of when you see that the safety net which is there doesn't produce any cover.'
>
> Participant 2: 'Well put. You compensate.'
>
> (Focus group with men)

21.6 Conclusion

This chapter highlights the overall challenges in relation to the right to work and the right to social protection, from the perspective of equality and non-discrimination, for ageing migrants in Sweden. It also highlights how socio-cultural processes connected to identity-based and discriminatory practices, can drive these challenges, impacting socio-economic outcomes and, to a degree, civic and social positionality for older migrants. Based on a case derived from a research project concerning migrants and pensions in a Swedish municipality, we can conclude that the system in Sweden in many cases uses positive discrimination and de facto equality to provide a more equal and non-discriminated right to social security. But the problems experienced by ageing migrants regarding social protection benefits, particularly the retirement pension, consequentially lies in the right to work and taxed wage income during the course of their working life trajectory. As the retirement pension is based on taxed wage income and years worked in Sweden, it is necessary to find ways to tackle discrimination and to achieve de facto equality regarding access to the formal labour market. The chapter connects socio-economic status and conditions of ageing migrants to civic, and broader forms of social exclusion, highlighting the impacts of these processes for person's sense of status in a society. This also requires policy initiatives to combat increasing cleavages between social groups, which are in this case propelled by migrants' experiences of structurally instituted exclusion during their working life, negatively impacting socio-economic outcomes in later life.

Finally, this chapter signals the importance of a future research agenda on the interaction of the various aspects of the working life trajectory of migrants and what that means for social exclusion in later life. It also highlights directions for a legislation on the right to work and the right to social security, envisioning equality and non-discrimination for ageing migrants in society.

Editors' Postscript

Please note, like other contributions to this book, this chapter was written before the COVID-19 pandemic of 2020. The book's introductory chapter (Chap. 1) and conclusion (Chap. 34) consider some of the key ways in which the pandemic relates to issues concerning social exclusion and ageing.

References

Alston, P., & Goodman, R. (2013). *International human rights. The successor to international human rights in context: Law, politics and morals*. Oxford: Oxford University Press.

Anderson, B. (2013). *Us and them? The dangerous politics of immigration control*. Oxford: Oxford University Press.

Arendt, H. (1979). *The origins of Totalitarism*. San Diego: Harvest.

Ben-Bassat, A., & Dahan, M. (2008). Social rights in the constitution and in practice. *Journal of Comparative Economics, 36*, 103–119.

Bolzman, C. (2012). Democratization of ageing: Also a reality for elderly immigrants? *European Journal of Social Work, 15*(1), 97–113.

Bommes, M. (2000). National welfare state, biography and migration. Labour migrants, ethnic Germans and the re-ascription of welfare state membership. In M. Bommes & A. Geddes (Eds.), *Immigration and Welfare, Challenging the borders of the welfare state* (pp. 90–108). Routledge/EUI studies in the Political Economy of Welfare.

Castles, S., de Haas, H., & Miller, M. J. (2014). *The age of migration: International population movements in the modern world.* Basingstoke: Palgrave Macmillan.

Esping-Andersen, G. (1990). *Three worlds of welfare capitalism.* Cambridge: Polity Press.

Friedman, J. (2007). Global systems, globalization, and anthropological theory. In I. Rossi (Ed.), *Frontiers of globalization research: Theoretical and methodological approaches* (pp. 109–132). New York: Springer Science+Business Media.

Hamacher, W., & Wetters, K. (2004). *The Right to Have Rights (Four-and-a-Half Remarks). The South Atlantic Quarterly, 103*, 343–356. https://www.muse.jhu.edu/article/169144.

Harrysson, L., & Werner, E. (2015). *Begriplig pensionsinformation för dem med små inkomster. En rapport från ett projekt om hur pensionsinformation begripliggörs bland migranter i Helsingborg. Lund.* Sweden: Research Reports in Social Work – Lund University, School of Social Work.

Harrysson, L., Werner, E., & Montesino, N. (2016). Preparations for retirement in Sweden: Migrant perspectives. *Critical Social Policy, 36*(4), 531–550. https://doi.org/10.1177/0261018316638081.

Held, D. (1995). *Democracy and the global order : From the modern state to cosmopolitan governance.* Cambridge: Polity Press.

International Labour Office. (2011). *Social security and the rule of law.* Geneva: International Labour Organization.

Lechner, F. J., & Boli, J. (2008). *World culture: Origins and consequences.* Oxford: Blackwell publishing.

Marshall, T. H. (2006). Citizenship and social class. In C. Pierson & F. Castles (Eds.), *The welfare state reader* (pp. 30–39). Cambridge: Polity Press.

Moeckli, D. (2010). Equality and non-discrimination. In D. Moeckli, S. Shah, & S. Sivakumaran (Eds.), *International human rights law* (pp. 189–208). New York: Oxford University Press.

Nussbaum, M. (2010). Patriotism and cosmopolitanism. In G. W. Brown & D. Held (Eds.), *The cosmopolitanism reader* (pp. 155–162). Cambridge: Polity.

Nussberger, A. (2007). Interpretation of international social security standards – Problems and prospects. In F. Pennings (Ed.), *International social security standards. Current views and interpretation matters* (pp. 33–51). Antwerpen\Oxford: Intersentia.

Pensionsmyndigheten. (2019a, 10 04). *Ny rapport: Äldre med låga inkomster 2018.* Retrieved from www.pensionsmyndigheten.se. https://www.pensionsmyndigheten.se/nyheter-och-press/pressrum/ny-rapport-aldre-med-laga-inkomster. Accessed 12 Aug 2019.

Pensionsmyndigheten. (2019b, Oct 04). *Pensionsmyndigheten.* Retrieved from https://www.pensionsmyndigheten.se/forsta-din-pension/om-pensionssystemet/sa-beraknas-din-pension-bas-belopp-och-varderegler Accessed 12 Jan 2020.

Pickett, K., & Wilkinson, R. (2009). *The spirit level: Why more equal societies almost always do better.* London: Allen & Unwin.

Sageant, M. (2018). *Discrimination and the law.* New York: Routledge.

Sen, A. (1992). *Inequality reexamined.* Oxford: Clarendon Press.

Smith, R. K. (2007). *Textbook on international human rights.* New York: Oxford University Press.

Therborn, G. (2012). The killing fields of inequality. *International Journal of Health Services, 42,* 579–589.

Woolfson, C., Fudge, J., & Thörnqvist, C. (2014). Migrant precarity and future challenges to labour standards in Sweden. *Economic and Industrial Democracy, 35*(4), 695–715.

Section VII
Interrelationships Between Different Domains of Exclusion

Chapter 22
Introduction: Framing Exclusion Interrelationships

Lena Dahlberg

22.1 Introduction

Multidimensionality is a key feature of social exclusion, that is, exclusion concerns different life domains, and disadvantages in one domain can be interrelated with disadvantages in other domains. Interrelationships across social exclusion domains have implications not only for the experience of the individual, but also for policy, since cutbacks or interventions addressing one domain may have additional effects on one or several other domains.

This section includes four chapters that examine interrelationships across social exclusion domains. These chapters place focus on older adults living in long-term care institutions; the relationship between exclusion from material resources and loneliness; how transport influences the multidimensionality of social exclusion; and homelessness among older adults.

The purpose of this chapter is to introduce interrelationships that can arise between different domains, within the multidimensionality of social exclusion in later life, and to broadly position the chapters presented in this section within this literature. The chapter starts with a brief reminder of some of the domains often considered in research on social exclusion. Thereafter, research on interrelationships in terms of cross-sectional and longitudinal associations across domains is presented. Finally, each of the chapters within the section are briefly introduced.

L. Dahlberg (✉)
School of Education, Health and Social Studies, Dalarna University, Falun, Sweden

Aging Research Center, Karolinska Institutet and Stockholm University, Stockholm, Sweden
e-mail: ldh@du.se

K. Walsh et al. (eds.), *Social Exclusion in Later Life*, International Perspectives on Aging 28, https://doi.org/10.1007/978-3-030-51406-8_22

22.2 Social Exclusion Domains

While key work by Burchardt et al. (2002), based on an analysis of the whole population, identified four domains of social exclusion – social interaction, political engagement, consumption, and production – researchers on exclusion in later life have critiqued the relevance and moved away from areas focused on labour market participation and economic production (*e.g.* Scharf et al. 2005). Instead, and as demonstrated by Walsh et al. in Chapter 1 of this volume, research related to ageing has typically emphasised domains that are more instrumental to the daily lives of older adults. This includes emphasis on the domain of neighbourhood and community (Scharf et al. 2005) as being crucial to addressing fundamental needs and staying independent in later life (Scharf et al. 2005; Van Regenmortel et al. 2018). Recent work has demonstrated that this domain can uniquely contribute to explain the variance in well-being of older adults (Dahlberg and McKee 2018).

Research on social exclusion of older adults has commonly considered exclusion from some or several of the following domains: material resources, social relations, civic participation, neighbourhood, services, and socio-cultural aspects of society (for overviews, see: Van Regenmortel et al. 2016; Walsh et al. 2017; Walsh et al. this volume), with a recent review identifying as many as 16 domains within the literature on social exclusion in older-age (Van Regenmortel et al. 2016). While some individuals may experience exclusion from one of these domains, others may be simultaneously excluded from two or more domains. This has been labelled multiple or deep exclusion (Scharf et al. 2005; Barnes et al. 2006; Levitas et al. 2007). As will be considered in the next section, some of the outcomes of these different forms of exclusion can be linked to each other and function as a part of other domain specific exclusionary processes.

22.3 Previous Research on Interrelationships

This research overview considers quantitative and not qualitative studies, with a focus on studies that have considered the multidimensional social exclusion construct rather than exclusion from, for example, just two domains. Quantitative approaches to researching multidimensionality include examining the number of domains on which older adults are excluded, clusters of different forms of exclusion, and the interrelationships across several domains.

In considering the first approach, exclusion from two or more domains have been found in 36% of people aged 60 years or older in deprived urban areas in England (Scharf et al. 2005), in 20% of a national sample of people aged 50 years or older in England (Barnes et al. 2006), and in 11% of people aged 55 years or older in Australia (Miranti and Yu 2015). This approach is based on a pre-defined threshold at which people are regarded as being socially excluded. The threshold for exclusion can be set in absolute terms by defining a level of activities or resources that can be considered as standard in the society in which people live (as in the studies by Scharf et al. and Miranti and Yu) or in relatives terms, for example, by defining a certain proportion of those least active as excluded (as done by Barnes et al.). Of course, the proportion of individuals identified as excluded is directly determined by the level at which this threshold is set (see Van Regenmortel et al. 2018).

A second approach to the study of multidimensionality of social exclusion is to examine clusters of different forms of exclusion indicators across the domains. Van Regenmortel et al. (2018) identified four clusters with, for example, one cluster that was comprised of people who had a higher probability of digital, civic and financial exclusion. Becker and Boreham (2009) explored social exclusion over time and found three dynamic clusters. Based on nine waves of data collection, they identified that between 44 and 68% of individuals had been in the same cluster at the previous wave of data collection, while 26–39% had been in a different cluster at the previous wave.

These approaches to researching social exclusion consider the coexistence of exclusion from different domains or the links between exclusion indicators, but not the interrelationship between exclusion from different domains. Interrelationships can be examined by analysing bivariate associations between domains. This approach has only been used in a small number of studies, mostly from the United Kingdom. The findings of these analyses are summarised in Table 22.1. Positive associations have been found between the majority of domain combinations, that is, being excluded on one domain increases the risk of exclusion from another domain. For example, a Swedish study with a sample of individuals aged 70 years or older found significant associations between all the exclusion domains analysed (Heap et al. in progress). While these associations were generally quite weak, stronger associations were found between exclusion from social relations and the other domains.

Relationships can also be reciprocal between more than two domains. While this specific dynamic is even less studied, interrelationships have been identified between social relations, civic activities and neighbourhood exclusion, and between civic activities, material consumption and financial products (Barnes et al. 2006).

Interrelationships across social exclusion domains can also operate over time, so that exclusion from one domain increases the risk of subsequent exclusions from another domain. This can be a cumulative process (see Silver and Miller 2003), where exclusion in one domain can lead to *additional* disadvantages in other domains (cf. the cumulative advantage/disadvantage theory, Dannefer 2003). Evidence for cumulative processes was found in a Swedish study of people aged 77–95 years at follow-up, particularly if the initial disadvantage concerned social relations (Heap and Fors 2015).

Longitudinal research on social exclusion in older adults is rare. That said, a study from Australia has shown that individuals experiencing social exclusion at one point in time have a considerably higher risk of experiencing exclusion again later (Miranti and Yu 2015). However, this research considered multiple exclusion over time and not interrelationships between exclusion from different domains. Based on a study of people aged 50 years or older in England, Kneale (2012) has

Table 22.1 Research findings on interrelationships across domains

	Material resources	Social relations	Civic activities	Services	Neighbourhood
Material resources	–				
Social relations	+ Barnes et al. (2006)	–			
	+ Heap et al. (in progress)				
	n.s. Kneale (2012)				
	+ Scharf et al. (2005)				
Civic activities	+ Barnes et al. (2006)	+ Barnes et al. (2006)	–		
	+ Heap et al. (in progress)	+ Heap et al. (in progress)			
	n.s. Kneale (2012)	+ Kneale (2012)			
	+ Scharf et al. (2005)	+ Scharf et al. (2005)			
Services	n.s. Barnes et al. (2006)	+ Barnes et al. (2006)	+ Barnes et al. (2006)	–	
	+ Scharf et al. (2005)	+ Scharf et al. (2005)	+ Scharf et al. (2005)		
Neighbourhood	+ Barnes et al. (2006)	+ Barnes et al. (2006)	+ Barnes et al. (2006)	n.s. Scharf et al. (2005)	–
	+ Heap et al. (in progress)	+ Heap et al. (in progress)	+ Heap et al. (in progress)		
	+ Scharf et al. (2005)	+ Scharf et al. (2005)	n.s. Scharf et al. (2005)		

Note: + positive association; n.s. non-significant association

identified to what extent people who were excluded from one domain had a higher risk of exclusion from another domain 6 years later. The analyses showed that exclusion from social relations more than doubled the risk of exclusion from the domains of financial products and from consumer goods, whereas exclusion from local amenities more than doubled the risk of exclusion from consumer goods at follow-up. Furthermore, exclusion from civic activities raised the risk of exclusion from social relations, and exclusion from financial products raised the risk of exclusion from cultural activities.

In summary, although there are individual studies of multidimensionality and the interrelationships between different domains, the amount of research with such focus is limited. In particular, there is a lack of longitudinal research and research covering different country settings.

22.4 Outline of This Section

This section includes four chapters that contribute to previous research by examining interrelationships across social exclusion domains. Chapter 23 focuses on exclusion among older adults who have lost part of their independence, namely those living in long-term care institutions. Here, social exclusion can be embedded in the culture of institutional care, such as via a task- rather than person-oriented approach, and an imbalance of power between residents and staff. In this chapter, interrelationships across three domains of social exclusion are examined: socio-cultural exclusion, exclusion from civic participation (separating civic exclusion out into the two merged domains – see chapters by Walsh et al. and Torres in this volume) and exclusion from social relations.

Chapter 24 examines the critical relationship between exclusion from material resources and loneliness as an outcome of exclusion from social relations. By isolating the effects of material deprivation on loneliness, the analyses show a strong and significant association between material deprivation between both the level of loneliness and increase in loneliness over time.

In Chap. 25, focus is placed on how transport influences the multidimensionality of social exclusion and cuts across most of the exclusion domains, not just access to services. It is argued that transport is not only a matter of individual choice but also a societal/structural issue and that age-related mobility – just as disability – is a construct of the intersection of demands and lack of support in the environment.

Finally, Chap. 26 focuses on perhaps one of the most extreme forms of social exclusion: homelessness. Through a review of gerontological research journals, the authors show that homelessness among older adults is related to all domains of social exclusion. While research usually considers interrelations across several domains, exclusion from services, amenities and mobility is the domain receiving most attention in research on homelessness.

While these chapters were written prior to the outbreak of the COVID-19 pandemic, the handling and consequences of the pandemic have made the topics examined even more pressing. Those excluded from social relations, material resources and/or neighbourhoods have not always been able to follow recommendations on social distancing, making them particularly vulnerable to the virus, while others face an increased risk of social isolation and loneliness. For example, physical distancing is difficult to achieve for people living in homelessness; older adults in institutions have become more dependent on staff to meet their social needs; and people living in the community have become dependent on paid or unpaid help from others.

References

Barnes, M., Blom, A., Cox, K., Lessof, C., & Walker, A. (2006). *The social exclusion of older people: Evidence from the first wave of the English Longitudinal Study of Ageing (ELSA): Final report*. London: Office of the Deputy Prime Minister, Social Exclusion Unit. http://www.ifs.org.uk/docs/odpm_social_exclusion.pdf.

Becker, E., & Boreham, R. (2009). *Understanding the risks of social exclusion across the life course: Older age*. London: Cabinet Office and National Centre for Social Research.

Burchardt, T., Le Grand, J., & Piachaud, D. (2002). Degrees of exclusion: Developing a dynamic, multidimensional measure. In J. Hills, J. Le Grand, & D. Piachaud (Eds.), *Understanding social exclusion* (pp. 30–43). Oxford: Oxford University Press.

Dahlberg, L., & McKee, K. J. (2018). Social exclusion and well-being among older adults in rural and urban areas. *Archives of Gerontology and Geriatrics, 79*, 176–184. https://doi.org/10.1016/j.archger.2018.08.007.

Dannefer, D. (2003). Cumulative advantage/disadvantage and the life course: Cross-fertilizing age and social science theory (Review). *Journals of Gerontology Series B-Psychological Sciences and Social Sciences, 58*(6), S327–S337. https://doi.org/10.1093/geronb/58.6.S327.

Heap, J., & Fors, S. (2015). Duration and accumulation of disadvantages in old age. *Social Indicators Research, 123*(2), 411–429. https://doi.org/10.1007/s11205-014-0744-1.

Heap, J., Lennartsson, C., McKee, K. J., Fritzell, J., & Dahlberg, L. (in progress). *Multidimensionality of social exclusion and associations across domains*.

Kneale, D. (2012). *Is social exclusion still important for older people?* London: International Longevity Centre – UK.

Levitas, R., Pantazis, C., Fahmy, E., Gordon, D., Lloyd, E., & Patsios, D. (2007). *The multi-dimensional analysis of social exclusion*. London: Social Exclusion Task Force.

Miranti, R., & Yu, P. (2015). Why social exclusion persists among older people in Australia (Article). *Social Inclusion, 3*(4), 112–126. https://doi.org/10.17645/si.v3i4.214.

Scharf, T., Phillipson, C., & Smith, A. E. (2005). Social exclusion of older people in deprived urban communities of England. *European Journal of Ageing, 2*(2), 76–87. https://doi.org/10.1007/s10433-005-0025-6.

Silver, H., & Miller, S. M. (2003). Social exclusion. The European approach to social disadvantage. *Indicators, 2*(2), 5–21. https://doi.org/10.1080/15357449.2003.11069166.

Van Regenmortel, S., De Donder, L., Dury, S., Smetcoren, A.-S., De Witte, N., & Verté, D. (2016). Social exclusion in later life: A systematic review of the literature. *Journal of Population Ageing, 9*(4), 315–344. https://doi.org/10.1007/s12062-016-9145-3.

Van Regenmortel, S., De Donder, L., Smetcoren, A.-S., Lambotte, D., De Witte, N., & Verté, D. (2018). Accumulation of disadvantages: Prevalence and categories of old-age social exclusion in Belgium. *Social Indicators Research, 140*(3), 1173–1194. https://doi.org/10.1007/s11205-017-1817-8.

Walsh, K., Scharf, T., & Keating, N. (2017). Social exclusion of older persons: A scoping review and conceptual framework. *European Journal of Ageing, 14*(1), 81–98. https://doi.org/10.1007/s10433-016-0398-8.

Chapter 23
Older People in Long-Term Care Institutions: A Case of Multidimensional Social Exclusion

Feliciano Villar, Rodrigo Serrat, Annette Bilfeldt, and Joe Larragy

23.1 Introduction

Residential care (or care homes) are communal living settings with various levels of health and psychosocial support aimed at improving the quality of life of residents. They include a range of different services provided by public, private (for-profit and not-for-profit), social- or health-care agencies and professionals. For the sake of simplicity, in this chapter we use the term "care homes" referring to a range of such facilities, differentiating among them where necessary.

If we define social exclusion broadly as the separation of individuals and groups from mainstream society (Moffatt and Glasgow 2009) it is evident that living in a care home involves challenges connected to a lack of opportunities to participate in key activities inside and outside of the institution. In this sense, care homes (and particularly those that follow what is described as a "traditional care culture") might be one of the remaining examples of what Goffman (1961) calls "total institutions", in which people are isolated from the wider community and lead an enclosed and regulated life formally monitored and controlled by professionals.

Such risks of exclusion might be exacerbated by the profile of the older population living in care homes. Older people living in care homes typically have multiple health and social care needs, with the prevalence of depression and dementia being particularly high. For example, up to 70% of care home residents in countries such as England (Alzheimer's Society 2016) or Norway (Selbaek et al. 2007) have been

F. Villar (✉) · R. Serrat
Department of Cognition, Development and Educational Psychology,
University of Barcelona, Barcelona, Spain
e-mail: fvillar@ub.edu

A. Bilfeldt
University of Greenland, Nuuk, Greenland

J. Larragy
Maynooth University, Kildare, Ireland

K. Walsh et al. (eds.), *Social Exclusion in Later Life*, International Perspectives
on Aging 28, https://doi.org/10.1007/978-3-030-51406-8_23

reported to have dementia. The presence of dependency and particularly of mental and physical health conditions increases the risk of social exclusion and the potential for violation of basic rights of people living in care homes (Cahill 2018).

Although in developed countries the quality of care offered by institutions has improved dramatically in recent decades, according to Alzheimer Disease International (2013) standards of care for those living in residential care are still far from perfect. It is on this basis that this chapter aims to explore the risks of social exclusion posed for older people living in a care home in relation to enjoy meaningful social relationships, to actively contribute to the institution and also to the wider community, and to exert control over their own life.

In focusing on these facets, the chapter will consider two domains of exclusion. We begin with exclusion from social relationships, and then follow by considering civic engagement and socio-cultural aspects, as components of the broad domain of civic exclusion [please see Walsh et al. this volume for a discussion]. We end the chapter by raising some brief conclusions concerning these areas, and their interrelationship, to advance work on this topic.

23.2 Exclusion from Social Relationships

Connecting with other people and having emotionally significant human relationships is a basic human need that must be maintained for older people living in care homes. Thus, social relationships have been repeatedly identified as essential to nursing home residents' quality of life (Roberts and Bowers 2015). Residents who do not have relevant social networks and are not socially engaged are at higher risk of depression and other negative health outcomes (Drageset 2004).

One might expect that care homes, being a communal living setting, could be a good place to enjoy varied and significant social relationships. After all, older people living in care homes are surrounded by other residents and by staff most of the day and, in fact, finding spaces to be alone and maintaining aspects of personal privacy has been repeatedly reported as one of the major problems older people living in institutions have to face (Pitkala 2016). Unfortunately, simply being in the same space and time with other people is not enough to address the emotional and existential dimensions of social relationships: on the contrary, the evidence suggests that loneliness is a prevalent phenomenon for people living in long-term care homes, where opportunities to meet the need for intimacy, closeness and touch are seriously restricted. For instance, in a study with older people without cognitive impairments living in nursing homes, Drageset et al. (2011) found that more than half experienced loneliness, and this is similar to the levels found in other studies exploring self-perceived loneliness among older people living in institutions (*e.g.* Nyqvist et al. 2013).

To understand why loneliness is so prevalent among older people living in care homes, several factors should be taken into account. Firstly, some studies have found that older people who have either lost significant social relations (*e.g.* through bereavement – see Urbaniak et al. this volume), or are experiencing loneliness in the community, are more likely to move into a care home (Hanratty et al. 2018). Secondly, many of the characteristics of care home users, such as being female, with low income, with disabilities and health conditions, or with cognitive impairments, are also risk factors for loneliness [see Morgan et al. this volume]. In addition, the transition to living in a care home might in itself cut off pre-existing social relations and reduce possibilities for replacing these relationships and establishing new bonds. For many residents, moving into a care home is a stressful event involving the loss of relatives and friends, and a diminished lifestyle, and might lead to a grief that makes it even more difficult to establish new significant relationships (Löfqvist et al. 2013). Moreover, residents might have problems making meaningful social connections without explicit support (Cipriani et al. 2006), a difficulty that is even greater if they experience mobility restrictions or, as in the case of dementia, communication impairments (Alzheimer Disease International 2013).

Apart from the lack of relationships with other care home users, studies focused on social relationships of older people living in institutional settings have emphasised the deficiency of communication and bonds with supporting staff. For instance, tight time schedules, frequent among staff working in care homes, might lead to a daily practice without dialogue and meaningful social contact between the resident and the employee, whereupon important knowledge about the resident's social and emotional needs is lacking (Andersen and Bilfeldt 2016). One study found that, aside from time spent receiving care, residents spent only two minutes within a six hour period interacting with other residents or staff (Alzheimer's Society 2007). This communicational isolation seems to be particularly severe for people with dementia [also see Andersen et al. this volume]. Using video recordings of daily life conversations in long-term care institutions for older people, Ward et al. (2008) estimated that people with dementia living in a care home spent just 10% of their awake time interacting with other people, with 75% of this time corresponding to interactions with visitors (mainly close relatives) and the remaining 25% corresponding to interactions with staff or other residents. In many care homes, interests of the staff seem to overshadow the wishes of the residents; and professionals rarely establish any communication with people with dementia beyond their assigned tasks, preferring to interact among themselves, even when the person with dementia was physically present (Doyle and Rubinstein 2013).

Labelling and depersonalising older people living in care homes (and particularly people with dementia) not only discourages communication and contributes to neglect, but also lowers the quality of the few interactions that they do have. Williams et al. (2016) highlight that in institutional settings contact between residents and staff tends to focus on instrumental care-related activities, trying to get the resident to cooperate in daily tasks, including activities of daily living, bodily functions, or health assessments. Consequently, talk is often initiated and directed by the caregiver and is often instructional, consisting of a set of short standardised imperative sentences and evaluative comments about the task being performed, with few opportunities for the resident to participate actively in the exchange (Allan and Killick 2014). This way of communicating exemplifies how staff prioritise getting through their work over addressing any of the emotional and social needs of the person that could be met by the interaction. Where residents are treated as frail bodies and objects it is overlooked that they are persons who are capable of expressing needs and possess a unique perspective on the world (Westerhof et al. 2013).

The consequence is a kind of extreme social exclusion and unequal interactions that disempower and disenable older people living in care homes, leading residents to experience lack of influence and autonomy (Bilfeldt et al. 2018) and confirming stereotypes of "persons-in-need". Older people may experience loneliness when they are increasingly limited in body with increased dependency on others (Paque et al. 2018). In the worst case, depersonalisation might lead to neglect or abuse whose consequences go far beyond relational or emotional outcomes (Phelan 2015).

Social and communicational neglect within these institutions is usually not intentional. Rather, it can happen due to the very nature of the institutional setting, the task-orientation of staff and the focus on efficiency. In this sense, the tendency towards "batch" treatment of residents is compelling and expedient from the perspective of the institution. This tendency is strong and reinforced by the context and day to day routine even of "well-run" care settings. Establishing a relationship between the resident and one or a few committed care personnel may be essential for feeling emotional closeness (Drageset et al. 2011) and requires that management staff and primary nurses should emphasise the psychosocial needs of the residents. Awareness of these constraints has been suggested as key to making a cultural shift within the care setting to enable and encourage opportunities for personal friendships and new emotional bonds to emerge.

Even where residents are provided with a variety of social programmes, these are again mostly planned and implemented using a "task-oriented" rigidly scheduled approach (Wiersma and Dupuis 2010), without input from residents. When residential care involves being catered to and entertained – like a continuous vacation – the routine may remove even minor challenges and stifle opportunities important for taking initiative, forming meaningful connections and achieving personal growth. A task-oriented approach obscures what is really needed, which is a space where residents can speak and be heard. Indeed, despite the ideals and best efforts of staff, residents often complain of a lack of meaning (Choi et al. 2008) and limited chances for reciprocity or contribution (Van Malderen et al. 2013).

23.3 Civic Engagement

Opportunities for civic engagement are extremely limited for those living in a care home (Leedahl et al. 2017). Although research on older people's civic engagement has grown steadily in recent decades (Serrat et al. 2020), care home residents are largely overlooked because the focus has been mainly on healthy, community-dwelling older people. This is ironic given that civic engagement has been associated with a wide range of positive outcomes, from higher levels of cognitive function or mental and physical health to reduced feelings of loneliness (Serrat et al. 2020).

Civic engagement, therefore, could be particularly relevant for older people living in care homes.

Civic engagement refers to ways in which "… an active citizen participates in the life of a community in order to improve conditions for others or to help shape the community's future" (Adler and Goggin 2005, p. 16). As a multidimensional concept, civic engagement entails both volunteering and political activities. Volunteering activities are aimed at improving conditions for others, with no explicit political intention, and could be carried out informally (referred to as informal volunteering; *e.g.* helping friends or relatives) or channelled through organizations (termed formal volunteering; *e.g.* participating in NGOs or community organizations). Political activity seeking to influence decision making processes, spans basic institutionalised activities directly related to government, *e.g.* voting or contacting representatives, and more advanced engagement outside the sphere of state politics in the form of non-institutionalised political activities, such as campaigning and participating in protest activities) (Serrat et al. 2020).

While volunteering activities may take place both inside and outside care homes, political activities are more likely to occur exclusively outside them. Indeed, when it comes to considering civic engagement among older people living in care homes, one should not overlook residents' councils as well as other similar mechanisms grouped under the label of client engagement (Petriwskyj et al. 2018). Enabling older people to voice grievances, and be heard in decision-making processes affecting their care environment, may even constitute important manifestations that can connect to wider political engagement.

The limited research on care home residents' engagement in civic activities has so far addressed three of these types of civic engagement: formal volunteering (*e.g.* Klinedinst and Resnick 2014), institutionalised political activities (particularly voting; *e.g.* Bonnie et al. 2018), and client engagement initiatives (*e.g.* O'Dwyer and Timonen 2010). In the following paragraphs we briefly review the main results of these streams of research.

Research on older residents' formal volunteering shows that they tend to participate less than community-dwelling older people, especially if they are among the oldest old or live with chronic health problems or disabilities (Resnick et al. 2013; Leedahl et al. 2017). Moreover, those who do engage civically are far more likely to do so inside rather than outside the care home (Resnick et al. 2013). The literature highlights a number of barriers for promoting greater engagement, from those which are related to residents' diminished personal resources (*e.g.* cognitive impairment), to practical issues (*e.g.* mobility, transportation) to contextual issues (*e.g.* staff attitudes towards residents' participation, ageism, and ableism) (Anderson and Dabelko-Schoeny 2010). Although the evidence on the effects of engagement in volunteering activities on residents' health and well-being is scarce and mixed, a small number of studies show positive impacts on life satisfaction (Yuen 2002) and feelings of usefulness (Klinedinst and Resnick 2014).

Moving to research on older residents' voting behaviour, this has been underpinned by ethical and legal discussions concerning the assessment and determination of voting competence among people with dementia (Appelbaum et al. 2005).

This debate highlights the complex tension between avoiding fraud and manipulation of residents with decreased cognitive capacity and preserving as far as possible their right to freely participate in the electoral processes (Bonnie et al. 2018). Although many national and international organisations advocate for assuring the effective and full participation of persons with disabilities in political and public life, research has shown that people with dementia tend to be intentionally or inadvertently disenfranchised (Karlawish et al. 2008). However, as Appelbaum et al. (2005) have demonstrated, most people with low to moderate cognitive impairment are cognitively able to vote, so dementia diagnosis by itself should never be an argument for disenfranchisement. Moreover, just as in the case of formal volunteering, organizational and contextual factors are important barriers to older residents' voting participation. In their study addressing voting behaviour among residents of care homes in Virginia (US), for instance, Bonnie et al. (2018) show that organizational policy and practices facilitating registration and voting have a positive effect on voter turnout among residents.

Finally, client engagement refers to initiatives allowing older people "…to have a voice – and control – in the services they receive as well as the policy that guides these" (Petriwskyj et al. 2018, p. 1351). These initiatives vary, both in scope, from participating in decisions about one's care to being involved in the management of the facility, and in depth, from mere consultation and discussion to collaboration, co-production, and true empowerment of residents. Research on client engagement initiatives have highlighted the difficulties associated with their implementation, including narrowing it to a mere consumerist approach (O'Dwyer 2013), or reinforcing tokenism and lack of influence of residents (*e.g.* O'Dwyer and Timonen 2010).

23.4 Socio-Cultural Exclusion

One important aspect of civic exclusion and broader processes of social exclusion for older people living in care homes relates to culture of care, and specifically how it can work to ameliorate or intensify socio-cultural aspects of exclusion. Cultures of care (Cassie and Cassie 2012; Fine 2015) involve a set of shared values, beliefs, expectations and practices (*i.e.*, a socio-cultural mindset) about what is supposed to be "good care" and which define both the responsibilities of staff and the position of older people ("users") in a care relationship. Thus, certain cultures of care could give rise, propagate and justify forms of exclusion, discriminatory practices and stigmatization of older people living in care homes. It is in that sense that we can talk about socio-cultural aspects of civic exclusion. These mechanisms can arise from or manifest within relationships with staff and others, and/or can drive experiences of exclusion across the social and civic lives of older people in residential facilities.

Traditionally, the culture of care in institutions for older people has been defined by task- or service-orientation whereby care is conceived as a service provided by professionals. Such professionals, coming from health and social fields, are within this system positioned as experts who have the necessary technical knowledge enabling them to determine what type of care is needed (that is to diagnose user needs and prescribe care) and how and to what degree it should be offered.

On this view, care involves a number of supporting tasks in some core areas, mainly related to basic activities of daily living (*e.g.* feeding, bathing and hygiene, mobility, etc.), security and avoidance of risks. In such cases, quality of care has to do with achieving certain outcomes, such as maximizing resident autonomy, reducing undesirable symptoms or states and increasing users' quality of life. This has led to the inclusion of psychosocial activities, both with recreational or therapeutic intention, among the tasks to be done in care homes. To assure quality, there is an emphasis on following protocols that define best practice processes, and on standardization of care, both of which contribute to care efficiency and the completion of care tasks with the least possible cost. That principle tends to involve a high degree of formalization, requiring employees to follow strict policies, schedules and procedures, and a rigid and markedly hierarchical division of responsibilities.

The New Public Management (NPM) quality control system allocates resources by the way of organizing principles aimed at cost reduction. The foundation of the allocation of resources in older adult care quality is becoming increasingly organised through principles that were originally developed for industrial production and whose main purpose has been the production of homogeneous services in a standardised way. Under these standards, the employee might end up in a paradoxical situation where care giving is conducted through homogeneous procedures instead of being conducted according to the individual needs of human beings. Increasingly, efficiency requirements and protocolization of services in detailed work descriptions lead to low priority being given to individual differences in needs and to the social dimensions of care (Szebehely 2005; Hjort 2009; Andersen and Bilfeldt 2016; Szebehely et al. 2017), with both excluded from the basis of work organization.

This technical and task-oriented culture of care often assumes that older people are merely passive care-receiving users. As Goffman (1961) would say, individuals' identities are stripped away, just to be thought of using standard (*e.g.* "patient", "resident") or diagnostic labels (*e.g.* "demented"). In other words, older persons are defined by their deficiencies, needs and vulnerabilities, which may be viewed as intrinsic and biomedical in nature with little susceptibility to change or improvement.

Such positioning of older people living in care homes as mere recipients of care accounts for some ageist practices contributing to social exclusion. One of the most studied examples of this is infantilisation, which is often manifest in the use of "elderspeak" by institutional staff (Williams et al. 2016). Elderspeak consists of speaking more slowly and using inappropriate terms of endearment, exaggerated intonation, simplified syntax, or questions that indicate a desired response (Brown and Draper 2003). However, as well-meaning as this may be, the use of elderspeak presupposes dependency and lack of competence, contributing to the construction of condescending and paternalistic relationships. Such a culture of care stigmatises older people and, in some cases, can lead to disruptive behaviors and resistance to care (Williams et al. 2017).

These sort of practices can contribute to what some authors, such as Sabat (2006), have called "excess disability", *i.e.*, dependency shaped by disabling cultural and environmental factors rather than physical or endogenous disease factors. Thus, defining older people as "dependent", with few or no opportunities for improvement, acts as a self-fulfilling prophecy and is linked to helplessness and learned dependency. In particular, where staff work under great pressure to perform certain care assignments in a short time, it may become expedient to presume a low level of functioning among residents and in turn restrict the opportunities to sustain and reinforce remaining competences (Stone and Bryant 2012). In some cases, older people may accommodate to such unsolicited support, and behave in a way that only confirms initial low expectations of functioning. In others, such dysfunctional interactions may elicit disruptive behaviors and expressions of discomfort that are interpreted as a symptom of disease, thereby reinforcing the initial presumption of a lack of competence (Scholl and Sabat 2008).

In any care relationship we find an imbalance of power between people living in care and those providing care (Roberts and Bowers 2015), which in turn could contribute to the marginalisation of older adult residents. Positioned as persons-in-need, older people living in institutions can develop very low expectations of their lives and about the support provided, causing them to lose autonomy and become dependent on others who determine their activities, and the rules governing daily life. Thus, the opportunities for people living in care homes to express themselves and let their voices be heard are dramatically diminished, even affecting older people's assessment of whether they are happy, and their ability to speak out if they are not.

23.5 Discussion

In this chapter we have explored the multidimensional and interrelated nature of exclusion in the context of institutional care settings for older people. First, we identified challenges in relation to fostering opportunities for continuity and evolution of the intimate, emotional and social facets of a person's life and relationships, which are either disrupted or intensified by admission to a residential care setting. A second dimension that typically gets lost in care settings, on admission, is continuity as a citizen of the care setting, and the opportunity for engagement (rather than merely an inmate, resident, consumer or user), both as a rights-bearer, and conceivably indeed as a duty-bearer. A third and probably broader dimension that underlies any form of exclusion in care homes has to do with the socio-cultural representations of care, whereby the individual may be dispossessed of a personal narrative by institutional and professional over-determining.

These three facets are related and reinforce each other to crystalise a social exclusion status that could be difficult to revert. For instance, a task-oriented culture of care that sees older people living in long-term care facilities exclusively through the lens of deficit may lead to relational and communicational patterns centered just on the completion of basic everyday activities, such as feeding or toileting, and forgetting socio-emotional needs that are not considered essential. In turn, such exclusion from social relationships hampers the capacity of controlling and deciding over their own life, and inhibits remaining capacities to reclaim and exert civic rights, promoting disempowerment. As a result, the initial views of older people as "people in need" and a task-oriented conception of care are reinforced.

However, there are ways to get out of these vicious circles. In recent decades we have witnessed increasing efforts to reverse such circumstances and substitute traditional biomedical and task-oriented protocols for a more holistic and individualised model of elder care, "person-centred care" (PCC). Rather than a single model, PCC is an approach with some core common assumptions considered as essential to provide quality care. Among them, most authors (*e.g.* Brooker 2004; Edvardsson et al. 2010; Doyle and Rubinstein 2013) mention: (1) the recognition of residents' personhood, exemplified in their life story, values and preferences, and their unique perspective of the world; and (2) the emphasis on empowerment of older people in the course of communication between caregivers and older people while performing daily care tasks, and on providing emotional (as distinct from instrumental or technical) support. The steady expansion of the PCC model in the latest decades, a model that has become the standard of good care at least in Western countries, is without a doubt a major breakthrough to reverse social exclusion in long-term care facilities.

While PCC models emphasise the concept of personhood to preserve the identity and reinforce the social bonds of older people living in long-term care facilities (and particularly, of those living with dementia), some authors have proposed to complement personhood with the concept of social citizenship, a more socially and politically oriented model that pays attention to issues of power, inclusion, and citizenship (*e.g.* Baldwin 2008; Bartlett and Connor 2010). The concept of social citizenship has a long pedigree since the publication of Marshall's seminal essay (Marshall 1950) in which he set out citizenship in more complete terms, encompassing civil rights, political rights and social rights. In the present context the concept is valuable in offering a paradigm that shifts the discourse around long-term care institutions by recognizing the challenge of realizing rights and citizenship in this rounded sense in the context of care homes for older people. It sets a norm, or goal, for which pathways to the realization of care tasks will need to be found, based on the notion that citizenship is the highest expression of human engagement. In the context of long- term care, the breach may be less of a problem in relation to meeting basic material dimensions of welfare, than in the areas of recognition of the older person's integrity, freedom, right to be self-governing and part of the "polity", whether defined in relation to the institutional context or the wider setting.

23.6 Conclusion

The exercise of rights as a citizen more generally, in the wider community and society, is critical to the individual. In fact, it is also key to the vindication of citizenship as the global principle of inclusion for a world where reaching deep old-age will become the norm. In sum, several domains of exclusion in later life, which may be accentuated in the residential care setting, could be addressed more effectively through the application of a coherent concept of citizenship.

Authors' Postscript

The outbreak in 2019 of the SARS CoV-2 (COVID-19) pandemic has had an unprecedented impact on long-term care institutions for older people in terms of the number of cases, the severity of these cases, and fatalities. Some of the decisions and measures discussed (or already taken) to cope with the pandemic in these institutions, such as the implementation of a particularly strict confinement and social distancing measures, the 'medicalisation' of these institutions that could make them more like hospitals and less like places to live, or the consideration of older people (and especially those living in care homes) as an at-risk group using a crude chronological criteria, might increase social exclusion in the domains outlined in this chapter. Decisive measures such as the advancement towards a person-centred model of care, the strengthening of social relationships both inside and outside the institution, or the consideration of these older residents as adult citizens whose opinions should be taken into account, are not guaranteed in post-pandemic times. And the risk of increased, rather than progressively reduced, social exclusion, is particularly at stake.

References

Adler, R., & Goggin, J. (2005). What do we mean by "civic engagement"? *Journal of Transformative Education, 3*, 236–253. https://doi.org/10.1177/1541344605276792.

Allan, K., & Killick, J. (2014). Communication and relationships: An inclusive social world. In M. Downs & B. Bowers (Eds.), *Excellence in dementia care* (pp. 240–255). London: Open University Press.

Alzheimer's Disease International. (2013). *World Alzheimer report 2013 'Journey of caring: An analysis of long-term care for dementia*. London: Alzheimer's Disease International. https://www.alz.co.uk/research/WorldAlzheimerReport2013.pdf.

Alzheimer's Society. (2007). *Home from home*. London: Alzheimer's Society.

Alzheimer's Society. (2016). *Fix dementia care: NHS and care homes*. London: Alzheimer's society. https://www.alzheimers.org.uk/sites/default/files/migrate/downloads/fix_dementia_care_nhs_and_care_homes_report.pdf.

Andersen, J., & Bilfeldt, A. (2016). Action research in nursing homes. *Action Research, 14*, 19–35. https://doi.org/10.1177/1476750315569082.

Anderson, K. A., & Dabelko-Schoeny, H. I. (2010). Civic engagement for nursing home residents: A call for social work action. *Journal of Gerontological Social Work, 53*, 270–282. https://doi.org/10.1080/01634371003648323.

Appelbaum, P. S., Bonnie, R. J., & Karlawish, J. H. (2005). The capacity to vote of persons with Alzheimer's disease. *The American Journal of Psychiatry, 162*, 2094–2100. https://doi.org/10.1176/appi.ajp.162.11.2094.

Baldwin, C. (2008). Narrative(,) citizenship and dementia: The personal and the political. *Journal of Aging Studies, 22*, 222–228. https://doi.org/10.1016/j.jaging.2007.04.002.
Bartlett, R., & Connor, D. O. (2010). *Broadening the dementia debate towards social citizenship*. Bristol: The Policy Press.
Bilfeldt, A., Mahler, M., & Soegaard Joergensen, M. (2018). Pårørendesamarbejde og psykisk arbejdsmiljø. In A. Bilfeldt et al. (Eds.), *Den ufærdige fremtid*. Aalbord: AAU.
Bonnie, R. J., Freedman, P., & Guterbock, T. M. (2018). Voting by senior citizens in long-term care facilities. *Election Law Journal: Rules, Politics, and Policy, 12*, 293–304. https://doi.org/10.1089/elj.2012.0187.
Brooker, D. (2004). What is person-centred care in dementia? *Reviews in Clinical Gerontology, 13*, 215–222. https://doi.org/10.1017/S095925980400108X.
Brown, A., & Draper, P. (2003). Accommodative speech and terms of endearment: Elements of a language mode often experienced by older adults. *Journal of Advanced Nursing, 41*, 15–21. https://doi.org/10.1046/j.1365-2648.2003.02500.x.
Cahill, S. (2018). *Dementia and human rights*. Bristol: Policy Press.
Cassie, K. M., & Cassie, W. E. (2012). Organizational and individual conditions associated with depressive symptoms among nursing home residents over time. *The Gerontologist, 52*, 812–821. https://doi.org/10.1093/geront/gns059.
Choi, N. G., Ransom, S., & Wyllie, R. J. (2008). Depression in older nursing home residents: The influence of nursing home environmental stressors, coping, and acceptance of group and individual therapy. *Aging and Mental Health, 12*, 536–547. https://doi.org/10.1080/13607860802343001.
Cipriani, J., Faig, S., Ayrer, K., Brown, L., & Johnson, N.C. (2006). Altruistic activity patterns among long-term nursing home residents. *Physical & Occupational Therapy in Geriatrics, 24*, 45–61. https://doi.org/10.1080/J148v24n03_04.
Doyle, P. J., & Rubinstein, R. L. (2013). Person-centered dementia care and the cultural matrix of othering. *The Gerontologist, 54*, 952–964. https://doi.org/10.1093/geront/gnt081.
Drageset, J. (2004). The importance of activities of daily living and social contact for loneliness: A survey among residents in nursing homes. *Scandinavian Journal of Caring Sciences, 18*, 65–71. https://doi.org/10.1111/j.0283-9318.2003.00251.x.
Drageset, J., Kirkevold, M., & Espehaug, B. (2011). Loneliness and social support among nursing home residents without cognitive impairment: A questionnaire survey. *International Journal of Nursing Studies, 48*, 611–619. https://doi.org/10.1016/j.ijnurstu.2010.09.008.
Edvardsson, D., Fetherstonhaugh, D., & Nay, R. (2010). Promoting a continuation of self and normality: Person-centred care as described by people with dementia, their family members and aged care staff. *Journal of Clinical Nursing, 19*, 2611–2618. https://doi.org/10.1111/j.1365-2702.2009.03143.x.
Fine, M. (2015). Cultures of care. In J. Twigg & W. Martin (Eds.), *Routledge handbook of cultural gerontology* (pp. 269–276). Abingdon: Routledge.
Goffman, E. (1961). *Asylums: Essays on the social situation of mental patients and other inmates*. Garden City: Anchor Books.
Hanratty, B., Stow, D., Collingridge Moore, D., Valtorta, N. K., & Matthews, F. (2018). Loneliness as a risk factor for care home admission in the English longitudinal study of ageing. *Age and Ageing, 47*, 896–900. https://doi.org/10.1093/ageing/afy095.
Hjort, K. (2009). Competence and development in the public sector: Development or dismantling of professionalism? In K. Illeris (Ed.), *International perspectives on competence development. Developing skills and capabilities* (pp. 112–123). London\New York: Routledge.
Karlawish, J., Bonnie, R., Appelbaum, P., Kane, R., Lyketsos, C., Karlan, P., et al. (2008). Identifying the barriers and challenges to voting by residents in nursing homes and assisted living settings. *Journal of Aging and Social Policy, 20*, 65–79. https://doi.org/10.1300/J031v20n01_04.
Klinedinst, N. J., & Resnick, B. (2014). Volunteering and depressive symptoms among residents in a continuing care retirement community. *Journal of Gerontological Social Work, 57*, 52–71. https://doi.org/10.1080/01634372.2013.867294.

Leedahl, S. N., Sellon, A. M., & Gallopyn, N. (2017). Factors predicting civic engagement among older adult nursing home residents. *Activities, Adaptation & Aging, 41*, 197–219. https://doi.org/10.1080/01924788.2017.1310581.

Löfqvist, C., Granbom, M., Himmelsbach, I., Iwarsson, S., Oswald, F., & Haak, M. (2013). Voices on relocation and aging in place in very old age—A complex and ambivalent matter. *The Gerontologist, 53*(6), 919–927. https://doi.org/10.1093/geront/gnt034.

Marshall, T. H. (1950). *Citizenship and social class, and other essays*. Cambridge: Cambridge University Press.

Moffatt, S., & Glasgow, N. (2009). How useful is the concept of social exclusion when applied to rural older people in the United Kingdom and the United States? *Regional Studies, 43*(10), 1291–1303. https://doi.org/10.1080/00343400903002697.

Nyqvist, F., Cattan, M., Andersson, L., Forsman, A. K., & Gustafson, Y. (2013). Social capital and loneliness among the very old living at home and in institutional settings: A comparative study. *Journal of Aging and Health, 25*, 1013–1035. https://doi.org/10.1177/0898264313497508.

O'Dwyer, C. (2013). Official conceptualizations of person-centered care: Which person counts? *Journal of Aging Studies, 27*, 233–242. https://doi.org/10.1016/j.jaging.2013.03.003.

O'Dwyer, C., & Timonen, V. (2010). Rethinking the value of residents ' councils: Observations and lessons from an exploratory study. *Journal of Applied Gerontology, 29*, 762–771. https://doi.org/10.1177/0733464809348002.

Paque, K., Bastiaens, H., Van Bogaert, P., & Dilles, T. (2018). Living in a nursing home: A phenomenological study exploring residents' loneliness and other feelings. *Scandinavian Journal of Caring Sciences, 32*, 1477–1484. https://doi.org/10.1111/scs.12599.

Petriwskyj, A., Gibson, A., & Webby, G. (2018). What does client "engagement" mean in aged care? An analysis of practice. *Ageing and Society, 38*, 1350–1376. https://doi.org/10.1017/S0144686X17000095.

Phelan, A. (2015). Protecting care home residents from mistreatment and abuse: On the need for policy. *Risk Management and Healthcare Policy, 8*, 215–223. https://doi.org/10.2147/RMHP.S70191.

Pitkala, K. H. (2016). Loneliness in nursing homes. *Journal of the American Medical Directors Association, 17*, 680–681. https://doi.org/10.1016/j.jamda.2016.04.007.

Resnick, B., Klinedinst, J., Dorsey, S., Holtzman, L., & Abuelhiga, L. S. (2013). Volunteer behaviour and factors that influence volunteering among residents in continuing care retirement communities. *Journal of Housing for the Elderly, 27*, 161–176. https://doi.org/10.1080/02763893.2012.754820.

Roberts, T., & Bowers, B. (2015). How nursing home residents develop relationships with peers and staff: A grounded theory study. *International Journal of Nursing Studies, 52*, 57–67. https://doi.org/10.1016/j.ijnurstu.2014.07.008.

Sabat, S. R. (2006). Mind, meaning, and personhood in dementia: The effects of positioning. In J. C. Hughes, S. J. Louw, & S. R. Sabat (Eds.), *Dementia: Mind, meaning, and the person* (pp. 287–302). Oxford: Oxford University Press.

Scholl, J. M., & Sabat, S. R. (2008). Stereotypes, stereotype threat and ageing: Implications for the understanding and treatment of people with Alzheimer's disease. *Ageing and Society, 28*, 103–130. https://doi.org/10.1017/S0144686X07006241.

Selbæk, G., Kirkevold, Ø., & Engedal, K. (2007). The prevalence of psychiatric symptoms and behavioural disturbances and the use of psychotropic drugs in Norwegian nursing homes. *International Journal of Geriatric Psychiatry, 22*, 843–849. https://doi.org/10.1002/gps.1749.

Serrat, R., Scharf, T., Villar, F., & Gómez, C. (2020). Fifty-five years of research into older people's civic participation: Recent trends, future directions. *The Gerontologist, 60*(1), e38–e51.

Stone, R. I., & Bryant, N. (2012). The impact of health care reform on the workforce caring for older adults. *Journal of Aging & Social Policy, 24*, 188–205. https://doi.org/10.1080/08959420.2012.659144.

Szebehely, M. (2005). Care as employment and welfare provision. Child care and elder care in Sweden at the dawn of the 21st century. In H. M. Dahl & T. R. Eriksen (Eds.), *Dilemmas of care in the Nordic welfare state. Continuity and change*. Aldershot: Ashgate.

Szebehely, M., Stranz, A., & Strandell, R. (2017). *Vem ska arbeta i framtidens äldreomsorg?* Stockholm: Department of Social Work, Stockholm Universitet.

Van Malderen, L., Mets, T., De Vriendt, P., & Gorus, E. (2013). The active ageing–concept translated to the residential long-term care. *Quality of Life Research, 22*, 929–937. https://doi.org/10.1007/s11136-012-0216-5.

Ward, R., Vass, A. A., Aggarwal, N., Garfield, C., & Cybyk, B. (2008). A different story: Exploring patterns of communication in residential dementia care. *Ageing & Society, 28*(5), 629–651.

Westerhof, G. J., van Vuuren, M., Brummans, B. H., & Custers, A. F. (2013). A Buberian approach to the co-construction of relationships between professional caregivers and residents in nursing homes. *The Gerontologist, 54*, 354–362. https://doi.org/10.1093/geront/gnt064.

Wiersma, E., & Dupuis, S. L. (2010). Becoming institutional bodies: Socialization into a long-term care home. *Journal of Aging Studies, 24*, 278–291. https://doi.org/10.1016/j.jaging.2010.08.003.

Williams, K. N., Ilten, T. B., & Bower, H. (2016). Meeting communication needs: Topics of talk in the nursing home. *Journal of Psychosocial Nursing and Mental Health Services, 43*, 38–45. https://doi.org/10.3928/02793695-20050701-05.

Williams, K. N., Perkhounkova, Y., Herman, R., & Bossen, A. (2017). A communication intervention to reduce resistiveness in dementia care: A cluster randomized controlled trial. *The Gerontologist, 57*, 707–718. https://doi.org/10.1093/geront/gnw047.

Yuen, H. K. (2002). Impact of an altruistic activity on life satisfaction in institutionalized elders: A pilot study. *Physical and Occupational Therapy in Geriatrics, 20*, 125–135. https://doi.org/10.1080/J148v20n03_08.

Chapter 24
Two Dimensions of Social Exclusion: Economic Deprivation and Dynamics of Loneliness During Later Life in Europe

Michal Myck, Charles Waldegrave, and Lena Dahlberg

24.1 Introduction

This chapter focuses on two domains of social exclusion: economic exclusion – in the form of material resources – and exclusion from social relations – in the form of loneliness. Usually, material resources are measured via indicators related to income or wealth, while social relations are measured via indicators of social contacts and social participation. Here we consider a more nuanced approach, on the one hand taking a comprehensive measure of material deprivation [also see Ogg and Myck, and Sumil-Laanemaa et al. this volume] and on the other using loneliness as a reflection, or outcome of exclusion from social relations (Burholt et al. 2019; see also Burholt and Aartsen, and Morgan et al. this volume). Based on longitudinal data from the Survey of Health, Ageing and Retirement in Europe (SHARE), the aim of this chapter is to examine the dynamics of loneliness and to investigate the causal relationship between material resources and loneliness. In doing this, we hope to better illuminate some of the interconnections between social and economic domains of exclusion. Despite the growing body of work on exploring links between economic and social factors in later life, we still lack the scientific insights to understand how outcomes and processes across these domains intersect in the exclusion of older adults.

The chapter starts with definitions of material deprivation and loneliness, and a review of previous research on the relationship between them and with other risk

---

M. Myck (✉)
Centre for Economic Analysis, CenEA, Szczecin, Poland
e-mail: mmyck@cenea.org.pl

C. Waldegrave
Family Centre Social Policy Research Unit, Lower Hutt, Wellington, New Zealand

L. Dahlberg
Dalarna University, Falun, Sweden

K. Walsh et al. (eds.), *Social Exclusion in Later Life*, International Perspectives on Aging 28, https://doi.org/10.1007/978-3-030-51406-8_24

factors that are relevant to understand this relationship. The following sections present data, methods and results. A discussion of the findings completes the chapter.

24.2 Material Deprivation and Loneliness in Ageing Populations

Material deprivation occurs when an individual or household is unable to (rather than chooses not to) afford a number of goods and services, *e.g.* unexpected expenses and payment arrears, adequate heating or a washing machine (Eurostat 2018). This concept differs from the measurement of poverty defined on the basis of personal or household income most often used in relation to national medians (Eurostat[1]). While current income as a measure of resources has its merits and has been a common reference for numerous studies, there is growing literature which shows that it may fail to accurately reflect the complexity of material conditions. From this perspective the important advantage of material deprivation measures which we use in this chapter, is that they reflect the combination of material resources and material needs which may be of high relevance for understanding the conditions in old-age.

Loneliness is understood to mean:

> 'the negative outcome of a cognitive evaluation of a discrepancy between (the quality and quantity of) existing relationships and relationship standards' (de Jong Gierveld et al. 2006, p. 495).

Recently, Tesch-Römer and Huxhold (2019) noted that loneliness is not necessarily a consequence of growing old, but depends on specific risk factors such as financial and material resources, and Fokkema et al. (2012) have underscored that "wealth and health are conditions for engaging in satisfying personal relationships and thus for the prevention and alleviation of loneliness" (p. 221). The literature on loneliness employs several measures to locate people's position within society, for example, demonstrating a relationship between loneliness and socio-economic position (Fokkema et al. 2012), income (De Jong Gierveld and Tesch-Römer 2012), poverty (Haushofer 2013), and low education and material deprivation (Gibney et al. 2019). Franzese (2015) found that material deprivation was more strongly correlated with health outcomes (especially mental health, including loneliness) than with income poverty.

Previous research also points to the importance of deprivation at neighbourhood level. Scharf et al. (2005) identified much higher rates of severe loneliness in deprived urban neighbourhoods than other English loneliness studies. A later comparison between deprived neighbourhoods in England and the Netherlands (Scharf and de Jong Gierveld 2008), drawing on the same English data, noted that similar mechanisms connected neighbourhood characteristics and loneliness in both studies; notably, older people in both countries who evaluated their neighbourhood

[1] https://ec.europa.eu/eurostat/web/products-datasets/product?code=tessi014

negatively tended to have higher loneliness scores. At country level, Nyqvist et al. (2019) found that welfare states, because of the provision of social protections, contribute to the absence of loneliness. The study found that the Nordic, Anglo-Saxon and Continental welfare regimes performed better than Southern and Eastern welfare regimes when it came to the absence of loneliness, suggesting that state provision of material resources can protect against loneliness. Hansen and Slagsvold (2015) investigated country differences in loneliness in Europe and found considerable between-country heterogeneity in late-life loneliness; especially among women, loneliness was strongly associated with lower socio-economic status.

The association between income inequality and loneliness was found in a study based on World Value Survey data from 43 countries, suggesting that poverty and income inequality have broad psychological consequences (Haushofer 2013). Similarly, based on SHARE data from 2013, Niedzwiedz et al. (2016, p. 29) found that the least wealthy older people had the highest risk of loneliness and concluded that there is a "need to consider social inequalities in loneliness as a public health issue among older people in Europe." Yet the questions concerning the causal effect of poor material conditions on loneliness and their magnitude – given the complexity of the relationship – remain to be convincingly addressed. Our approach in this chapter aims to provide a contribution to this debate.

24.2.1 Other Relevant Risk Factors

In order to isolate the effect of material deprivation on loneliness, it is necessary to control for factors known to be associated with both material deprivation and loneliness. There is ample evidence that social contacts are protective against loneliness (*e.g.* Dykstra et al. 2005; Donovan et al. 2017), and being married or living with a partner is especially important for loneliness (*e.g.* Pikhartova et al. 2016) with recently widowed individuals at increased risk of loneliness (*e.g.* Dahlberg et al. 2015; Pikhartova et al. 2016). Cross-sectional studies have found that having no or fewer children is associated with loneliness (Cohen-Mansfield et al. 2016). Moreover, widowhood is also an important factor related to old-age poverty (Tinios et al. 2011; Bover et al. 2014), though on the other hand poverty and financial hardship among older people are often found to be higher in larger households (Lyberaki and Tinios 2008; Bover et al. 2014), most probably due to the fact that family solidarity and co-residence often act as a support mechanism to those with lowest resources.

Self-perceived health, co-morbidity, reduced health status and functional limitations have been found to be associated with both a higher risk of loneliness in older people (*e.g.* Cohen-Mansfield et al. 2009; Pikhartova et al. 2016; Hawkley and Kocherginsky 2017) and poor material conditions (Adena and Myck 2014; Bover et al. 2014; Franzese 2015).

Finally, an increased risk of loneliness has been found in women, although this association is usually non-significant when variables such as health and social factors are taken into account (*e.g.* Dahlberg et al. 2015; Hawkley and Kocherginsky 2017). Similarly, some studies have found higher age to be associated with loneliness in bivariate but not in multivariable analyses (*e.g.* Dahlberg et al. 2015; Pikhartova et al. 2016). However, the evidence regarding age is inconsistent in that other studies have not found this association (*e.g.* Warner and Adams 2016). These findings indicate that although loneliness may be more common in women and in people of higher ages, this can be explained by other factors such as the higher likelihood of loss of partner and other social relations, health problems and functional limitations in these groups. Analysis of SHARE data also suggests that age and being female is positively correlated with the risk of falling into financial hardship, although the key determinants of material conditions among older people are having labour market or retirement income and being in good health (Bover et al. 2014).

24.3 SHARE Data: Descriptive Statistics

For the purpose of our analysis we use the data from SHARE, a multidimensional panel study focused on individuals aged 50 years and older and covering key aspects of their lives such as health, labour market activity and retirement, material conditions as well as family and social relations (see *e.g.* Börsch-Supan et al. 2013). In our analysis we use information drawn from waves 5 and 6 of the survey, administered in 2013 and 2015 respectively. This is supplemented with additional retrospective data on childhood conditions from wave 3, when a full special life history interview was conducted, and wave 5 – from an additional module for those who did not participate in wave 3. The reason why we focus on these two waves is because the survey in wave 5 contained a special module specifically focused on broad aspects of well-being in later life and covering detailed data on material conditions. This allows us to use an indicator for material deprivation based largely on these extra variables. Additionally, both of these waves include a measure of loneliness, which enables the analysis of the relationship between loneliness and material conditions at a given point in time and over time. The analysis thus covers two waves of SHARE data and spans over 13 European countries which participated in SHARE in both of these waves: Austria, Germany, Sweden, Spain, Italy, France, Denmark, Switzerland, Belgium, Czech Republic, Luxembourg, Slovenia and Estonia. The final sample sizes used in the analysis of levels and changes in loneliness, together with basic descriptive statistics, are presented in Table 24.1. The respective total samples consist of 30,072 and 18,954 individuals.

In Table 24.1 we show the gender composition of the sample, the proportion of respondents living with a partner, the proportion of those reporting poor health status and the proportion of those working at the time of wave 5. There is large cross-country heterogeneity in particular with regard to the latter two characteristics. While only 3.0% of the sample report poor health in Switzerland, as many as 22.4% do so in Estonia, and rates of paid employment vary from 17.7% in Austria to 45.1%

Table 24.1 Basic descriptive statistics, SHARE wave 5: demographics, health, work and material deprivation

			General demographics and descriptive statistics (levels sample)				Material deprivation (levels sample)	
	Number of observations, analysis in levels	Number of observations, analysis in changes	% females	% with partner	% in poor health	% working in W5	% in highest deprivation quintile	% in second highest quintile
Austria	1843	1327	52.3%	71.0%	6.4%	17.7%	7.8%	15.0%
Germany	3114	1870	47.9%	79.7%	8.7%	36.9%	12.5%	15.8%
Sweden	2533	1729	49.3%	76.5%	5.0%	32.0%	4.5%	10.0%
Spain	3039	2093	48.3%	82.0%	11.8%	25.5%	23.4%	26.1%
Italy	2429	1324	49.5%	81.1%	9.2%	22.4%	32.3%	23.2%
France	2127	1295	51.0%	70.5%	10.9%	24.4%	16.6%	20.7%
Denmark	2607	2092	48.5%	78.2%	4.5%	45.1%	3.3%	9.2%
Switzerland	1687	1238	46.0%	78.1%	3.0%	37.4%	4.7%	15.2%
Belgium	3031	1854	48.1%	74.2%	5.2%	27.5%	8.7%	15.6%
Czech Rep	2521	1122	55.4%	72.7%	14.2%	19.3%	20.0%	27.6%
Luxembourg	859	520	47.7%	81.3%	5.7%	26.4%	4.8%	12.8%
Slovenia	1609	1074	52.9%	78.3%	14.5%	18.2%	24.9%	25.2%
Estonia	2673	1416	57.0%	72.3%	22.4%	32.6%	48.2%	28.3%
Total	30,072	18,954	50.4%	76.5%	9.7%	28.7%	17.2%	19.1%

Notes: poor health based on self-reported health status (declared as poor), quintiles of material deprivation based on a continuous material deprivation measure (see Myck et al., 2015) for the W5 sample of countries included in the analysis in Denmark.[2] We also present the proportion of the specific country samples who are in the highest and the second highest quintiles of material deprivation – measured via the material deprivation index constructed on the basis of the additional survey items available in the SHARE Survey in wave 5.

The index aggregates a set of binary indicators on whether a person is deprived of a specific item applying weights related to how a given item affects individual welfare (see Adena et al. 2015; Bertoni et al. 2015; Myck et al. 2015).[3] The final deprivation index takes values from zero to one, with higher values implying higher levels of deprivation. There is a number of advantages of using such indices to measure material conditions, especially in an international context. In particular, the indices are comparable across countries, since they refer to the same list of items, and they are comprehensive measures capturing a broader concept of material conditions compared to income or assets with a specific focus on the material needs of older people. In the analysis, we use information on the respondents' position in the distribution of material deprivation and focus on the top two quintiles – those in the highest 20% and the second highest 20% of material deprivation. There is very high variation in the proportion of respondents who face material deprivation in different countries. The proportion of individuals who belong to the highest quintile of material deprivation in the full SHARE sample in wave 5 varies from 3.3% in Denmark to as much as 48.2% in Estonia [see Sumil-Laanemaa et al. this volume for a discussion of this variation by welfare clusters]. Similarly, 9.2% and 28.3% of respondents are located in the second quintile of the overall material deprivation distribution in the two countries respectively. Our measure of loneliness is based on three items in the SHARE survey available in waves 5 and 6 which are based on the following questions [as also used by Morgan et al. this volume]:

- How much of the time do you feel you lack companionship?
- How much of the time do you feel left out?
- How much of the time do you feel isolated from others?

Each of these questions has three response categories: "Often", "Some of the time" or "Hardly ever or never". On the basis of these three questions we identify people as being in mild or severe loneliness depending on whether they report: "Some of the time" or "Often" to either of the three questions, respectively.

In columns 2 and 3 of Table 24.2, we present the levels of mild and severe loneliness across countries in the sample used for the levels analysis. About a quarter of

---

[2] Note that the rates are not adjusted for age composition and some of this variation may be related to this because countries refresh their panel samples at different stages. We control for age in all our detailed analysis.

[3] The items relate to: (a) affordability of: meat/fish/chicken, fruits/vegetables, an unexpected expense, a week-long vacation once a year, regular grocery shopping; (b) keeping living costs down by: reducing heating, wearing worn-out shoes, wearing worn-out clothes, not replacing glasses, postponing dentist, postponing doctor; (c) having payment arrears (d) experiencing insufficient resources to do things that one would like to do. See: Bertoni, Cavapozzi, Celidoni, & Trevisan, 2015.

Table 24.2 Loneliness in SHARE: levels in wave 5 and changes between waves 5 and 6

	Levels: at (t-1), wave 5		Change: becoming lonely between (t-1) and (t)	
	Mild loneliness	Severe loneliness	Mild loneliness	Severe loneliness
Austria	0.207	0.037	0.146	0.014
Germany	0.311	0.072	0.214	0.027
Sweden	0.243	0.053	0.223	0.019
Spain	0.174	0.066	0.161	0.044
Italy	0.295	0.130	0.262	0.043
France	0.266	0.100	0.184	0.031
Denmark	0.145	0.035	0.097	0.012
Switzerland	0.220	0.034	0.177	0.014
Belgium	0.261	0.106	0.185	0.035
Czech Rep	0.413	0.126	0.343	0.072
Luxembourg	0.286	0.092	0.165	0.032
Slovenia	0.246	0.059	0.288	0.039
Estonia	0.331	0.112	0.226	0.070
Total	0.263	0.080	0.199	0.034

the entire SHARE sample in these 13 countries in wave 5 reported mild loneliness – with rates varying between 14.5% in Denmark to 33.1% in Estonia. Eight per cent of the sample experience severe loneliness, with lowest rates in Switzerland, Denmark and Austria (between 3.4% and 3.7%) and highest rates in Estonia, Czech Republic and Italy (from 12.6% to 13.0%). In columns 4 and 5 we present the proportion of respondents among those who in wave 5 report no loneliness, and who in wave 6 report either mild or severe loneliness. Nearly 20% of all respondents who did not report loneliness at the time of wave 5, report falling into mild loneliness and 3.4% into severe loneliness over the two-year period. The highest proportion of those who fall into severe loneliness are once again found in Estonia (7.0%) and the Czech Republic (7.2%).

In Fig. 24.1, we present the distribution of the populations for a selection of six of the thirteen countries we use for analysis, conditional on their loneliness and material deprivation status. Each population is divided into six categories. The first three include people who do not report loneliness and:

- are in the bottom three quintiles of material deprivation (Category 1)
- are in the second highest quintile of material deprivation (Category 2)
- are in the highest quintile of material deprivation (Category 3)

While the last three categories include those who report mild or severe loneliness and similarly:

- are in the bottom three quintiles of material deprivation (Category 4)
- are in the second highest quintile of material deprivation (Category 5)
- are in the highest quintile of material deprivation (Category 6)

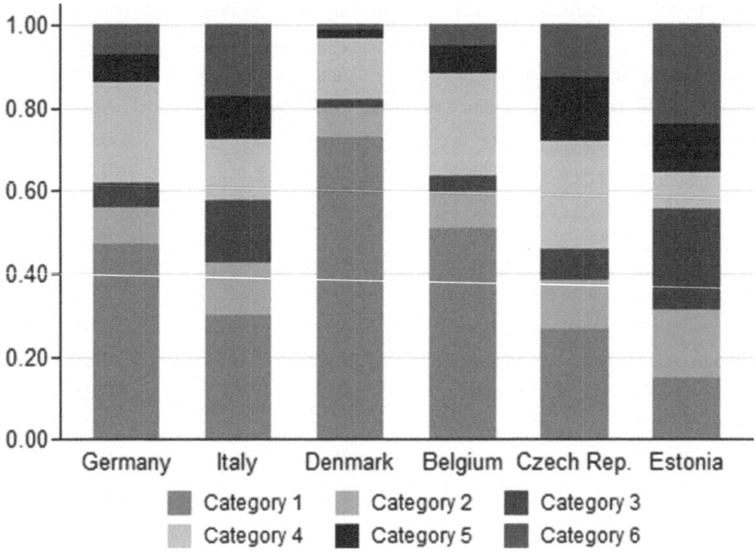

Fig. 24.1 Proportion of respondents by combination of loneliness and material deprivation. Selected countries. (Notes: Sample proportions (weighted) on y-axis; Categories 1–6 – see main text)

The categories reflect the differences between the scale of reported loneliness in the respective countries, and within these we can distinguish the scale of material deprivation. The top three categories (4–6) cover respondents who declare some degree of loneliness. If we treat loneliness and material deprivation as reflections of two different aspects of social exclusion, we can see a significant overlap between the two dimensions. For example, in Estonia nearly 24% of the SHARE sample report some degree of loneliness and at the same time fall into the highest quintile of material deprivation. In Italy this proportion is as high as 17.2%, while the proportion in Belgium and Denmark is 4.9% and 1.0% respectively.

24.4 Data Analysis

The main focus of our analysis is to relate poor material conditions to loneliness in later life and to try to identify if material conditions have causal implications for the dynamics of loneliness. Generally the relationship could be summarised in the following equation:

$$L_{i,t} = \beta_1' X_{i,t} + \gamma' mc_{i,t} + \varepsilon_{i,t} \tag{24.1}$$

where $L_{i,t}$ is a measure of loneliness of individual i at time t, $X_{i,t}$ are his or her characteristics, $mc_{i,t}$ is the individual indicator (or a vector of indicators) of poor material conditions, *i.e.* our key variable of interest, and $\varepsilon_{i,t}$ is an individual, t-specific residual. Naturally, the above specification is unable to identify the causal role of material conditions on loneliness due to the potential endogeneity of the former with respect to the latter, since loneliness at time t might be caused by poor material conditions and vice versa. In addition, there may be factors in $\varepsilon_{i,t}$ which are correlated with both material conditions and loneliness which would result in a biased estimation of the coefficient on $mc_{i,t}$. We take several steps to reduce this bias. Firstly, we control for an extensive set of potential risk factors identified in previous research and making use of the richness of the SHARE data. In the $X_{i,t}$ vector of variables we include those related to physical health, family relations, as well as childhood conditions drawn from life history interviews of the survey. Second, apart from examining the basic relationship in levels, as presented in Eq. 24.1, we take advantage of the panel nature of the SHARE survey and look at the correlation of material conditions and other factors with dynamics of loneliness. This is done by taking a sample of respondents who did not show any signs of loneliness in wave 5 (see Table 24.1) and examining the role of various factors on the probability of falling into loneliness by wave 6 (see Table 24.2). With this approach – through the differences in loneliness scores between the waves – we account for some of the so called "fixed effects" which might affect both material conditions and loneliness and as a result bias the examined relationship (for another application of this approach see Myck et al. 2019).

The vector of control variables in the levels specifications, which are based on wave 5 data, includes such characteristics as: gender, age polynomial, years of education, living in a rural area, work status, a set of controls for physical health, for having a partner, the size of the household, number of sons, number of daughters, number of children living close to the respondent (within 5 km radius), as well as indicators for: ever having siblings, having a living sister, brother, mother and father. The set of controls which cover characteristics from retrospective interviews related to the situation of the respondent at the age of 10 includes such information as accommodation conditions, number of books at home, relative performance at school in native language and maths, vaccinations and health status during childhood. Naturally, we also control for country-fixed effects. Additionally, the specifications in changes are extended to include information on: leaving work, losing a partner and changes in the size of the household between waves 5 and 6. Standard errors are clustered at the country level and estimates are conducted using linear probability models. The dependent variables are binary indicators for reporting either any loneliness (mild or severe) or severe loneliness.

24.5 Results: Material Deprivation and Loneliness

Results of our analysis are presented in Table 24.3 in four specifications. Specifications one and two present the relationship in levels of loneliness, as reported in wave 5 of SHARE, while specifications three and four show the results in changes between waves 5 and 6 (from reporting no expressions of loneliness in

Table 24.3 Results: correlates of levels of and changes in loneliness

	Levels: at (t-1), wave 5		Change: becoming lonely between (t-1) and (t)	
	Mild or severe loneliness	Severe loneliness	Mild or severe loneliness	Severe loneliness
	1	2	3	4
Female	0.0142	−0.0021	−0.0111	−0.0057
	(0.0132)	(0.0037)	(0.0091)	(0.0060)
Age	−0.0589***	−0.0283**	−0.0369*	−0.0103
	(0.0120)	(0.0084)	(0.0141)	(0.0064)
Age squared	0.0120**	0.0058*	0.0109*	0.0039*
	(0.0031)	(0.0026)	(0.0042)	(0.0014)
Years of education	0.0023*	0.0006	−0.0000	−0.0001
	(0.0009)	(0.0006)	(0.0009)	(0.0002)
Lives in rural area	0.0049	−0.0006	0.0204	0.0027
	(0.0119)	(0.0056)	(0.0115)	(0.0024)
Material deprivation: quintile 1	0.1072***	0.0820***	0.0479*	0.0204*
	(0.0103)	(0.0099)	(0.0167)	(0.0068)
Material deprivation: quintile 2	0.0451***	0.0210***	0.0398**	0.0105**
	(0.0077)	(0.0033)	(0.0104)	(0.0032)
Works in W5	−0.0391***	−0.0201***	−0.0250*	−0.0044
	(0.0090)	(0.0045)	(0.0108)	(0.0054)
Leaves work by W6			0.0124	0.0096
			(0.0118)	(0.0046)
Has partner in W5	−0.1825***	−0.0826***	−0.0847***	−0.0113
	(0.0203)	(0.0127)	(0.0143)	(0.0058)
Loses partner by W6			0.3219***	0.1635***
			(0.0329)	(0.0331)
No people in HH, W5	−0.0104*	−0.0054	−0.0056	−0.0029
	(0.0047)	(0.0033)	(0.0033)	(0.0015)
No people in HH, lower in W6			0.0200	0.0166**
			(0.0095)	(0.0050)
Joint tests for significance of:				
Health variables	***	***	***	***
Family variables	**	***	*	**
Childhood variables	***	***	***	**
Observations	30,072	30,072	18,954	18,954
Adjusted R^2	0.121	0.086	0.074	0.054

Notes: Specification 1: declaring "Often" or "Some of the time" in any of the three SHARE loneliness items in wave 5 (see text for details); Specification 2: declaring "Often" in any of the three SHARE loneliness items in wave 5; Specifications 3 and 4 – declarations as in Specifications 1 and 2 at the time of wave 6, conditional on declaring "Hardly ever or never" for all three items in wave 5. Additional, unreported, variables include country fixed effects and time between surveys (in months). Age measured as (age-50)/10

Standard errors in parentheses; $^{*}p < 0.05$, $^{**}p < 0.01$, $^{***}p < 0.001$

wave 5). In each case, the first specification shows the relationship for any loneliness, mild or severe, and the second for severe loneliness. In Table 24.3 we only report a selection of coefficients with the remaining ones shown only with respect to the joint significance of the entire group of factors divided into health, family and childhood variables. In all specifications we control for the level of material deprivation through the indicators of belonging to either the first or second quintile of the distribution.

24.5.1 The Role of Control Factors

The results show a very clear and consistent pattern. First of all we see a significant effect of age in all specifications, and while the coefficients on age is negative the curvature of the relationship picked up by controlling for age squared shows that, while age initially is associated with lower loneliness – or lower probability of falling into loneliness – at a certain point, the relationship turns negative and loneliness begins to grow for older-ages. Detailed analysis of the two coefficients suggests that this tipping point is around the age of between 64 and 67 years. Neither the gender of the respondent nor his or her education seems to have a consistently significant effect on the levels of loneliness. We also find no correlation between loneliness and living in a rural area. Working at the time of wave 5 is associated with lower levels of loneliness and reduces the probability of falling into mild or severe loneliness but has no effect on the probability of falling into severe loneliness, and we find no effect of leaving work after wave 5 on the probability of reporting loneliness 2 years later. Partnership status and the experience of losing one's partner between waves 5 and 6 is strongly and significantly correlated with the level and change in loneliness. In the latter case, the probability of falling into severe loneliness grows by 16.4 percentage points (pp), and reporting any expression of loneliness in wave 6 grows by as much as 32.2 pp. among those who lost their partner. While the overall household size does not seem to reduce the probability of falling into loneliness, a reduction of household members between waves 5 and 6 increases the probability of falling into severe loneliness by 1.6 pp. In all specifications we find that the groups of variables related to physical health, extended family as well as childhood conditions are all significantly related to both levels and changes in loneliness [also see Morgan et al. this volume].

24.5.2 Loneliness and Material Deprivation

Turning to the role of material conditions, our results show that being located in the highest or the second highest quintile of the material deprivation distribution is strongly associated with both the level of loneliness (specifications 1 and 2) and with falling into loneliness in wave 6 conditional on not reporting loneliness 2 years earlier. Being in the highest quintile of the distribution is associated with a nearly 4.8 pp. higher probability of falling into loneliness in wave 6 and with a 2.0 pp. higher probability of falling into severe loneliness (compared to those in the bottom three quintiles). Given that, as we saw in Table 24.1, the average probability of falling into severe loneliness is only 3.3%, this suggests a potentially very important role of material conditions in affecting the level of loneliness among older people. The probability of falling into severe loneliness among those in the second highest quintile of the material deprivation distribution is also higher (by 1.1 pp) compared to those further down the deprivation scale (*i.e.* those less deprived) and the effect is also statistically significant.

24.6 Discussion

This chapter primarily focused on two domains of social exclusion: economic exclusion – in the form of material resources – and exclusion from social relations – in the form of loneliness. The aim was to examine the dynamic effect of material exclusion on loneliness, through an analysis of the longitudinal data from the Survey of Health, Ageing and Retirement in Europe (SHARE).

The finding that older people living in materially deprived conditions is strongly associated with loneliness adds to the growing body of evidence, cited earlier in this chapter, on this critical risk factor. This finding was strong, both in terms of the cross-sectional analysis for the earlier wave, and the dynamic analysis between the two waves for those who were not lonely during 2013 but became lonely in 2015. Being located in the highest or the second highest quintile of the material deprivation distribution is strongly associated with both the level of loneliness and with falling into loneliness in wave 6 demonstrating increasing negative impacts over time. The analysis focussed on the highest two deprivation quintiles to highlight the impact of material deprivation on the levels of loneliness for older people experiencing lower living standards. This result supports earlier findings of Cohen-Mansfield et al. (2009) who also found that poor material conditions have implications for the onset of loneliness.

The variables used as controls in this research largely confirmed previous studies, presented earlier in this chapter. Having a partner is protective against loneliness and losing a partner is strongly associated with an increase in loneliness. Growing older and having a reduction in the number of people in one's household between the two waves are both associated with loneliness, but not as strongly. Being in work correlates with lower levels of loneliness, but we find no relationship between work (and leaving it) and becoming severely lonely between the waves. Gender, education and living in a rural area did not demonstrate consistently significant effects. However, the overall grouping of variables on physical health and childhood conditions confirmed earlier research findings with physical health being protective and negative childhood conditions providing a risk.

Given the robust links of loneliness to overall negative morbidity and mortality outcomes (Holt-Lunstad et al. 2015), our research findings provide important pointers for developing our understanding of causal relations in a complex reality of overlapping domains of exclusion. The results demonstrate the implications of material exclusion on changes in the degree of loneliness and as such, the effect of economic related factors, in this case material resources, on social relations. Poor material conditions may influence people's welfare directly, but on top of this they seem to affect the standard of living also through negative impacts on social relations and other domains further down the line.

24.7 Conclusion

The findings raise a number of important questions about the role of poor living conditions on loneliness and social exclusion more generally. For example, does material deprivation lead some older people to being shy about initiating and sustaining relationships because they feel they have nothing that is attractive to give others? Does a lower standard of living lead to negative psychological responses such as a loss of self-worth and a sense of shame that may inhibit social connection and deepen the experience of loneliness? Do lower living conditions create affordability stress as older people endeavour to balance their budgets between food, housing, utilities and other goods and services to such an extent that they find it difficult to afford socially connecting activities? Future research can explore these questions to illuminate further the interrelationships between the economic and social domain of exclusion in later life.

The results also raise important policy issues. The cost of loneliness on health and welfare budgets is considerable (Public Health England 2017). An increased investment in material living standards may therefore lead to lower healthcare and welfare costs over time and a better life in a number of dimensions for people currently living in materially deprived conditions.

Editors' Postscript

Please note, like other contributions to this book, this chapter was written before the COVID-19 pandemic of 2020. The book's introductory chapter (Chap. 1) and conclusion (Chap. 34) consider some of the key ways in which the pandemic relates to issues concerning social exclusion and ageing.

Data Acknowledgement This paper uses data from SHARE Waves 3, 5 and 6 (DOIs: https://doi.org/10.6103/SHARE.w3.600, https://doi.org/10.6103/SHARE.w5.600, https://doi.org/10.6103/SHARE.w6.600; Börsch-Supan, 2017), see Börsch-Supan et al. (2013) for methodological details. The SHARE data collection has been primarily funded by the European Commission through FP5

(QLK6-CT-2001-00360), FP6 (SHARE-I3: RII-CT-2006-062193, COMPARE: CIT5-CT-2005-028857, SHARELIFE: CIT4-CT-2006-028812) and FP7 (SHARE-PREP: N°211,909, SHARE-LEAP: N°227,822, SHARE M4: N°261,982). Additional funding from the German Ministry of Education and Research, the Max Planck Society for the Advancement of Science, the U.S. National Institute on Aging (U01_AG09740-13S2, P01_AG005842, P01_AG08291, P30_AG12815, R21_AG025169, Y1-AG-4553-01, IAG_BSR06–11, OGHA_04–064, HHSN271201300071C) and from various national funding sources is gratefully acknowledged (see www.share-project.org).

References

Adena, M., & Myck, M. (2014). Poverty and Transitions in Health in Later Life. *Social Science and Medicine, 116*, 202–210.

Adena, M., Myck, M., & Oczkowska, M. (2015). Material deprivation – in SHARE Wave 5 data: A contribution to a better understanding of differences in material conditions in later life. In A. Börsch-Supan, T. Kneip, H. Litwin, M. Myck, & G. Weber (Eds.), *Ageing in Europe: Supporting policies for an inclusive society* (pp. 25–38). Berlin: De Gruyter.

Bertoni, M., Cavapozzi, D., Celidoni, M., & Trevisan, E. (2015). Assessing the material deprivation of older Europeans. In A. Börsch-Supan, T. Kneip, H. Litwin, M. Myck, & G. Weber (Eds.), *Ageing in Europe: Supporting policies for an inclusive society* (pp. 49–56). Berlin: De Gruyter.

Börsch-Supan, A. (2017). *Survey of Health, Ageing and Retirement in Europe (SHARE) Waves 3, 5 and 6*. Release version: 6.0.0. SHARE-ERIC.

Börsch-Supan, A., Brandt, M., Hunkler, C., Kneip, T., Korbmacher, J., Malter, F., et al. (2013). Data resource profile: The Survey of Health, Ageing and Retirement in Europe (SHARE). *International Journal of Epidemiology, 42*(4), 992–1001. https://doi.org/10.1093/ije/dyt088.

Bover, O., Brugiavini, A., & Weber, G. (2014). Anatomy of financial hardship. In A. Brugiavini & G. Weber (Eds.), *Longer-term consequences of the great recession on the lives of Europeans* (pp. 4–37). Oxford: Oxford University Press.

Burholt, V., Winter, B., Aartsen, M., Constantinou, C., Dahlberg, L., Feliciano, V., et al. (2019). 156 A critical review and development of a conceptual model of exclusion from social relations for older people. *European Journal of Ageing, 17*, 3–19. https://doi.org/10.1007/s10433-019-00506-0.

Cohen-Mansfield, J., Hazan, H., Lerman, Y., & Shalom, V. (2016). Correlates and predictors of loneliness in older-adults: a review of quantitative results informed by qualitative insights. *International Psychogeriatrics, 28*(4), 557–576. https://doi.org/10.1017/s1041610215001532.

Cohen-Mansfield, J., Shmotkin, D., & Goldberg, S. (2009). Loneliness in old age: longitudinal changes and their determinants in an Israeli sample. *International Psychogeriatrics, 21*(6), 1160–1170. https://doi.org/10.1017/s1041610209990974.

Dahlberg, L., Andersson, L., McKee, K. J., & Lennartsson, C. (2015). Predictors of loneliness among older women and men in Sweden: A national longitudinal study. *Aging and Mental Health, 19*(7), 409–417. https://doi.org/10.1080/13607863.2014.944091.

de Jong Gierveld, J., & Tesch-Römer, C. (2012). Loneliness in old age in Eastern and Western European societies: theoretical perspectives. *European Journal of Ageing, 9*(4), 285–295. https://doi.org/10.1007/s10433-012-0248-2.

de Jong Gierveld, J., van Tilburg, T. G., & Dykstra, P. A. (2006). Loneliness and social isolation. In A. Vangelisti & D. Perlman (Eds.), *Cambridge handbook of personal relationships*. Cambridge: Cambridge University Press.

Donovan, N. J., Wu, Q., Rentz, D. M., Sperling, R. A., Marshall, G. A., & Glymour, M. M. (2017). Loneliness, depression and cognitive function in older US adults. *International Journal of Geriatric Psychiatry, 32*(5), 564–573. https://doi.org/10.1002/gps.4495.

Dykstra, P. A., van Tilburg, T. G., & de Jong Gierveld, J. (2005). Changes in older adult loneliness: Results from a seven-year longitudinal study. *Research on Aging, 27*(6), 725–747. https://doi.org/10.1177/0164027505279712.

Eurostat. (2018). *Glossary: Material deprivation*. https://ec.europa.eu/eurostat/statistics-explained/index.php/Glossary:Material_deprivation.

Fokkema, T., Gierveld, J. D., & Dykstra, P. A. (2012). Cross-national differences in older adult loneliness. *Journal of Psychology, 146*(1–2), 201–228. https://doi.org/10.1080/00223980.2011.631612.

Franzese, F. (2015). Slipping into poverty: effects on mental and physical health. In A. Börsch-Supan, T. Kneip, H. Litwin, M. Myck, & G. Weber (Eds.), *Ageing in Europe: Supporting policies for an inclusive society* (pp. 139–148). Berlin: De Gruyter.

Gibney, S., Moore, T., & Shannon, S. (2019). Loneliness in later life: a cross-sectional survey analysis of place-based factors in Ireland. *Quality in Ageing and Older Adults, 20*(2), 80–96. https://doi.org/10.1108/qaoa-04-2018-0015.

Hansen, T., & Slagsvold, B. (2015). Late-life loneliness in 11 European countries: results from the generations and gender survey. *Social Indicators Research, 124*(1), 1–20.

Haushofer, J. (2013). *The Psychology of Poverty: Evidence from 43 Countries*. Cambridge, MA: Massachusetts Institute of Technology.

Hawkley, L. C., & Kocherginsky, M. (2017). Transitions in loneliness among older adults: A 5-year follow-up in the National Social Life, Health, and Aging Project. *Research on Aging*, Published online ahead of print 17 March 2017. https://doi.org/10.1177/0164027517698965.

Holt-Lunstad, J., Smith, T. B., Baker, M., Harris, T., & Stephenson, D. (2015). Loneliness and social isolation as risk factors for mortality: A meta-analytic review. *Perspectives on Psychological Science, 10*(2), 227–237. https://doi.org/10.1177/1745691614568352.

Lyberaki, A., & Tinios, P. (2008). Poverty and Persistent Poverty: Adding Dynamics to Familiar Findings. In A. Börsch-Supan et al. (Eds.), *Health, Ageing and Retirement in Europe (2004–2007). Starting the Longitudinal Dimension*. Mannheim: Mannheim Research Institute for the Economics of Aging.

Myck, M., Najsztub, M., & Oczkowska, M. (2015). Measuring social deprivation and social exclusion. In A. Börsch-Supan, T. Kneip, H. Litwin, M. Myck, & G. Weber (Eds.), *Ageing in Europe. Supporting policies for an inclusive society* (pp. 67–78). Berlin: De Gruyter.

Myck, M., Oczkowska, M., & Najsztub, M. (2019). Implications of social and material deprivation for changes in health of older people *Journal of Aging and Health*, (January), 1–25.

Niedzwiedz, C. L., Richardson, E. A., Tunstall, H., Shortt, N. K., Mitchell, R. J., & Pearce, J. R. (2016). The relationship between wealth and loneliness among older people across Europe: Is social participation protective? *Preventive Medicine, 91*, 24–31. https://doi.org/10.1016/j.ypmed.2016.07.016.

Nyqvist, F., Nygard, M., & Scharf, T. (2019). Loneliness amongst older people in Europe: a comparative study of welfare regimes. *European Journal of Ageing, 16*(2), 133–143. https://doi.org/10.1007/s10433-018-0487-y.

Pikhartova, J., Bowling, A., & Victor, C. (2016). Is loneliness in later life a self-fulfilling prophecy? *Aging & Mental Health, 20*(5), 543–549. https://doi.org/10.1080/13607863.2015.1023767.

Public Health England. (2017). *Commissioning cost-effective services for promotion of mental health and wellbeing and prevention of mental ill-health*. London: PHE Publications.

Scharf, T., & de Jong Gierveld, J. (2008). Loneliness in urban neighbourhoods: an Anglo-Dutch comparison. *European Journal of Ageing, 5*(2), 103–115. https://doi.org/10.1007/s10433-008-0080-x.

Scharf, T., Phillipson, C., & Smith, A. E. (2005). Social exclusion of older people in deprived urban communities of England. *European Journal of Ageing, 2*(2), 76–87. https://doi.org/10.1007/s10433-005-0025-6.

Tesch-Römer, C., & Huxhold, O. (2019). Social Isolation and Loneliness in Old Age. *Oxford Research Encyclopedias. Subject: Developmental Psychology*. https://oxfordre.com/psychology/view/10.1093/acrefore/9780190236557.001.0001/acrefore-9780190236557-e-393#acrefore-9780190236557-e-393-div1-2.

Tinios, P., Lyberaki, A., & Georgiadis, T. (2011). Explaining Persistent Poverty in SHARE: Does the Past Play a Role? In A. Börsch-Supan et al. (Eds.), *The Individual and the Welfare State* (pp. 19–29). Berlin\Heidelberg: Springer.

Warner, D. F., & Adams, S. A. (2016). Physical disability and increased loneliness among married older adults: The role of changing social relations. *Society and Mental Health, 6*(2), 106–128. https://doi.org/10.1177/2156869315616257.

Chapter 25
Beyond Accessibility: Transport Systems as a Societal Structure Supporting Inclusion in Late-Life

Anu Siren

25.1 Introduction

In their review, Walsh et al. (2017) identify transport mobility as an area in which older adults can experience social exclusion. However, transport is a cross-cutting mechanism in social exclusion: while it is interrelated with economic exclusion, it also constitutes an important element in community and spatial exclusion, as well as in exclusion from social relations, services [see Draulins and Lamura, and Cholat and Dacanto this volume] and civic participation. Thus, transport both allows people to access the destinations and services they want or need and helps them maintain social relations, participate in society, and maintain their sense of citizenship and belonging in their community (Davey 2007; Musselwhite 2018).

In this chapter, I advance the idea of a transport system as part of the societal structures that construct and shape mobility opportunities and barriers, and, in turn, social inclusion or exclusion. I argue that a transport system is a societal structure that can support good ageing and the social inclusion of older adults, and that some major problems in, and barriers to, transport mobility for older adults are the consequences of ageist or otherwise non-age-acknowledging policies and priorities.

This chapter begins with an overview of the relation between transport mobility and well-being in late-life. Next, I discuss transport as a societal structure affecting late-life inclusion and analyse the mismatch between current structures and actual needs. Finally, I discuss the interconnections between transport and other domains of social inclusion/exclusion.

A. Siren (✉)
The Danish Center for Social Science Research, Copenhagen, Denmark
e-mail: anu@vive.dk

K. Walsh et al. (eds.), *Social Exclusion in Later Life*, International Perspectives on Aging 28, https://doi.org/10.1007/978-3-030-51406-8_25

25.2 Transport Mobility and Well-Being in Late-Life

Transport mobility is an important part of older individuals' well-being. Early scholarship has defined an individual's ability to manage transportation as one of the main areas in instrumental activities of daily living (Lawton and Brody 1969), and research has shown that the ability to leave the home and independently move about are among the essential aspects of well-being in late-life (Farquhar 1995). Research has also found that mobility loss in late-life causes depression and feelings of social isolation (*e.g.* Fonda et al. 2001; Qin et al. 2019).

Mobility is a highly appreciated value in our society, partly because it enables people to engage in social relations and obtain a feeling of proximity (Urry 2002), and partly because it enables people to access the necessities of contemporary life, *e.g.* work, shopping and leisure activities. Mobility and travel greatly regulate inclusion and exclusion in terms of social interaction, out-of-home activities and experiences, and civic power.

Nevertheless, mobility carries more than merely instrumental value and entails more than the necessities or preconditions for access and social encounters. Mobility plays an important part in constructing the self in social and other settings and in giving people pleasure and enjoyment (Musselwhite and Haddad 2010). Indeed, in their model of the different levels of older adults' mobility needs, Musselwhite and Haddad *(ibid.)* emphasise the affective and aesthetic needs related to travel, arguing that these needs have received only a minimum of awareness from policy makers and transport planners.

Because transport mobility in late-life entails both reaching desirable or necessary destinations or services and obtaining social connectedness, we need to extend our view beyond accessibility issues. Accessibility problems caused by barriers to transport, such as the lack of access to shopping or services, can be targeted through single-domain interventions, such as online shopping, telemedicine and care at home. However, to prevent the loss of social inclusion and citizenship (due to unmet instrumental, affective or aesthetic needs) caused by lack of transportation requires a broader understanding of transport as a social structure.

25.3 Transport as a Societal Structure

Transportation is a culturally and socially shaped dynamic system in which the users and the infrastructure are inter-related. The way that the transportation system is designed, arranged and managed reflects both our societal values and everyday life. In principle, a transport system is an arena open to all members of society, with everyone being able to arrange his or her travel in the most convenient and preferable way. According to contemporary travel models, transport is the medium needed for individuals to satisfy their travel demand (*e.g.* Axhausen and Gärling 1992). However, if transport is discerned as a space that both constructs and is constructed, one can challenge its commonly understood meaning as a mere platform for activities.

Foucault, as one of the first scholars to analyse public spaces, power relations and related meanings, has argued that constructed and built spaces hold different meanings for different users (*e.g.* Foucault 1977). In his view, a built space such as transport systems not only regulates and constructs social relations and interactions between people but also produces cultural meanings. De Certeau (1984) has analysed space both as an intersection of mobile elements and as a platform for spatial practices. He argues that the meanings of a given space are specifically constructed in the process of practicing spatial actions.

Given the constructed and constructing nature of the transport system, questions involving power, inclusion and exclusion arise. Who is to construct and design the system, and for whom? How does the system influence the lives of different groups of people? Can it, indeed, be an arena for everyone if the opportunities for influencing its construction are not equal?

Older adults' marginal position in transport policy and planning may be a consequence of the predominant focus on utilitarian travel demand in transport planning scholarship. A conventional tenet in transportation research is that travel is the manifest choice derived from an individual's activities (*e.g.* Axhausen and Gärling 1992) and that therefore the most common activities in a society are the most important for planning that society's transport system. Older adults' travel and mobility needs tend to be less utilitarian, less predictable and more discretionary. Parkhurst et al. (2014) have argued that the economy-efficiency approach – dominant in transport policy and planning – prioritises travel that creates net benefits within the formal economy (*i.e.* work- related and commercial travel). Discretionary travel, *i.e.* trips made for social purposes or for the sake of travel itself, receives lesser priority.

25.4 Transport and Social Exclusion in Late-Life

Previous studies have provided evidence on how lack of transport is a direct barrier to participation in activities and social encounters. Availability of transport has been found to regulate older adults' employment (Anderson et al. 2013), participation in education (Patterson et al. 2016), grocery shopping (Hare et al. 2001), participation in cultural and religious activities (Johnson et al. 2011; Sowa et al. 2016).

Other studies have identified factors contributing to the likelihood of having transport disadvantage that leads or adds to social exclusion in old-age. Older adults who lack a driver license, are in poorer health, are older or women, and have lower income, lower levels of mobility and higher levels of unfulfilled mobility needs (Siren and Hakamies-Blomqvist 2004). People living in rural areas have a likelihood of transport disadvantage (Higgs and White 1997), mainly because they depend solely on private car transportation (Glasgow and Blakely 2000; see also Cholat and Dacanto this volume). Nevertheless, as Engels and Liu (2011) point out, older adults in metropolitan areas with insufficient public transport can also be highly dependent on cars, leading to transport disadvantage among those with no option of driving (or of being driven by others).

In general, the lack of a driving option is problematic from a social inclusion standpoint, and particularly so in North America and Australia, where stopping driving can be associated with a significant decrease in social integration (Mezuk and Rebok 2008). Haustein and Siren (2014) have shown that older adults without a driving option experienced limited mobility, and this disparity remained even if those involved lived near public transport.

Some research has more closely analysed how transport mobility contributes to inclusion in older-age. Davey (2007) has suggested that different types of mobility have different implications for inclusion. While necessity travel, for example for health care or grocery shopping, is experienced as more "legitimate", discretionary travel for enjoyment or "leisure" is viewed as less legitimate. Consequently, older adults without personal transportation are hesitant to ask family or friends for rides for discretionary purposes.

25.5 Structural Lag and Transport

The traditional view in transport mobility research – that travel is "reasoned" behaviour (*e.g.* Bamberg et al. 2003) – emphasises individual choice as the main regulator of personal travel. From this viewpoint, all people in principle have the same choice-making opportunities: although choice-based models recognise that a number of factors influence the array of choices (*e.g.* car access, spatial context, or physical limitations), these models locate these factors in the domain of the individual. In other words, these models view limitations in the array of choices as a unique set of features for each individual, rather than features of a constructed institution—in this case, the transport system.

However, just as social studies on disability argues that disability, rather than being a biological fact, is a construct of the intersection of demands and lack of support in the environments people live in (Wendell 1996, p. 58), one can view age-related mobility problems as socially constructed through systems, policies, and priorities in the transport area. Some mobility limitations emerge only in the intersection of current structures and the needs of system users, a problem that demands a better understanding and acknowledgement of the interplay between structures and individuals. If one lays aside the conventional assumption that the mobility problems of older adults are caused solely by the effects of old-age (*e.g.* physical frailty), one might realise that they are also the outcome of a mismatch between the transportation system and the transport needs and experiences of older adults.

In 1994, Riley and her colleagues introduced the concept of "structural lag" to describe the mismatch between structures and people's capabilities, needs and aspirations, in a context of rapid social change. They argued that:

> 'While the twentieth century has experienced a revolution in human development and ageing, there has been no comparable revolution in the role structures of society to keep pace with the changes in the ways people grow up and grow old. The lag involves not only institutional and organizational arrangements, but also the many aspects of culture that, in addition to being internalised by people, are built into role expectations and societal mores and laws'. (Riley et al. 1994, p. 16–17)

The concept of structural lag is useful for investigating the area of transport and late-life. In the past 100 years, throughout the industrialised world, transport systems, mobility patterns and societal demands for mobility have changed tremendously (Siren and Sørensen 2015). Mobility and travel are essential parts of contemporary life (Urry 2002), people today travel more than ever, and mobility is deeply embedded in western culture and people's everyday lives. For older adults, the travel patterns have changed even more rapidly across time than for other groups.

Improved health conditions, active lifestyles, increased access to cars and, for some groups, higher income and education create greater possibilities and needs for more varied activities and extended travelling than for the previous generations of older adults. These expectations are especially associated with the baby boomer generation (Coughlin 2009).

Studies have demonstrated higher travel activity, driver licensing rates, car access and car use in each successive cohort of older adults (*e.g.* Newbold et al. 2005; Hjorthol et al. 2010). Older people's travel has increased in the social/leisure category in particular (Arentze et al. 2008) and for car trips in general (*e.g.* Newbold et al. 2005; Delbosc and Currie 2011).

Given the tremendous change in older adults' travel, the question arises as to whether the structures surrounding late-life mobility have adapted to the change. The answer is largely no. Transport-related structures and norms still lag behind rapidly changing late-life. While older adults are increasingly encouraged to age actively and productively by, for example extending their working lives (Walker 2002), the transport policies are not aligned with these goals. Driver licenses in many countries expire at age 55–70 years as a default and require renewal if the driver wishes to continue driving (Siren and Haustein 2015). The free or subsidised public transport entitlements for older adults are often valid only in during off-peak hours (Mackett 2014), indicating that older adults are expected to have travel needs at different times than everyone else.

Among the policies affecting older adults' mobility opportunities, the one most obviously dated is the age-related regulation of driver licenses. While for mature drivers the chronological age is only a weak predictor of safe driving performance, licensing policies based on age are widely used in most European countries and many US and Australian states (Langford et al. 2004; Dickerson et al. 2014; Siren and Haustein 2015). In their review, Siren and Haustein (2015) conclude that the policies are coercive because they require both frequent renewals and proof of driver fitness in connection with renewal. Siren and Haustein (ibid.) also note that having these types of coercive policies signal that society finds car-driving by older citizens a questionable, even suspect, activity, and they may encourage people to give up driving even when they are still fit to drive.

Rather than being evidence-based, these age limits of renewal and medical assessment are usually intuitive and set ad hoc. They are not based on any current knowledge on age or crash propensity or risk (Langford et al. 2006), nor on epidemiological knowledge on the age-related incidence of diseases influencing driving skills (*e.g.* Alzheimer's Disease International 2008). Rather, they reflect the aspirations, behaviours and capabilities of older adults in terms of the way "old-age" was viewed 50 or 60 years ago.

25.6 Adjusting the Structures to Alleviate the Lag

The World Health Organization's "age-friendly movement" (WHO 2007) has encouraged age-friendly adjustments to transportation systems, with a focus on, for example availability, affordability, age-friendly design, safety and comfort. However, perhaps because these guidelines have a global focus, they have not been implemented in wider social policies on local or national levels, especially in western industrialised societies. Moreover, as these guidelines do not directly address the societal implications of late-life mobility, they have been mostly used in isolated small-scale initiatives such as redesigning buses (Broome et al. 2013) or improving public transport service in particular communities (*e.g.* Shiau and Huang 2014).

Since 2008 older adults in Britain have been entitled to a pass enabling them to travel by bus during off-peak hours. The objectives of introducing the concessionary pass were social, aimed at improving the lives of older people by improving their access to services and increasing social inclusion. From the perspective of structural lag, the concessionary bus pass does not appear to be an active adjustment of structures to shifting demographics or emerging needs. Rather, it appears to be a social benefit compensating for the individual deficits bundled under an assumed common denominator, "old-age". Mackett (2014) argues that while bus travel among older adults has increased and that the overall impacts are positive, the bus pass is being used only by a small group of eligible users, partly due to the availability of high-quality bus services across Britain.

The private car is the safest and most convenient mode of transport for older adults (OECD 2000), and it plays an important role in their everyday mobility. Nevertheless, licensing policies tend to work against driving in late-life. Ageism, vested interests and biased conceptions of the ageing process all contribute to society's eagerness to regulate older drivers' rights to drive (O'Neill 2012). While scholars have called for more evidence-based policies (Desapriya et al. 2012; Salmi et al. 2014), no major change has yet occurred in measuring the returns on the societal investments made for these policies.

Only few countries have reviewed their policies on licensing and age in response to changing demographics and travel patterns. Sweden, which has never had age-based licensing, reviewed its policy in 2018 and the potential safety gains of implementing driver license regulations (Skyving et al. 2018). The analysis, based on all Swedish road accidents involving older adult drivers with medical conditions, showed no potential safety gains from screening for these conditions. Consequently, Sweden decided to continue without age-based regulations. Although Denmark used to have age-based policies, it decided to remove them in 2017 after a review. According to parliamentary documents (Folketinget 2017), the change was based on a review of research evidence, assessment of the costs associated with having all older drivers screened for driving fitness, the administrative burden of licensing offices (given the large cohorts of older drivers), and the financial and psychological burden on older adults having to undergo the screening. While the overall rationale was economic, based on cost-benefit analyses, additional political motives might have included the growing voting population of older voters.

In the US, seeking individual transport solutions for non-driving older adults is more common than in Europe. Independent Transport Network (ITN) America, started specifically as a response to a transportation system incapable of meeting the needs of an ageing population (Freund 2003). In many ways, the ITN concept is a non-profit predecessor of Uber, Lyft and sharing economy-based services alike. ITN provides a sharing-economy platform for (predominately volunteer and mainly mature) drivers to provide transportation services for older and visually impaired adults that no longer are able to drive themselves. Interestingly, such a bottom-up service appears to capture the need for actively adjusting structures to match changing needs better and more quickly than any public policy. While not directly transferable to transport contexts outside the US, such sharing economy- or local community-driven models might work in rural and other car-dependent areas in Europe if they were modified to the local context (see also Shergold and Parkhurst 2012).

25.7 Interconnections Between the Domains of Social Exclusion and Knowledge Gaps

As a review of the international literature shows, transport is a cross-cutting element in social exclusion and in some cases can serve as a principal driver of exclusionary experiences in late-life. Access to transportation has direct implications for economic inclusion and exclusion (*i.e.* being able to access work) and inclusion in or exclusion from social relations, services and civic participation. Economic exclusion and exclusion from social relations in turn influence transport accessibility, as personal transport requires financial or social resources or both (*e.g.* paying for transport, keeping a car, asking people for rides) [see Cholat and Dacanto for a discussion of these factors in relation to reverse mobilities].

Understanding the interconnections with the spatial dimensions of exclusion is critical, as rural areas have a more restricted palette of transport options, combined with longer distances between settled areas and service centres, and lower population density. A framework for understanding rural transport disadvantage has been suggested by Marr (2015). His main argument is that transport disadvantage is not dichotomous but rather a continuum, and that various factors, such as demographic characteristics or socio-economic status, determine the levels of disadvantage in rural areas. Similarly, Grant et al. (2010) have argued that the planning strategies for increasing transport possibilities for older adults need to go beyond mere density. They found that the walking behaviour among older adults was not solely influenced by physical design; rather, an interconnection existed between physical walkability and neighbourhood socio-economic characteristics.

Because of the intersecting domains of exclusion, Audirac (2008) argues that (spatial) planning has the potential to reduce several types of old-age related social exclusion. However, to fully integrate the various domains related to social exclusion, we need to look beyond accessibility and the instrumental value of transport. As this chapter has demonstrated, a transport system is not merely a travel platform derived from individual choices. The priorities that shape the transport system and guide planning, design and policies are based on culturally and socially shaped ideas within a society.

We thus need to take a closer look at the goals and priorities in transport, analysing not only the origins of these ideas but also their implications for different demographic groups. Do initiatives for greener transport favour some groups at the cost of others? Does an efficient transport system mainly serve the needs of those belonging to the formal economy? We also need to ask whether we should view transport systems as a societal welfare structure, aimed at producing benefits beyond the transport sector or formal economy. If transport is understood in this way, planning may become a tool for reducing social exclusion – but only if the stated goals are set beyond accessibility, to include wider social inclusion, belonging and civic participation.

25.8 Conclusion

The current framing of transport-related social exclusion predominantly takes place within the planning of transport services and physical environments. While planning for accessibility is important, the lack of a broader conceptual understanding of transport-related social exclusion is clear, and the gerontological scholarship and wider understanding of social exclusion more generally is scarce. To fully understand the role of transport in late-life social exclusion, we must go beyond the transport system and view transport-related social exclusion as a societal issue, because various domains (*e.g.* social participation) are interrelated with transport. We need also to look beyond mere designs and services to focus on structures, including ageist legislation that causes transport-related exclusion, such as coercive and ageist driver licensing policies.

Mobility has great impacts on people's lives, with quantifiable gains from late-life mobility, in terms of psychological, physical and community benefits (Spinney et al. 2009). Sadly, transport deficits are often viewed simply as an outcome of exclusion from specific services. In this chapter, I have demonstrated the multidimensionality of transport-related exclusion and transport's interrelations with other domains of exclusion. Policymakers and scholars alike need to acknowledge these cross-sectoral benefits and relations, and to consider the role of transport systems beyond the mere equipment for and logistics of transporting people and goods.

Editors' Postscript

Please note, like other contributions to this book, this chapter was written before the COVID-19 pandemic of 2020. The book's introductory chapter (Chap. 1) and conclusion (Chap. 34) consider some of the key ways in which the pandemic relates to issues concerning social exclusion and ageing.

References

Alzheimer's Disease International. (2008).*The prevalence of dementia worldwide*. http://www.alz.co.uk/adi/pdf/prevalence.pdf.

Anderson, K. A., Richardson, V. E., Fields, N. L., & Harootyan, R. A. (2013). Inclusion or exclusion? Exploring barriers to employment for low-income older adults. *Journal of Gerontological Social Work, 56*(4), 318–334. https://doi.org/10.1080/01634372.2013.777006.

Arentze, T., Timmermans, H., Jorritsma, P., Olde Kalter, M.-J., & Schoemakers, A. (2008). More grey hair—But for whom? Scenario-based simulations of elderly activity travel patterns in 2020. *Transportation, 35*(5), 613–627. https://doi.org/10.1007/s11116-008-9170-z.

Audirac, I. (2008). Accessing transit as universal design. *Journal of Planning Literature, 23*(1), 4–16.

Axhausen, K. W., & Gärling, T. (1992). Activity-based approaches to travel analysis: Conceptual frameworks, models, and research problems. *Transport Reviews, 12*(4), 323–341. https://doi.org/10.1080/01441649208716826.

Bamberg, S., Ajzen, I., & Schmidt, P. (2003). Choice of travel mode in the theory of planned behavior: The roles of past behavior, habit, and reasoned action. *Basic and Applied Social Psychology, 25*(3), 175–187. https://doi.org/10.1207/S15324834BASP2503_01.

Broome, K., Worrall, L., Fleming, J., & Boldy, D. (2013). Evaluation of age-friendly guidelines for public buses. *Transportation Research Part A: Policy and Practice, 53*, 68–80. https://doi.org/10.1016/j.tra.2013.05.003.

Coughlin, J. F. (2009). Longevity, lifestyle, and anticipating the new demands of aging on the transportation system. *Public Works Management & Policy, 13*(4), 301–311. https://doi.org/10.1177/1087724X09335609.

Davey, J. A. (2007). Older people and transport: Coping without a car. *Ageing and Society, 27*(1), 49–65. https://doi.org/10.1017/S0144686X06005332.

De Certeau, M. (1984). *Practice of everyday life*. Berkeley: University of California Press.

Delbosc, A., & Currie, G. (2011). Transport problems that matter – Social and psychological links to transport disadvantage. *Journal of Transport Geography, 19*(1), 170–178. https://doi.org/10.1016/j.jtrangeo.2010.01.003.

Desapriya, E., Ranatunga, Y., & Pike, I. (2012). We need evidence based tools to identify medically at risk drivers. *BMJ, 345*, e7087–e7087. https://doi.org/10.1136/bmj.e7087.

Dickerson, A. E., Meuel, D. B., Ridenour, C. D., & Cooper, K. (2014). Assessment tools predicting fitness to drive in older adults: A systematic review. *American Journal of Occupational Therapy, 68*(6), 670–680. https://doi.org/10.5014/ajot.2014.011833.

Engels, B., & Liu, G.-J. (2011). Social exclusion, location and transport disadvantage amongst non-driving seniors in a Melbourne municipality, Australia. *Journal of Transport Geography, 19*(4), 984–996. https://doi.org/10.1016/j.jtrangeo.2011.03.007.

Farquhar, M. (1995). Elderly people's definitions of quality of life. *Social Science & Medicine, 41*(10), 1439–1446. https://doi.org/10.1016/0277-9536(95)00117-P.

Folketinget. (2017). *L 201 Forslag til lov om ændring af færdselsloven*. Copenhagen: Folketinget.

Fonda, S. J., Wallace, R. B., & Herzog, A. R. (2001). Changes in driving patterns and worsening depressive symptoms among older adults. *The Journals of Gerontology Series B: Psychological Sciences and Social Sciences, 56*(6), S343–S351.

Foucault, M. (1977). *Discipline & Punish: The birth of the prison*. London: Penguin Books.

Freund, K. (2003). Independent transportation network: The next best thing to driving. *Generations, 27*(2), 70–71.

Glasgow, N., & Blakely, R. M. (2000). Older nonmetropolitan residents' evaluations of their transportation arrangements. *Journal of Applied Gerontology, 19*(1), 95.

Grant, T. L., Edwards, N., Sveistrup, H., Andrew, C., & Egan, M. (2010). Inequitable walking conditions among older people: Examining the interrelationship of neighbourhood socioeconomic status and urban form using a comparative case study. *BMC Public Health, 10*, 677–692. https://doi.org/10.1186/1471-2458-10-677.

Hare, C., Kirk, D., & Lang, T. (2001). The food shopping experience of older consumers in Scotland: Critical incidents. *International Journal of Retail & Distribution Management, 29*(1), 25. https://doi.org/10.1108/09590550110366343.

Haustein, S., & Siren, A. (2014). Seniors' unmet mobility needs - how important is a driving licence? *Journal of Transport Geography, 41*, 45–52. https://doi.org/10.1016/j.jtrangeo.2014.08.001.

Higgs, G., & White, S. D. (1997). Changes in service provision in rural areas. Part 1: The use of GIS in analyzing accessibility to services in rural deprivation research. *Journal of Rural Studies, 13*(4), 441.

Hjorthol, R. J., Levin, L., & Siren, A. (2010). Mobility in different generations of older persons. The development of daily travel in different cohorts in Denmark, Norway and Sweden. *Journal of Transport Geography, 18*(5), 624–633.

Johnson, V., Currie, G., & Stanley, J. (2011). Exploring transport to arts and cultural activities as a facilitator of social inclusion. *Transport Policy, 18*(1), 68–75. https://doi.org/10.1016/j.tranpol.2010.06.001.

Langford, J., Fitzharris, M., Newstead, S., & Koppel, S. (2004). Some consequences of different older driver licensing procedures in Australia. *Accident Analysis & Prevention, 36*(6), 993–1001. https://doi.org/10.1016/j.aap.2003.11.003.

Langford, J., Methorst, R., & Hakamies-Blomqvist, L. (2006). Older drivers do not have a high crash risk – A replication of low mileage bias. *Accident Analysis and Prevention, 38*(3), 574–578.

Lawton, M. P., & Brody, E. M. (1969). Assessment of older people: Self-maintaining and instrumental activities of daily living. *The Gerontologist, 9*(3 Part 1), 179–186. https://doi.org/10.1093/geront/9.3_Part_1.179.

Mackett, R. (2014). Has the policy of concessionary bus travel for older people in Britain been successful? *Case Studies on Transport Policy, 2*(2), 81–88. https://doi.org/10.1016/j.cstp.2014.05.001.

Marr, E. (2015). Assessing transportation disadvantage in rural Ontario, Canada: A case study of Huron County. *Journal of Rural & Community Development, 10*(2), 100–120.

Mezuk, B., & Rebok, G. W. (2008). Social integration and social support among older adults following driving cessation. *Journals of Gerontology Series B: Psychological Sciences & Social Sciences, 63B*(5), S298–S303.

Musselwhite, C. (2018). Community connections and Independence in later life. In E. Peel, C. Holland, & M. Murray (Eds.), *Psychologies of ageing* (pp. 221–252). Cham: Palgrave Macmillan Ltd.

Musselwhite, C., & Haddad, H. (2010). Mobility, accessibility and quality of later life. *Quality in Ageing and Older Adults, 11*(1), 25–37. https://doi.org/10.5042/qiaoa.2010.0153.

Newbold, K. B., Scott, D. M., Spinney, J. E. L., Kanaroglou, P., & Páez, A. (2005). Travel behavior within Canada's older population: A cohort analysis. *Journal of Transport Geography, 13*(4), 340–351. https://doi.org/10.1016/j.jtrangeo.2004.07.007.

O'Neill, D. (2012). More mad and more wise. *Accident Analysis & Prevention, 49*, 263–265. https://doi.org/10.1016/j.aap.2012.01.010.

OECD. (2000). *Transport and ageing of the population*. Paris: Organization for Economic Cooperation & Development.

Parkhurst, G., Galvin, K., Musselwhite, C., Phillips, J., Shergold, I., & Todres, L. (2014). Beyond transport: Understanding the role of mobilities in connecting rural elders in civic society. In C. Hennesey, R. Means, & V. Burholt (Eds.), *Countryside connections: Older people, community and place in rural Britain* (pp. 125–157). Bristol: Policy Press.

Patterson, R., Moffatt, S., Smith, M., Scott, J., Mcloughlin, C., Bell, J., & Bell, N. (2016). Exploring social inclusivity within the University of the Third age (U3A): A model of collaborative research. *Ageing & Society, 36*(8), 1580–1603. https://doi.org/10.1017/S0144686X15000550.

Qin, W., Xiang, X., & Taylor, H. (2019). Driving cessation and social isolation in older adults. *Journal of Aging and Health*, 1–19. https://doi.org/10.1177/0898264319870400.

Riley, M. W., Kahn, R. L., & Foner, A. (1994). *Age and structural lag*. New York: Wiley.

Salmi, L. R., Leproust, S., Helmer, C., & Lagarde, E. (2014). Assessing fitness to drive in the elderly and those with medical conditions: Guidelines should specify methods and evidence. *Injury Prevention, 20*(3), 210–212. https://doi.org/10.1136/injuryprev-2013-040972.

Shergold, I., & Parkhurst, G. (2012). Transport-related social exclusion amongst older people in rural Southwest England and Wales. *Journal of Rural Studies, 28*(4), 412–421. https://doi.org/10.1016/j.jrurstud.2012.01.010.

Shiau, T. A., & Huang, W. K. (2014). User perspective of age-friendly transportation: A case study of Taipei City. *Transport Policy, 36*, 184–191. https://doi.org/10.1016/j.tranpol.2014.08.010.

Siren, A., & Hakamies-Blomqvist, L. (2004). Private car as the grand equaliser? Demographic factors and mobility in Finnish men and women aged 65+. *Transportation Research Part F: Traffic Psychology and Behaviour, 7*(2), 107–118.

Siren, A., & Haustein, S. (2015). Driving licences and medical screening in old age: Review of literature and European licensing policies. *Journal of Transport and Health, 2*(1), 68–78. https://doi.org/10.1016/j.jth.2014.09.003.

Siren, A., & Sørensen, C. H. (2015). Immense changes in traffic – Considerable stability in discourses: Road speed in Danish parliamentary documents 1900-2010. *Transport Policy, 40*, 1–7. https://doi.org/10.1016/j.tranpol.2015.02.005.

Skyving, M., Forsman, Å., & Dukic Willstrand, T. (2018). *Samband mellan sjukdomar och äldre bilförares inblandning i trafikolyckor*. Stockholm: Transportstyrelsen.

Sowa, A., Golinowska, S., Deeg, D., Principi, A., Casanova, G., Schulmann, K., Ilinca, S., Rodrigues, R., Moreira, A., & Gelenkamp, H. (2016). Predictors of religious participation of older Europeans in good and poor health. *European Journal of Ageing, 13*(2), 145–157. https://doi.org/10.1007/s10433-016-0367-2.

Spinney, J. E. L., Scott, D. M., & Newbold, K. B. (2009). Transport mobility benefits and quality of life: A time-use perspective of elderly Canadians. *Transport Policy, 16*(1), 1–11. https://doi.org/10.1016/j.tranpol.2009.01.002.

Urry, J. (2002). Mobility and proximity. *Sociology, 36*(2), 255–274. https://doi.org/10.1177/0038038502036002002.

Walker, A. (2002). A strategy for active ageing. *International Social Security Review, 55*(1), 121–139.

Walsh, K., Scharf, T., & Keating, N. (2017). Social exclusion of older persons: A scoping review and conceptual framework. *European Journal of Ageing, 14*(1), 81–98. https://doi.org/10.1007/s10433-016-0398-8.

Wendell, S. (1996). *The rejected body: Feminist philosophical reflections on disability*. New York: Routledge/Taylor & Francis Group.

WHO. (2007). *Global age-friendly cities: A guide*. Geneva: WHO.

Chapter 26
Homelessness Trends in Ageing Literature in the Context of Domains of Social Exclusion

Nilufer Korkmaz-Yaylagul and Ahmet Melik Bas

26.1 Introduction

Homelessness is a contemporary phenomenon that has emerged in all modern societies, due to individual and structural factors regardless of the level of a nation's wealth. Homeless individuals are described as people sleeping on the streets, in temporary shelters and those who live in precarious housing (Crane and Warnes 1997; Craig and Timms 2000; Zufferey and Kerr 2004). Several different terms such as "homeless" "rough sleepers" and "street people" are used in the literature. As such, the diversity of the terms used can be problematic when defining the focus and scope of research and indeed participant selection on the topic. Independent of the definition used, homelessness creates disadvantages such as poverty, exclusion, victimisation, abuse, susceptibility to diseases and an inability to access services. Homeless people are not homogenous, they may have different features, different backgrounds and distinct needs. Age is an important factor affecting the needs and conditions of homeless groups. Older homeless, as a part of a new ageing population, are increasing in number and facing more disadvantages compared to other age groups experiencing homelessness. Recent restrictions in social welfare policies, increasing poverty rates and lack of appropriate housing supply have made homelessness more visible amongst older people, which in turn has resulted in an increase in research on homelessness in later life (Warnes and Crane 2000; Anderson 2003; Woolrych et al. 2015).

Grenier et al. (2016a) revealed in their literature review that homelessness is defined in the literature as encompassing three different groups. First, transitional

N. Korkmaz-Yaylagul (✉)
Faculty of Health Sciences, Department of Gerontology, Akdeniz University, Antalya, Turkey
e-mail: niluferyaylagul@akdeniz.edu.tr

A. M. Bas
Chiba University, Chiba, Japan

K. Walsh et al. (eds.), *Social Exclusion in Later Life*, International Perspectives on Aging 28, https://doi.org/10.1007/978-3-030-51406-8_26

homeless are individuals who live in shelters for less than 1 month. This group consists of younger individuals with less physical and mental health, and addiction problems compared to other homeless groups. Second, episodically homeless are mainly young individuals with high levels of mental and physical health, and addiction problems. This group use shelters periodically and often end up staying in hospitals, prisons, detoxification centres and on the streets. Third, chronically homeless are often older individuals who need shelter for longer periods, and who have more disabilities compared to other groups. The possibilities to turn back to work or find a new job is more difficult compared to younger individuals, with unemployment significantly contributing to the higher proportion of older adults (those 50 years and over) chronically homeless (Caton et al. 2005; Grenier et al. 2016b).

Alcohol and drug addiction, mental health problems, family conflicts, domestic violence, street culture, prostitution, imprisonment, begging, street-level drug dealing are among the extensive list of risk factors for homelessness in later life (Bowpitt et al. 2011; Fitzpatrick et al. 2013). Individuals might lose their social, physical and mental well-being as a result of the vicious cycle of deteriorating life conditions. Inability for self-help and seeking help, might increase problems cumulatively and might result in the deterioration of family relations, health and self-care permanently (Wolch et al. 1988; Rothwell et al. 2017). Besides the onset of traumatic circumstances, such as war and natural disasters, significant life changes such as loss of work and bereavement might also result in homelessness (Crane et al. 2005). However, all older individuals facing such risks do not necessarily end up as being homeless.

Older homeless adults are not a homogenous group. Fitzpatrick et al. (2011) proposed homelessness as a multidimensional form of exclusion. However, research assessing the extent of evidence linking homelessness in later life to the multidimensionality of old-age exclusion is scarce, if not non-existent. To uncover this connection, it is necessary to present how social exclusion, as a multidimensional concept, and homelessness in later life are connected in the international scientific literature. This research aims to reveal the intensity of the intersectional patterns of multidimensionality of old-age exclusion and homelessness in the ageing literature and to visualise these cross-sectional patterns, which can point to the possible interrelationships between different forms of disadvantage for older homeless adults.

We will begin by reviewing the general literature on older adult homelessness, including key determinants and risk factors, and will present an overview of the representation of social exclusion in research on homelessness. We will then outline our methodological approach to reviewing the literature. This is followed by a presentation of our analysis of exclusion and homelessness in the ageing literature.

26.2 Homelessness in Older-Age and Multidimensional Social Exclusion

Homelessness in old-age first began to emerge as a research topic in the 1980s with the changes in social welfare policies, and the scientific interest in homelessness in later life has been growing since. One strand of literature focused on the impact of rough living conditions associated with homelessness on the ageing process. Some researchers draw attention to higher prevalence of chronic diseases and disabilities among older homeless adults as well as to lower opportunities of re-entering the labour force (Cohen et al. 1988; Crane et al. 2005; Shinn et al. 2007). Another strand of literature focuses on earlier experiences of older homeless adults. Researchers reveal that older homeless individuals can sometimes possess devastating childhood experiences, addictions or mental health problems (Susser et al. 1993; Herman et al. 1997; Caton et al. 2000). Susser et al. (1993) assert the cumulative risk factors at different stages of life in relation to homelessness in old-age. Research shows that a lower education profile, a history of imprisonment, poverty and violence at younger age adds to traumatic life transitions and increases the possibility of being homeless in later life (Metraux and Culhane 2006; Grenier et al. 2016b). Moreover, life transitions in older-age such as widowhood, loss of next of kin, divorce, loss of work and poverty were also highlighted as factors specific for older homelessness (Crane and Warnes 1997; Cohen 1999; Norman and Pauly 2013).

The older homeless population are particularly of interest due to the complexity and distinctiveness of their needs. The need for proper nutrition and care increases with older-age, as well as the need for adequate and safe residential conditions (Johnson and McCool 2003; Abbott and Sapsford 2005). Older homeless adults, especially older women and transgender individuals, are also more likely to be prone to being victims of crime (Cohen et al. 1992; Salem et al. 2014; Grenier et al. 2016b). While older homeless individuals are more vulnerable to diseases, health services are difficult to access for this group. Therefore, health care needs of older homeless adults are often not sufficiently addressed (Power and Hunter 2001). This is compounded by their reluctance to request or access services and other benefits (Watson et al. 2016). Older homeless adults are reluctant to stay in shelters because of crowd, noise and fear of violence. Warnes and Crane (2000) highlights that even though the services targeting older homeless have been improved in the US and Australia since 1980s, older homeless individuals as a distinct group are not widely acknowledged in policy and practice. Factors suggested to be driving this lack of awareness include the priority often given to younger homeless populations and the deficiencies in the reporting of homelessness in later life.

Researchers have increasingly looked to adopt social exclusion as a concept in homelessness research (Kennett 1999; Anderson 2003). Social exclusion and homelessness can be considered mutually nurtured. Social exclusion is described as the deficiency of accessing different resources such as financial resources, services, social relations, and participation in society, causing inequality. Exclusion from each of these resources constitute social exclusion as a multidimensional process.

According to Horsell (2006), social exclusion occurs in three processes: disadvantages related to social, economic and political conditions; the process of disadvantage; and the outcome of processes of marginalisation. Social and economic struggles might cause homelessness; during homelessness support systems and resources may diminish; and lastly individuals may become prone to marginalisation and stigmatisation (Norman and Pauly 2013).

26.3 Method

The main question that the research targets to address gaps concerning the connections between social exclusion and homelessness is: How are old-age exclusion domains represented in the older homelessness literature?

The first step of the research involved determining the sample selection criteria. The main inclusion/exclusion criteria were: peer-review articles in geriatrics and gerontology journals published in English: articles focused on older adults (50 years and over); articles focused on homelessness. Research posters, research reports and grey literature were excluded. All gerontology and geriatrics journals were searched for this material. The SCImago Journal & Country Rank portal enables access to all journals relevant to geriatrics and gerontology. In total, 105 journals were extracted, however, 10 were excluded as they were non-English journals. The key words: "homeless", "street people", and "rough sleepers" were used for the title review. Out of the 95 journals, 59 articles (across 25 journals) were found to be relevant to homelessness in old-age. Accordingly, these 59 articles were adopted as the final research sample. The review was carried out from September 2018 to August 2019.

The structured review process consists of two phases; a summative content analysis (SCA) and a social network analysis (SNA). SCA is a form of qualitative analysis that helps to quantify keywords to comprehend the focus of the content (Hsieh and Shannon 2005). In the research, SCA is employed to identify how intensely articles on homelessness concentrate on the domains of social exclusion. In contrast, SNA is an interdisciplinary method to analyse a wide range of subjects such as kinship structures, science citations, and contacts among members (Scott 1988). In this chapter, SNA is used to reveal the patterns and trends of the dataset between articles and social exclusion domains. To provide an example: while article A might have keywords under *neighbourhood and community* and *social relations* domains, article B might have keywords under all domains. SNA enables the visualisation of multiple relations of multiple factors concurrently. SNA also assists the development of a network visualization to simplify the complexity of links between social exclusion domains and the networks of different articles constituting the research sample in this research. The reason why this chapter has adopted SCA and SNA is that classical review techniques would not fully facilitate the sort of elaboration on interconnections and relationships that can be ascertained and visualised using these methods.

Old-age exclusion has a multidimensional nature including multiple domains. Therefore, social exclusion domains must be determined in order to reveal social exclusion patterns in the homelessness literature. Walsh et al. (2017) classify the

Table 26.1 Domain specific key words

Domains of old-age exclusion	Key words
Neighbourhood and community	Neighbourhood, community, place, crime, safety, social cohesion
Social relations	Social relations, social connections, social resources, social network, loneliness, isolation
Services, amenities, and mobility	Service(s), utilities, utilisation, transport, mobility
Material and financial resources	Poverty, low income, deprivation, material resources, financial resources
Socio-cultural aspects of society	Burden, image, attitudes, symbolic, identity, cultural, ageism
Civic participation	Civic, voting, volunteer, responsibility, political, participation

Source: Walsh et al. (2017)

exclusion domains as: (1) *neighbourhood and community*; (2) *social relations*; (3) *services, amenities, and mobility*; (4) *material and financial resources*; (5) *socio-cultural aspects of society*, and (6) *civic participation*. Each domain is represented by domain-specific words (see Table 26.1). Those keywords determined by Walsh et al. (2017) have been used for the summative content analysis in this research. Frequencies of domain specific key words were counted for each domain, and the intensity of each domain was extracted for multidimensionality, using a data-charting form created in Microsoft Excel.

Data was imported into Gephi – the Yifan Hu Proportional algorithm for visualisation. Data visualization depicted the intensity to which articles address the social exclusion domains.

26.3.1 Limitations

The research sample consists of gerontology and geriatrics journals published in English only. Related articles in journals outside of this field, books and research reports, and journals published in other languages were excluded.

26.4 Findings

26.4.1 Sample Characteristics

Out of the 59 articles identified from 25 journals, *The Gerontologist* (n = 15) was the dominant publication source. Articles were published on this topic from 1961–2019. Yet, no article was published between 1961 and 1983. Assuming Lovald's review

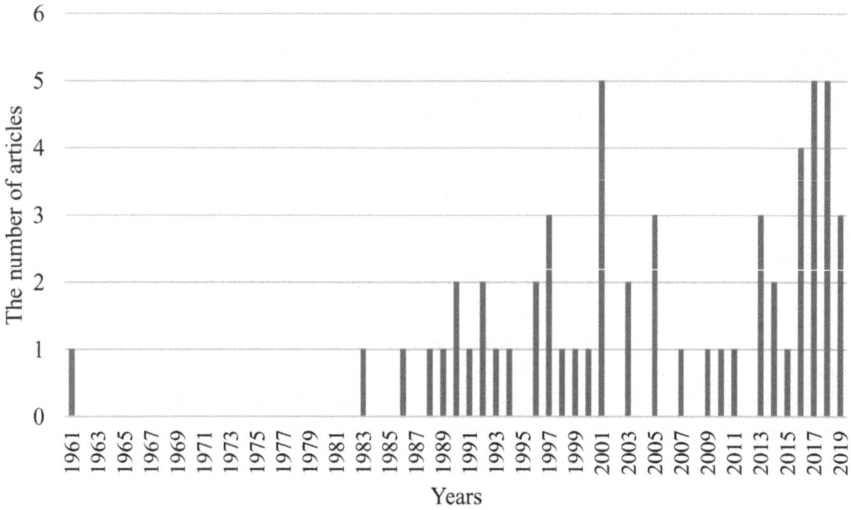

Fig. 26.1 Distribution of articles by years

(1961) was an exception, it would not be wrong to say that homelessness became a research interest in parallel with the emergence of restrictions in housing and social policies and global demographic ageing patterns during the 1980s (Grenier et al. 2016a) and this trend was accelerated in 2000s due to a rising interest in global ageing (Fig. 26.1).

Factors causing homelessness and the concept of homelessness was discussed the most (n = 16) in old-age homelessness research. Reflecting the range of risk factors associated with homelessness, and the ambiguity surrounding the concept itself, it is not surprising that these topics were most evident within the reviewed literature.

Homelessness and health was the second most common theme (n = 15), and is likely to be due to the higher incidence of diseases in older-age for homeless individuals. The remaining papers comprised topics related to services for homelessness such as health care and meal provision (n = 11), shelters such as emergency and temporary housing (n = 9) and coping strategies and planning for special needs (n = 4). The least discussed subjects were mortality, addictions, socio-cultural aspects and nutrition, with only one article on each of these subjects.

26.4.2 Old-Age Exclusion Domains in Homelessness Literature

Summative content analysis was conducted to reveal the connections of old-age exclusion domains in the sample. Domain specific keywords constituting each domain have been counted for all 59 articles and the total number of domain specific

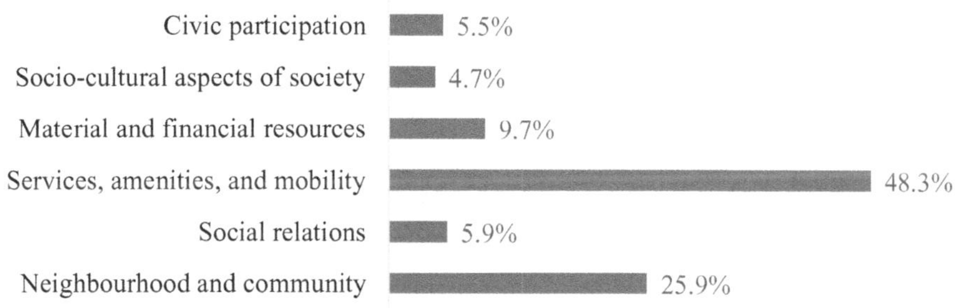

Fig. 26.2 Distribution of domains of old-age exclusion

key words was found to be n = 2685. Approximately half of the articles about homelessness in the gerontology and geriatrics literature referred to the services, amenities and mobility domains of social exclusion and about a quarter referred to the neighbourhood and community domains. Social relations, material and financial resources, socio-cultural aspects of society, and civic participation domains comprised the remaining quarter (see, Fig. 26.2).

The domain specific keywords of all six old-age exclusion domains were counted separately, after revealing the distribution of domains of old-age exclusion. "Service", was the most frequent identified domain specific keyword (n = 1085; 40.4%). Followed by community (n = 366; 13.6%), place (n = 177; 6.6%), utilisation (n = 111; 4.1%), poverty (n = 108; 4.1%), financial resources (n = 87; 3.2%); isolation (n = 70; 2.6%), neighbourhood (n = 57; 2.2%), and social network (n = 45; 2%). The remaining 27 keywords were present in less than 2 per cent, of articles. The least repeated words were the ones representing the socio-cultural aspects of social exclusion.

26.5 Multidimensionality

In order to determine multidimensionality, two categories were established; related and unrelated. In the absence of domain specific keywords, the article was coded as unrelated. On the other hand, if one or more domain specific keywords existed in the article, it was coded as related. Domain specific keywords in all the articles were counted for all the domains separately and all were found to be related to one or more old-age exclusion domains. Eleven articles (18.6%) were found to be related to all six domains. Twenty (33.9%) were related to five domains, sixteen (27.1%) to four domains, ten (16.9%) to three domains. None of the articles were relevant to two domains and only two (3.4%) were relevant to one domain. Almost all articles (n = 58; 98.3%) were related to *services, amenities, and mobility*. Fifty-six articles (94.9%) were linked to *neighbourhood and community*, 50 articles (84.7%) were related to *material and financial resources*, 37 articles (62.7%) were related to

Table 26.2 Multidimensional nature of old-age exclusion in homelessness literature

	Neighbourhood and Community		Social relations		Services, amenities, and mobility		Material and financial resources		Socio-cultural aspects of society		Civic participation	
	n	%	n	%	n	%	n	%	n	%	n	%
Multidimensionality (n = 59)	56	94,9	37	62,7	58	98,3	50	84,7	33	55,9	28	47,4

social relations, 33 articles (55.9%) were related to *socio-cultural aspects of society* and 28 articles (47.4%) were related to *civic participation* (see, Table. 26.2).

Services, amenities, mobility and *neighbourhood and community domains* represent the main trends in older homelessness literature. All articles, except one (which had only one network), had two or more networks with old-age exclusion domains, 11 articles had networks with all domains, 20 articles had networks with five domains, 16 articles with four, 10 articles with three and 2 articles with only one domain. This finding might reveal the multidimensional nature of social exclusion and homelessness. This multidimensionality has resulted with multiple networks as it is difficult to isolate in social exclusion and homelessness research one domain only.

26.5.1 Multidimensional Patterns of Old-Age Exclusion

The data discussed above gathered from the summative content analysis revealed the multidimensionality of old-age exclusion. However, it did not reveal the density of the connection between articles and old-age exclusion domains virtually. In order to illustrate these connections, social network analysis was conducted and the pattern obtained was visualised using GEPHI software (Fig. 26.3).

Edge and Node matrixes were used to import the data to GEPHI. In this research, nodes were identified as network members (59 articles and six old-age exclusion domains). Edges were identified as a network showing the connection of the literature with old-age exclusion domains. The thickness of the edge (line) was directly related with the frequency of network members. A thicker edge was indicating a higher frequency of old-age exclusion domains in articles. These matrixes were created in Excel and were imported into GEPHI. There were 65 nodes (59 articles and six social exclusion domains) and 263 edges (total number of the connections between articles and social exclusion domains). To visualise this data, the Yifan Hu Proportional algorithm in GEPHI was applied.

The sum of all frequencies identified the weight of nodes regarding old-age exclusion domains. The old-age exclusion domain nodes grew and located towards the centre with increasing frequency. While article nodes with lower frequencies were more decentralised and heterogeneous, article nodes with multiple connections with the old-age exclusion domain nodes and with a higher frequency

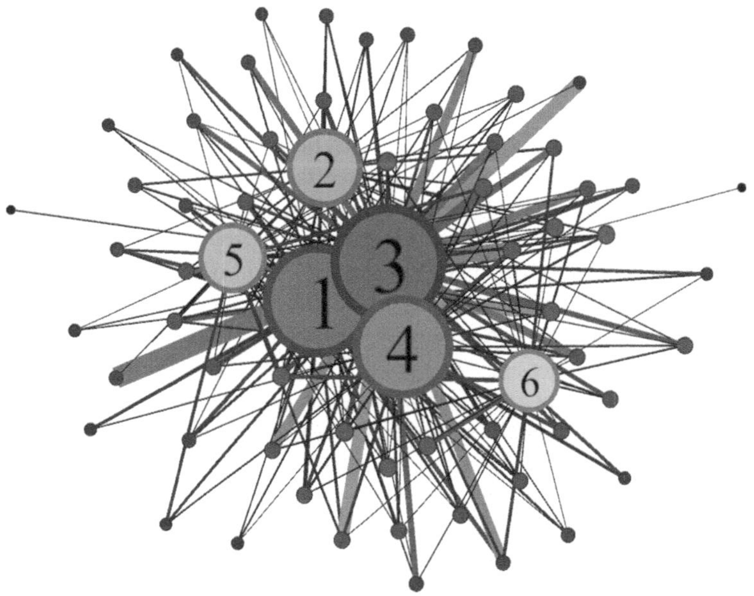

Fig. 26.3 Networks of domains of old-age exclusion in homelessness literature (1. Neighbourhood and community; 2. Social relations; 3. Services, amenities, and mobility; 4. Material and financial resources; 5. Socio-cultural aspects of society; 6. Civic participation)

represented stronger connections with the network and the pattern of network was more centralised in the resulting figure (see Fig. 26.3).

Figure 26.3 enabled a clear visualisation of the least and most addressed old-age exclusion domains in the old-age homelessness literature according to the size of nodes and thickness of edges. The most centralised zone in the figure was *services, amenities and mobility*. The nodes representing *neighbourhood and community*, and *material and financial resources* are located near the centre. These three domains were partially positioned in the centre, constituting the old-age exclusion domain with the highest density regarding homelessness. *Socio-cultural aspects* and *civic participation* however were found to have the least density and were located further from the centre.

26.6 Conclusion

Homeless older adults are among the main groups exposed to social exclusion. Older homeless individuals are more vulnerable in terms of social exclusion compared to homeless adults of other age groups. The disadvantages of older homeless is discussed in the literature (Sullivan 1991; Burns and Sussman 2018). Researchers focused on the prevention of exclusion by proper service provision and revealed that the deficiency in support systems increases the risk for older homelessness

(Warnes and Crane 2000; Manthorpe et al. 2013). The high frequency of the domain of services, amenities, and mobility found in this research can be explained in connection with this. Research articles were concentrating on service provision gaps mainly for health and social services.

The multidimensionality of old-age exclusion in homelessness literature appeared partly in this research, focused on *services, amenities and mobility*; *neighbourhood and community* and *material and financial resources* domains. These domains were found to be interconnected according to SNA analysis. *Socio-cultural aspects of society*, *civic participation* and *social relations* exclusion domains however were less frequently researched.

Even though the articles comprising the sample in this research were specifically on homelessness in older-age but not on old-age exclusion, old-age exclusion domains were strongly prevalent in all articles. These findings show clearly that homelessness in old-age is crossing social exclusion ontologically. Parallel to our result, homelessness experiences in old-age were discussed as a social exclusion process, concentrating on problems and solutions. The reasons that this was the case however could not be highlighted. It is not possible to address multidimensionality in old-age homelessness research unless political, economic and social macro processes causing exclusion are addressed. Old-age homelessness is a worldwide phenomenon and the number of old-age homeless is increasing due to the rising cost of housing, global economic and localised recessions, poverty and global ageing. This trend is expected to be reflected in the international literature even more in the future.

This research has focused only on whether old-age exclusion key words exist in articles and the number of key words in each article. Accordingly, we can only conclude on frequencies and unfortunately cannot elaborate in depth about the connections between homelessness and the different domains of exclusion, the interconnection between these domains and about the impacts involved. Further research will be valuable to explore these connections in detail.

Editors' Postscript

Please note, like other contributions to this book, this chapter was written before the COVID-19 pandemic of 2020. The book's introductory chapter (Chap. 1) and conclusion (Chap. 34) consider some of the key ways in which the pandemic relates to issues concerning social exclusion and ageing.

References

Abbott, P., & Sapsford, R. (2005). Living on the margins: Older people, place and social exclusion. *Policy Studies, 26*(1), 29–46.

Anderson, I. (2003). Synthesizing homelessness research: Trends, lessons and prospects. *Journal of Community & Applied Social Psychology, 13*(2), 197–205.

Bowpitt, G., Dwyer, P., Sundin, E., & Weinstein, M. (2011). Comparing men's and women's experiences of multiple exclusion homelessness. *Social Policy and Society, 10*(4), 537–546.
Burns, V. F., & Sussman, T. (2018). Homeless for the first time in later life: Uncovering more than one pathway. *The Gerontologist, 59*(2), 251–259.
Caton, C. L., Hasin, D., Shrout, P. E., Opler, L. A., Hirshfield, S., Dominguez, B., & Felix, A. (2000). Risk factors for homelessness among indigent urban adults with no history of psychotic illness: A case-control study. *American Journal of Public Health, 90*(2), 258.
Caton, C. L., Dominguez, B., Schanzer, B., Hasin, D. S., Shrout, P. E., Felix, A., et al. (2005). Risk factors for long-term homelessness: Findings from a longitudinal study of first-time homeless single adults. *American Journal of Public Health, 95*(10), 1753–1759.
Cohen, C. I. (1999). Aging and homelessness. *The Gerontologist, 39*(1), 5–15.
Cohen, C. I., Teresi, J. A., & Holmes, D. (1988). The physical well-being of old homeless men. *Journal of Gerontology, 43*(4), 121–128.
Cohen, C. I., Onserud, H., & Monaco, C. (1992). Project rescue: Serving the homeless and marginally housed elderly. *The Gerontologist, 32*(4), 466–471.
Craig, T., & Timms, P. (2000). Facing up to social exclusion: Services for homeless mentally ill people. *International Review of Psychiatry, 12*(3), 206–211.
Crane, M., & Warnes, T. (1997). *Homeless truths: Challenging the myths about older homeless people*. London: Help the Aged.
Crane, M., Byrne, K., Fu, R., Lipmann, B., Mirabelli, F., Rota-Bartelink, A., et al. (2005). The causes of homelessness in later life: Findings from a 3-nation study. *The Journals of Gerontology Series B: Psychological Sciences and Social Sciences, 60*(3), 152–159.
Fitzpatrick, S., Johnsen, S., & White, M. (2011). Multiple exclusion homelessness in the UK: Key patterns and intersections. *Social Policy and Society, 10*(4), 501–512.
Fitzpatrick, S., Bramley, G., & Johnsen, S. (2013). Pathways into multiple exclusion homelessness in seven UK cities. *Urban Studies, 50*(1), 148–168.
Grenier, A., Barken, R., & McGrath, C. (2016a). Homelessness and aging: The contradictory ordering of 'house' and 'home'. *Journal of Aging Studies, 39*, 73–80.
Grenier, A., Barken, R., Sussman, T., Rothwell, D., Bourgeois-Guérin, V., & Lavoie, J. P. (2016b). A literature review of homelessness and aging: Suggestions for a policy and practice-relevant research agenda. *Canadian Journal on Aging/La Revue canadienne du vieillissement, 35*(1), 28–41.
Herman, D. B., Susser, E. S., Struening, E. L., & Link, B. L. (1997). Adverse childhood experiences: Are they risk factors for adult homelessness? *American Journal of Public Health, 87*(2), 249–255.
Horsell, C. (2006). Homelessness and social exclusion: A Foucauldian perspective for social workers. *Australian Social Work, 59*(2), 213–225. https://doi.org/10.1080/03124070600651911.
Hsieh, H. F., & Shannon, S. E. (2005). Three approaches to qualitative content analysis. *Qualitative Health Research, 15*(9), 1277–1288.
Johnson, L. J., & McCool, A. C. (2003). Dietary intake and nutritional status of older adult homeless women: A pilot study. *Journal of Nutrition for the Elderly, 23*(1), 1–21.
Kennett, P. (1999). Homelessness, citizenship and social exclusion. In P. Kennett & A. Marsh (Eds.), *Homelessness: Exploring the new terrain* (pp. 37–60). Bristol: Policy Press.
Lovald, K. A. (1961). Social life of the aged homeless man in skid row. *The Gerontologist, 1*(1), 30–33.
Manthorpe, J., Cornes, M., O'Halloran, S., & Joly, L. (2013). Multiple exclusion homelessness: The preventive role of social work. *The British Journal of Social Work, 45*(2), 587–599.
Metraux, S., & Culhane, D. P. (2006). Recent incarceration history among a sheltered homeless population. *Crime & Delinquency, 52*(3), 504–517.
Norman, T., & Pauly, B. (2013). Including people who experience homelessness: A scoping review of the literature. *International Journal of Sociology and Social Policy, 33*(3/4), 136–151.
Power, R., & Hunter, G. (2001). Developing a strategy for community-based health promotion targeting homeless populations. *Health Education Research, 16*(5), 593–602.

Rothwell, D. W., Sussman, T., Grenier, A., Mott, S., & Bourgeois-Guérin, V. (2017). Patterns of shelter use among men new to homelessness in later life: Duration of stay and psychosocial factors related to departure. *Journal of Applied Gerontology, 36*(1), 71–93.

Salem, B. E., Nyamathi, A., Brecht, M. L., Phillips, L. R., Mentes, J. C., Sarkisian, C., & Stein, J. A. (2014). Constructing and identifying predictors of frailty among homeless adults—A latent variable structural equations model approach. *Archives of Gerontology and Geriatrics, 58*(2), 248–256.

Scott, J. (1988). Social network analysis. *Sociology, 22*(1), 109–127.

Shinn, M., Gottlieb, J., Wett, J. L., Bahl, A., Cohen, A., & Baron Ellis, D. (2007). Predictors of homelessness among older adults in new York City: Disability, economic, human and social capital and stressful events. *Journal of Health Psychology, 12*(5), 696–708.

Sullivan, M. A. (1991). The homeless older woman in context: Alienation, cutoff and reconnection. *Journal of Women & Aging, 3*(2), 3–24.

Susser, E., Moore, R., & Link, B. (1993). Risk factors for homelessness. *Epidemiologic Reviews, 15*(2), 546–556.

Walsh, K., Scharf, T., & Keating, N. (2017). Social exclusion of older persons: A scoping review and conceptual framework. *European Journal of Ageing, 14*, 81–98. https://doi.org/10.1007/s10433-016-0398-8.

Warnes, A. M., & Crane, M. A. (2000). The achievements of a multiservice project for older homeless people. *The Gerontologist, 40*(5), 618–626.

Watson, J., Crawley, J., & Kane, D. (2016). Social exclusion, health and hidden homelessness. *Public Health, 139*, 96–102.

Wolch, J. R., Dear, M., & Akita, A. (1988). Explaining homelessness. *Journal of the American Planning Association, 54*(4), 443–453.

Woolrych, R., Gibson, N., Sixsmith, J., & Sixsmith, A. (2015). "No home, no place": Addressing the complexity of homelessness in old age through community dialogue. *Journal of Housing for the Elderly, 29*(3), 233–258.

Zufferey, C., & Kerr, L. (2004). Identity and everyday experiences of homelessness: Some implications for social work. *Australian Social Work, 57*(4), 343–353.

Section VIII
Policy and Social Exclusion in Later Life

Chapter 27
Introduction: Policy to Reduce Late-Life Social Exclusion – From Aspirations to Action

Norah Keating and Maria Cheshire-Allen

27.1 Introduction

This chapter, as with others in this section, was written prior to the COVID-19 pandemic and to the ways in which it placed older persons' vulnerability to social exclusion in stark relief. Early in the pandemic we saw swift policy action focussed on older persons. In some countries, people over age 70 were held to stricter rules of self-isolation. In others, nursing homes were locked down. Such policies afford protection on one hand but remove agency on the other. COVID-19 highlighted the values stances that continue to place older people as conditional citizens.

For those of us who devote our professional lives to understanding social challenges of population ageing, who see inequities and embrace a social justice agenda, in the end we must ask—*so what*? How can this knowledge we have created, the networks we have developed and our theoretical insights make a difference in the lives of older people?

From the outset, the mission of Reducing Old-Age Social Exclusion (ROSEnet) was to create shared understandings of late-life exclusion that would be foundational to the development of meaningful policy and practice. It is an ambitious agenda, given the goal of reducing exclusion across broad contexts of peoples' lives that intersect and that evolve and diverge across the life course.

Policy is the most macro of these contexts. It is within the policy environment that we can come to understand values about age and ageing, about who is seen to

N. Keating (✉)
University of Alberta, Edmonton, Canada

Swansea University, Swansea, Wales, UK
e-mail: nkeating@ualberta.ca

M. Cheshire-Allen
Swansea University, Swansea, Wales, UK

K. Walsh et al. (eds.), *Social Exclusion in Later Life*, International Perspectives on Aging 28, https://doi.org/10.1007/978-3-030-51406-8_27

be deserving of full citizenship and about how these cultural ways of knowing frame courses of action within a society. Chapter authors in this section of the book speak to these big policy questions and to the global and regional aspirations that underlie the approaches to late-life social exclusion. Others address the actions needed and those that have been taken toward legislation and regulations to reduce exclusion.

The purpose of this chapter is to consider social exclusion as a policy framework for population ageing and older persons, highlighting key debates and where we should embrace them in more than just rhetoric. We introduce the six chapters in this section that provide important narratives on these debates and actions.

27.2 Social Exclusion as a Policy Framework

Policy experts have argued that "the most difficult policy questions tend to have at least some element of disagreement about what is valuable and how things ought to be" (Muers 2018, p. 14). This statement resonates given the longstanding discussions about population ageing and the value of older people. Early theorising placed older people as conditional citizens—dependent, burdensome and unproductive—where policy levers such as mandatory retirement were consistent with moving older people out of the mainstream. But such certainty about appropriate action was soon challenged. Concepts such as ageism began to populate the lexicon of ageing. Butler's (1969, p. 243) provocative statement naming ageism as "a form of bigotry we tend to overlook" is an example of powerful voices that have a hallmark of ageing policy discourses for 50 more than years. We've come a long way, though the policy terrain remains uncertain.

Social exclusion moves the lens firmly away from discourses of burden to a view of older people as full citizens with rights of access to societal resources that are not contingent on age. Its values-stance and focus on a large and growing group of older adults could be a touchstone for the decisions that governments will undertake and the values that drive those decisions. It reminds us that while the visible elements of public policy are embodied in "constitutions, legislative acts, and judicial decisions" (Peters 2015, p. 3), it is the symbols, narratives and language that define "what is fair, what constitutes right and wrong…and similar ethical matters" (Muers 2018, p. 7). Together these two elements of policy (the values and the actions on which they are based) determine the extent to which the lives of older persons are improved across the life domains articulated in this framework.

We believe that social exclusion is a timely and relevant approach to the development of meaningful policy and practice. It allows for an examination of policy drivers as well as policy actions and it places onto public agendas the contemporary values-debates that so often lead to the policy dilemmas that Muers describes. An important question is the extent to which the particular values underpinning social exclusion are likely to be broadly embraced and enacted. There are promising signals. In her analysis of EU social policy development undertaken several years ago, Daly (2008) noted that social exclusion had been taken up as a template for social policy development. She argued though that its implementation had foundered, in a setting of weak pressure from relevant constituents, vague targets and lack of clarity on desirable outcomes. At that time, she saw little political commitment "to address the kind of problems that the concept of social exclusion originated to characterize" (p. 16).

27.3 Policy Challenges and Contemporary Public and Political Debates

It's perhaps not surprising that the (EU) social policy process and its links to social exclusion have been uneven and its pathways unclear [see Walsh et al. this volume]. In some ways it seems a classic example of the policy development process: "recursive and discontinuous and involving many steps and dynamic factors over a considerable period of time" (Pawson 2011, p. 10). Nonetheless, the past decade has seen impressive levels of endorsement of values around reducing social exclusion.

United Nations agencies have been instrumental in redefining the values discourse. The World Report on Ageing and Health (World Health Organization 2015) took as its major premise that older persons should expect to live in ways that they consider important to them. The United Nations 2030 Agenda for Sustainable Development (2015), has a similar vision though a broader reach: to leave no one behind. Both have goals of realising human rights for all. Both place the onus on governments to reduce inequities that can lead to exclusion. Both have been adopted by countries around the world.

At the same time that thought leaders are changing the values agenda, strategies toward action are increasingly prominent. Pressure from relevant constituents is becoming more organized and sustained through organizations such as AGE Platform Europe (https://www.age-platform.eu/), a European network of NGOs that promotes interest and raises awareness of issues of concern to older persons in the EU. AGE Platform members are organizations of older people. They too have as their vision "an inclusive society for all ages".

What then is the place of evidence in the policy process? Chapters in this book have illustrated the impressive accumulation of knowledge across broad domains of late-life exclusion. Evidence matters. It matters in reducing risk of unnecessary harm and in achieving important policy goals (Parkhurst 2017). Policy theorists caution against assuming a direct relationship between sound scientific knowledge and the adoption of a particular public policy action (Cairney 2016). The relative power of evidence is always muted by values, political agendas and competition among multiple social goals (Parkhurst 2017; Fisher 2019).

27.4 Outline of This Section

Chapters in this section of the book establish many of the important issues and debates around social exclusion: values and beliefs about the place of older people in society; aspirational versus legislative documents to address social exclusion; and evidence of structural sources of social exclusion.

Conboy (Chap. 28) and Kucharczyk (Chap. 33) each provide critical analyses of some of international policy documents that delineate contemporary values and principles to address social exclusion. Conboy addresses macro policy issues that are foundational to the UN Sustainable Development Goals and the 2030 agenda for Sustainable Development. She lays out the processes and barriers between governments signing on to a global agenda to "Leave no one behind" and actions that might affect the lives of older people. Kucharczyk analyses the European Pillar of Social Rights (EPSR), a set of social rights and principles to improve lives of the Europeans through more equality, inclusion and well-being. The rights-based approach makes EPSR a powerful tool for harmonization of policy instruments, though increased political commitment and accountability are needed for it to succeed.

Ogg (Chap. 29) and Grigorieva et al. (Chap. 30) address approaches to pension reform and their likelihood of increasing risks of late-life economic exclusion. Ogg examines European pension systems in the context of new social risks resulting from shifting political systems, rapid technological change, and economic uncertainties. He highlights issues including extended working life that increase likelihood of economic exclusion in old-age. Grigorieva et al. undertake a comparative analysis of pension reform and the structure of social services in post-Soviet Russia and Ukraine. They come to a stark conclusion that the intersections of low income, chronic illnesses and poor access to services including social care may lead to deep exclusion of older people in both countries.

Although both address specific domains of exclusion, both Andersen et al. (Chap. 31) and Leppiman et al. (Chap. 32) also speak to the values that influence change. Andersen et al. undertake a micro policy analysis of how nursing home design can reduce spatial and community exclusion. Their four settings illustrate different approaches to connecting with the local community. They emphasise the importance of residents as a heterogeneous group with different needs, values and capabilities. Leppiman et al. discuss digitalisation and its potential both to improve lives of older people through access to services and information and to exclude them. They use the example of Estonia and Finland to illustrate how what they call values-based technology development could enhance well-being of older people.

27.5 From Aspirations to Action

In many ways, social exclusion has come of age. Its values are embedded in global social agendas and its language in regional policy frameworks. Actions to reduce exclusion are emerging with steady pressure from constituencies such as older persons organisations. Articulation of an explicit social exclusion conceptual framework and evidence to support it have created a solid foundation to inform social action. Chapters in this section have identified gaps between aspirations and action and have identified both opportunities and barriers to address them.

References

Age Platform Europe. *The voice of older persons at EU level*. https://www.age-platform.eu/

Butler, R. N. (1969). Age-ism: Another form of bigotry. *The Gerontologist, 9*(4), 243–246. https://doi.org/10.1093/geront/9.4_Part_1.243.

Cairney, P. (2016). *The politics of evidence-based policy making*. London: Palgrave Macmillan.

Daly, M. (2008). Whither EU social policy? An account and assessment of developments in the Lisbon social inclusion process. *Journal of Social Policy, 37*(1), 1–19. https://doi.org/10.1017/S0047279407001468.

Fischer, F. (2019). *Politics, values, and public policy: The problem of methodology*. New York: Routledge.

Muers, S. (2018). *Culture, values and public policy*. IPR report, Institute for Policy Research, University of Bath. https://www.bath.ac.uk/publications/culture-values-and-public-policy/attachments/ipr-culture-values-and-public-policy.pdf

Parkhurst, J. (2017). *The politics of evidence: From evidence-based policy to the good-governance of evidence*. Abingdon: Routledge.

Pawson, R. (2011). Conclusion: Flying the tattered flag of enlightenment. In *Evidence-based policy* (pp. 167–182). London: SAGE Publications Ltd. https://doi.org/10.4135/9781849209120.

Peters, B. G. (2015). *Advanced introduction to public policy*. Cheltenham: Edward Elgar Ltd. ISBN 978-1-78195-576-5.

United Nations. (2015). *Transforming our world: The 2030 agenda for sustainable development*. New York.

World Health Organization. (2015). *World report on ageing and health*. Geneva: WHO.

Chapter 28
Older-Age Exclusion and the 2030 Agenda for Sustainable Development

Patricia Conboy

28.1 Introduction

The 2030 Agenda for Sustainable Development incorporating 17 Sustainable Development Goals (SDGs) was adopted by United Nations Member States in 2015 as a transformative agenda for economic, social and environmental development. Critically, from the perspective of older-age exclusion, the commitments of the 2030 Agenda are global, applicable in all countries; explicitly inclusive of people of all ages, therefore incorporating older people; and are founded on a central pledge to "Leave no one behind", aiming to reach the furthest behind first (United Nations 2015). Given these parameters, the 2030 Agenda has the potential to advance the recognition and rights of older people through bringing them into the mainstream of development policy and practice at global and national levels. The purpose of this chapter is to explore how far the potential of the 2030 Agenda has been realised as a global framework to address multidimensional older-age exclusion.

28.2 Exploring Older-Age Exclusion

In this chapter, older-age is understood as the latter stages of the life course (HelpAge International 2016), with older-age exclusion defined as a multidimensional process leading to inequities for older people in access to resources, power and rights in six domains conceptualised by Walsh et al. (2017). The domains cover material resources; social relations; civic and political participation; services; neighbourhood and community; and, of central importance in this chapter, socio-cultural aspects of society [see Torres et al. this volume for a discussion]. The socio-cultural

---

P. Conboy (✉)
HelpAge International, London, UK
e-mail: Patricia.Conboy@helpage.org

K. Walsh et al. (eds.), *Social Exclusion in Later Life*, International Perspectives on Aging 28, https://doi.org/10.1007/978-3-030-51406-8_28

domain [referred to in the wider book under the term civic exclusion – see Walsh et al. this volume] embraces ageism, symbolic exclusion and identity exclusion. Ageism is identified as treating people unfairly because of their age (HelpAge International 2019b). Symbolic exclusion is defined as "negative representations such as when older people are portrayed as marginal or valueless" and identity exclusion as the transfer of a partial identity to an individual or a group as their sole identity, dismissing or ignoring their multiple and distinctive identities (Grenier and Guberman 2009).

In focusing on the socio-cultural aspects of exclusion, this chapter considers whether and how ageing and older people are recognised in the framing, implementation, monitoring and reporting of the 2030 Agenda. It does so through a selective review of the grey literature published between 2015 and 2019, including UN reports, selected national government and civil society reports, related websites and conference reports. The emphasis is on experience in low- and middle-income countries and Sub-Saharan Africa in particular where countries face extreme challenges in implementing the SDGs. Two thirds of African countries are in the "low human development" category and continue to struggle with healthcare and education and the SDG funding gap is estimated at between $5 billion and $1.2 trillion annually (SDG Center for Africa 2019).

28.3 The Sustainable Development Goals

The Sustainable Development Goals (SDGs) aim to eradicate extreme poverty by 2030, to realise the human rights of all and to ensure that all human beings can fulfil their potential in dignity and equality and in a healthy environment (see Fig. 28.1). They are broader in scope and ambition than the UN Millennium Development Goals (MDGs) which preceded the 2030 Agenda and expired in 2015. With their breadth and focus on an integrated approach, the SDGs do offer opportunities to address both specific dimensions of exclusion and the interaction between multiple domains of exclusion for people of all ages. The detail of the SDGs is articulated in 169 specific targets and 230 indicators intended to track progress on their implementation (Inter-Agency and Expert Group on Sustainable Development Indicators 2016).

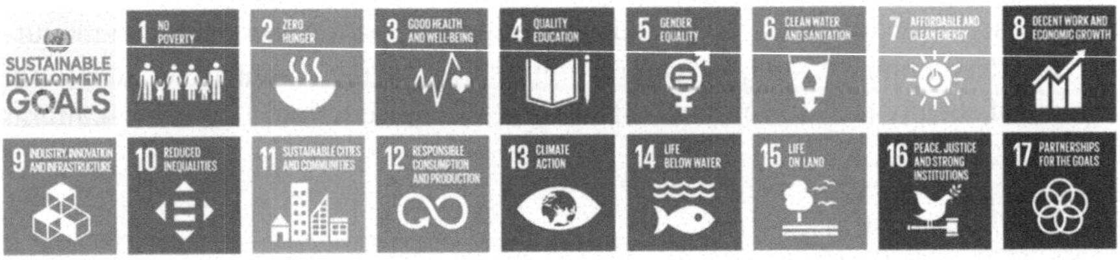

Fig. 28.1 The sustainable development goals

The 2030 Agenda provides a global framework for action which UN Member States then implement at a national level. Member States participate in the SDG process on a voluntary basis, each determining the scope and nature of their involvement and national approaches to implementation, monitoring and reporting on progress. Governments are invited to submit Voluntary National Reviews (VNRs) to the High-Level Political Forum (HLPF), the central platform for annual review and follow-up of the 2030 Agenda and the SDGs. While UN guidance is provided, national governments choose what they include in the VNRs.

28.4 Significance of the 2030 Agenda for Sustainable Development

The 2030 Agenda shapes the global conversation on development. If older people and ageing are recognised in the 2030 Agenda, they form part of a global conversation between key policymakers and influencers. If not, older people are in effect "left behind". This is of particular relevance to policy agendas in low- and middle-income countries where, in contrast with high-income countries, the issue of demographic ageing has received less political attention. All of the UN entities have aimed to align their strategic programmes of work with the Agenda and the SDGs (United Nations, Economic and Social Council 2018). These include bodies such as the regional economic commissions and multilateral agencies such as the United Nations Development Programme (UNDP), the World Health Organization (WHO) and the World Bank. National and institutional donor agencies and aid programmes also align their strategies and their funding priorities with selected elements of the 2030 Agenda.

The overall effects apply to the period to 2030 *and beyond* in that the SDGs are likely to be succeeded by a new UN development agenda. While the MDGs did not recognise older people and ageing, the SDGs do offer space for recognition. Whether or not this space is extended and mainstreamed in a post-2030 UN agenda will be influenced by the degree to which older-age exclusion becomes part of global and national policy agendas up to 2030.

There are other pressing reasons why the 2030 Agenda is significant. It is an immediate driver of global action on policies relevant to older people. Health is an example, with SDG3 promoting access to affordable and quality health services for all under the banner of universal health coverage (UHC). While there are stated commitments across the UN, national governments and civil society to UHC, policies and programmes, the risk of omission of older people from UHC implementation remains high. There are similar patterns across other policy areas of significance such as gender equality, access to income and employment, and disability inclusion.

As with any other global framework, the 2030 Agenda absorbs energy and attention within the matrix of processes involving governments, multilateral entities, civil society organisations and other stakeholders who constitute "the development system". As well as VNRs (47 in 2019), there are policy audits, budgetary analyses, new committees and consultations with stakeholders. When there are failures to address the issues of key population groups, there is an opportunity cost in terms of misplaced energy. From the perspective of older people, this channelling of energy represents paradoxically both an opportunity for age mainstreaming and a risk of deepening multidimensional exclusion. It can be said with reasonable confidence that most older people are unaware of commitments by their governments to the delivery of the 2030 Agenda and the SDGs. The corollary is that they are missing out on chances to hold governments to account for delivery on commitments that would make a material difference to enjoyment of their rights and quality of life in older-age.

28.5 Older-Age Exclusion in Low- and Middle-Income Countries

While growing old is not a new human experience, the way people are ageing is new. People are living longer and in larger numbers and, globally, later life has become a less predictable and more fluid part of the life course. The scale of the challenge countries face in adapting to the demographic transitions they are now experiencing is immense. The largest share of the world's older people (37%) live in Eastern and South Eastern Asia and this is the region where the speed of population ageing is fastest (UNDESA 2019). Though the share of older people in Sub-Saharan Africa looks small by comparison (5%), the numbers involved are large. There are 31.9 million people aged 65 and over living in Sub-Saharan Africa. Notably, while the 2030 Agenda presents a call to transform our world, it does not incorporate consideration of demographic ageing in its founding documents (United Nations 2015).

In terms of older-age exclusion, there are difficulties in characterising the experience of older people across regional and national settings where political, cultural, socio-economic and demographic landscapes are extraordinarily diverse and varied. However, there are sufficient data to establish that older persons do experience systematic, multidimensional exclusion as conceptualised by Walsh et al. (2017) in the form of lack or denial of rights, resources, goods and services as they age. Worldwide, 68% of people above retirement age receive an old-age pension. In Sub-Saharan Africa, 22.7% do so and in Southern Asia the figure is 23.6% (ILO 2017). In terms of access to health and care services and supports, older people are under-served. As an illustration, in most high-income countries, under half of people living with dementia have received a diagnosis. From the limited data available in LMIC settings, it is estimated that no more than 5–10% of people living with dementia have received a diagnosis, and specialist continuing care is extremely limited (HelpAge and AARP 2018). There is also sufficient evidence available from consultations with older people to establish that they do experience ageism in countries of all levels of development (Ayalon and Tesch-Römer 2018; Phoenix and Parravani 2019).

In terms of trajectories of older-age exclusion, the interaction between demographic ageing and other mega trends such as the growth of artificial intelligence and digital technologies, migration trends, rising inequalities and climate change will have a bearing on how people age in future decades. For example, a person in the Asia Pacific region is five times more likely to be affected by disasters than anywhere else in the world and those disasters have a disproportionate impact on older people (HelpAge International 2019c).

28.6 Framing a Whole Population Group as Vulnerable

Where older people are identified in Agenda 2030, they are primarily included with other groups characterised as "vulnerable", including children, persons with disabilities and refugees (United Nations 2015; Republic of Rwanda 2019; SDGs Kenya Forum 2019; United Republic of Tanzania 2019). How a group or issue is presented or framed affects the ways in which people react and respond to that group or issue. Frames are ways of thinking that shape the way people see the world. A frame effect is said to occur when people react differently to a social or scientific issue as a result of the way it is framed, for example whether it is presented as a loss or a gain, or a problem that affects individuals or society (Frameworks Institute 2019).

The framing of a whole population group, in this case older people, as vulnerable solely on the basis of their chronological age raises serious questions. It is factually inaccurate. Older populations are characterised by both diversity and inequality. It is unscientific in that, as research evidence has demonstrated, the relationship between chronological age and human functioning and capacity is far from straightforward (Beard and Bloom 2015). It is at odds with the evidence available to us of older people's own views and preferences. In consultations across a range of low- and middle-income settings, older people have consistently identified their preferences and priorities. These include voice, visibility, respect, participation, an emphasis on autonomy, independence and choice in living their lives, and on recognition of their rights (Sleap 2019a, b). Older people seek equality and parity of esteem with others and inclusion in the mainstream, not special treatment as a distinct group outside the mainstream of society. This "vulnerability" framing also contradicts the framing of the 2030 Agenda as a transformative vision for society rooted in human rights principles.

While the concept of "vulnerable groups" has been used to argue for the protection of human rights of groups, such as members of the Roma community, asylum seekers and people with impaired health or abilities in European courts of law, risks associated with use of the concept have been identified in a critical assessment (Peroni and Timmer 2013). Concerns relate to the potential danger of reinforcing vulnerability "by essentialising, stigmatising, victimising and paternalising" a group. Essentialising occurs when significant differences within the group are obscured and they are homogenised regardless of, for example, health or cognitive status, individual preferences and aspirations. Stigmatising occurs when the term "vulnerable" carries connotations of harm or injury for the members of the group themselves. Paternalising occurs when the agency and autonomy of members of the group is denied and protection is imposed on them (Peroni and Timmer 2013, pp. 1070–73). A further nuance relates to the perspective from which protection is provided. From a charity perspective, support is available to the "deserving" poor and groups seek to establish that they deserve support. In the case of older people, this sometimes takes the form of the contribution argument which focuses on quantifying their economic contributions as carers, grandparents, volunteers, community development activists and such. In these attempts to counter the "burden" narrative that dominates discourse on population ageing, proponents of the contribution argument may, in the view of the author, unwittingly deepen the socio-cultural exclusion of older people (European Commission 2015).

The categorisation of older people as a vulnerable group in the 2030 Agenda, while reflective of mainstream approaches in the development sector, is misguided. It undermines the rights of older people. It also reinforces the failure to identify ageism as a key driver of the discrimination and exclusion evident in the design and implementation of laws, policies, and programmes that should serve people equally across the life course. A further irony is that, while the pledge to "Leave no one behind" has opened the space for identification and inclusion of groups typically at high risk of exclusion, the way in which this space has been used to reinforce the categorisation of older people as a vulnerable group is proving counterproductive. It fails to identify older people as rights holders and governments as duty bearers in their regard. Yet this is precisely the breakthrough that is required if older-age exclusion is to be addressed effectively globally and nationally.

28.7 Implementation of the 2030 Agenda and the Sustainable Development Goals

The explicit recognition of older people and ageing in the SDGs is limited. With SDG1, promoting the eradication of poverty and SDG3, promoting health and well-being, the goals clearly refer to people of all ages. Otherwise, the only explicit references to older people are in SDG2.2 which focuses on malnutrition among older people and SDG11 on sustainable cities and communities which identifies the need to consider older people in widening access to public transport and access to green spaces. Generalised statements about people "of all ages" are meaningless when older people are effectively eliminated from delivery of the SDGs, as happens when benchmarks are age-capped. For example, while SDG 5.6 advocates universal access to sexual and reproductive health and rights, the indicators measuring the goal are capped at 49 years. Evidence about the *implementation* of the SDGs is largely derived from the reports of the UN Secretary General to the HLPF and the VNRs submitted by individual Member States. With the exception of a single ageing-specific report to the General Assembly, based on research commissioned by the UN Focal Point on Ageing, the coverage of older people in these documents is patchy and superficial. In general, the evidence that is available is descriptive rather than analytical with little detail on the implementation of policies or the outcomes for older people (UN 2019).

Findings from a recent Tanzanian study illustrate the importance of more granular analysis of policy implementation at national levels (HelpAge International and AARP 2019). While national policy in Tanzania provides for free access to public health services for people aged 60 and over by means of a waiver scheme, there are significant gaps in implementation. These include reluctance on the part of some health service providers at local levels to extend free services. This is due to a conflicting policy demand to recover local costs from service users. The result is an incentive to prioritise patients who can pay for services. In addition, older people themselves are not always sure about their right to the services or how to exercise this right. Issues on which they need support include accessing the waiver cards that would establish their age and entitlement to a health service, and a process for making complaints or seeking redress when they were denied access to services or receive a poor service, for example partial filling of prescriptions for medicines. These findings also point to the value of a multidimensional analysis of older-age exclusion in illustrating how forms of discrimination reinforce each other in different domains; in this example, material, political, services and socio-cultural domains.

28.8 Evidence from the National Level in Low- and Middle-Income Settings

The evidence base on the implementation of policy on ageing and older people in low- and middle-income countries is thin, and even more sparse in terms of tracking policy implementation associated with the influence of the SDGs. In a review of experience from small-scale SDG pilot programme interventions in eight countries, it was found that national partners faced a number of common challenges when advocating for the recognition of older people in the SDGs. Critically, these included a broad lack of awareness among policymakers, civil society groups and older people about the links between ageing and sustainable development issues (HelpAge International 2019a). What this meant in practice was that, for some countries preparing their VNRs, ageing was not considered or that government focal points on ageing were not consulted. Even when awareness was raised and stakeholders appeared sympathetic, this did not necessarily trigger action due to competing priorities or staff being moved to other departments. Partners reported that, when trying to establish themselves in key policy spaces, they found that the person in government working on ageing was not always involved in the SDG process and those working on the SDGs were not aware of the links with ageing. There were additional challenges in some governments where the ownership of SDGs rested with multiple departments without a central coordination structure. This made it difficult for civil society partners with limited resources to engage with all the key players. The complexity of these implementation processes is another barrier to older people's participation in the 2030 Agenda.

28.9 Visibility of Older People and Ageing in Monitoring and Reporting of the SDGs

An analysis of statistical reporting on progress of the SDGs at global level illustrates the near invisibility of older people and ageing in the process (United Nations 2019). The indicators presented are those for which data are available. In the case of older people, reporting is confined to social protection floors under SDG1. The targets and indicators for which data on older people are **not** reported due to underlying deficiencies in the data include malnutrition, HIV infection, mortality attributed to non-communicable diseases (NCDs), access to universal health coverage, to education and lifelong learning, gender equality, employment and unemployment, coverage by mobile phone network, deaths due to disasters, experience of sexual violence and access to legal identity. This goes against the commitment of SDG17 to increase the availability of reliable data disaggregated by income, gender, age, disability, ethnicity, migratory status and other characteristics. While the 2030 Agenda has led to a proactive focus on data development and disaggregation and there are positive initiatives on ageing-related statistics, such as the establishment of the Titchfield City Group (Pullinger 2018), there is a systemic bias towards addressing data gaps for younger age groups. Age data gaps and discriminatory age caps will continue to hinder the monitoring of older-age exclusion in the 2030 Agenda.

28.10 Mainstreaming of Ageing and of Older People

It is evident from this review that the potential of the 2030 Agenda as a framework to address multidimensional older-age exclusion is not being maximised. If anything, the findings about framing and visibility of older people suggest the risk of deepening socio-cultural exclusion over the lifetime of the 2030 Agenda. How then to address these concerns in practice?

The development of coherent policy on ageing is not straightforward. Beard and Bloom (2015) have highlighted several of the challenges, including the complexity of the changes that constitute and affect ageing; the loose correspondence between chronological ageing and functional ability and capacity; and the inter-individual variability and diversity of older populations. They point out that the variability is not random and that, while some heterogeneity in health and function is genetically determined, the major proportion is strongly affected by the cumulative effect of health behaviours and inequities across the life course. Other issues identified include the rigid use of a policy framework typically based on a three-stage life cycle of student, working life and retirement which "reinforces ageist stereotypes and prevents the flexible forms of participation older people are increasingly seeking" (Beard and Bloom 2015). In their conceptualisation of old-age exclusion, Walsh et al. (2017) have identified key domains and also pointed to unique features of older-age exclusion including the accumulation of disadvantage over the life course and the greater susceptibility of some older people to marginalisation. While these dimensions are typically well understood by academics, professionals and practitioners in the fields of gerontology, geriatrics and ageing, they are not well embedded in many arenas of the policy world.

28.11 The Gap Between Knowledge on Ageing and Policy Action on Ageing

The reality is that there are knowledge translation gaps between the professional "ageing" world and significant policy arenas including that of the 2030 Agenda. While there is concerted action to influence policy on ageing, the responses of political leaders fall short (Stakeholder Group on Ageing 2019). There are bodies of research knowledge and empirical experience that stakeholders could use better to influence policy design on older-age exclusion. These include an extensive literature on the process of knowledge translation incorporating the steps between the creation of new scientific knowledge, its synthesis, dissemination, exchange and application to yield useful outcomes for society (Straus et al. 2009). Dissemination and exchange, stemming as they do from research evidence, include but go beyond communications strategies (Barwick et al. 2014). Traditional approaches to communications strategies based on publication of a research report, launch and press release will have no impact on policy implementation, but the communications world is vibrant with new strategies, platforms and approaches that can boost the effectiveness of knowledge translation processes (Cast from clay 2018).

28.12 Policymaking is a Political Process

There is also an extensive literature on policy implementation, identifying the political nature of the policymaking process (Tilley et al. 2017; Viennet and Pont 2017). Barr and Crawford (2005) describe the three legs of the policy reform tripod as policy design, political implementation and administrative/technical implementation. A case study based on empirical experience of advocacy for a universal social pension in Malawi illustrates the political dimensions of policy influencing (Juergens 2019). This advocacy has been led by a Malawi network of older persons' organisations, MANEPO, and directed towards Ministries, parliament and the media. A feasibility study, developed jointly by the Malawi Ministry for Social Welfare and a civil society partner, provided evidence and direction for their advocacy, enabling a shared understanding and consensus among the key stakeholders. As an effective national champion, MANEPO's leader played a critical role in terms of his understanding of national political dynamics, his connections to politicians, media, editors and parliamentarians, and his nuanced understanding of the legislative process. Another key factor was the development of effective partnerships between the national network, civil society and multilateral partners to augment technical capacity and share strategic intelligence. They were successful in achieving the drafting of a draft Social Pension Bill immediately before the 2019 General Election. Advocacy activities require financial support and the fourth enabling factor was sustained and flexible funding from Irish aid.

28.13 Technical/Administrative Implementation

While the 2030 Agenda advocates an integrated approach to economic, social and environmental policy, little guidance is given on the technical and administrative challenges of cross-sectoral policymaking. Traditionally, government departments work within silos and dedicated budget lines. Policymakers must break new ground to implement cross-cutting approaches. In terms of multidimensional older-age exclusion, it is precisely these kinds of cross-cutting approaches that are required but hard to achieve. Typical issues include political failure to build support for national policy commitments among frontline and regional staff; to establish effective processes for multisectoral coordination; and to support implementation with action plans and budgets. One place where there is practical knowledge emerging is New Zealand, which has implemented a well-being budget breaking down traditional silos of government to agree a limited number of well-being priorities backed up by evidence on policy impacts (Government of New Zealand 2019).

28.14 Conclusion

This chapter has explored how far the potential of the 2030 Agenda is being realised to address multidimensional older-age exclusion. A broad review has been conducted across the breadth of a global framework. The strength of this approach has been that it provides an overview for diverse interest groups at a crucial time for the 2030 Agenda. There have been 5 years to bed down the SDGs, but there is still a decade in which to make improvements. The limitation has been that broad brushstrokes have been applied to issues and contexts that are inherently complex and diverse with inevitable losses of nuance and subtlety and limits to explanatory power.

In terms of socio-cultural older-age exclusion, the key question was whether older people and ageing were recognised in the framing, implementation, monitoring and reporting of the 2030 Agenda. The finding is that recognition of ageing and older people is limited across each of these dimensions. Where there is explicit recognition, it takes place primarily within the framing of older people as a vulnerable group rather than as rights holders on an equal footing with people of other ages. The major shift required in this context is the recognition of older people as rights holders, of States as duty bearers and the extension of a rights-based approach to policy design and implementation to counteract multidimensional social exclusion. Unless there is a major shift in the coming decade, the pledge that the 2030 Agenda and the SDGs should be met for "all nations, peoples … and segments of society" will not be achieved in the case of older people, and the risks of failure are highest for older people in low- and middle-income countries.

Failure is not inevitable. With the political commitment of key stakeholders, it is possible to make more effective use of the 2030 Agenda to address older-age exclusion at all levels. Partnership working with older people is essential. Other tools are available, as discussed in this chapter. These include a conceptual framework of older-age exclusion to support more effective policy influencing, design and implementation within the system; the more systematic use of relevant bodies of research knowledge and empirical experience, including those related to knowledge translation and policy implementation; and the use of more innovative communication strategies. In terms of research/policy networks aiming to advance knowledge sharing and policymaking regarding multidimensional older-exclusion, a Eurocentric perspective is insufficient. The participation of researchers, policymakers and older people from low- and middle-income countries would greatly strengthen impact in relation to the 2030 Agenda. Finally, recognition by multilateral and bilateral aid agencies of multidimensional older-age exclusion in the context of the 2030 Agenda would increase strategic impact and enable financial support for the policy influencing that needs to be done over the next decade.

Author's Postscript

The near invisibility of older people in statistical reporting on the SDGs at global level has already been identified as a concern in this chapter. During the pandemic, 80 per cent of surveyed national statistical offices (NSOs) in low- and middle-income countries (LMICs) reported that they were struggling to operate due to financial constraints and 90 per cent suggested that they were struggling to meet international reporting requirements (UNSD and World Bank 2020). Even before the pandemic, many NSOs struggled to produce good quality age-disaggregated data on older women and men in development and humanitarian contexts. The crisis has compounded those problems. In the main, the numbers of cases and fatalities from COVID-19 were being reported, but the production of data disaggregated by age and sex was much more limited (Mihnovits 2020). In addition, gaps in reliable data and evidence on underlying health conditions, access to essential health services and cause of death among older people will become even more pressing concerns for policymakers at both global and national levels as countries aim to recover and "to build back better" through the framework of the 2030 Agenda for Sustainable Development. Multilateral and donor agencies must ensure their pandemic response includes funding and technical support to NSOs in LMICs to sustain collection, analysis and reporting of timely data on ageing and older people during emergencies.

Acknowledgements This chapter benefitted from contributions by Alex Mihnovits, Flavia Galvani, Florian Juergens, Roseline Kihumba, Verity McGivern, Mark Gorman, Mariana Rudge and Camilla Williamson, HelpAge International, Professor Thomas Scharf, University of Newcastle, and Professor Kieran Walsh, NUI Galway.

References

Ayalon, L., & Tesch-Römer, C. (2018). *Contemporary perspectives on ageism*. https://link.springer.com/content/pdf/10.1007%2F978-3-319-73820-8.pdf. Accessed 8 Dec 2019.

Barr, N., & Crawford, I. (2005). *Financing higher education: Answers from the UK*. London/New York: Routledge.

Barwick, M., Phipps, D., Myers, G., Johnny, M., & Coriandoli, R. (2014). Knowledge translation and strategic communications: Unpacking differences and similarities for scholarly and research communications. *Scholarly and Research Communications, 5*, 1–14. https://doi.org/10.22230/src.2014v5n3a175.

Beard, J., & Bloom, D. (2015). Towards a comprehensive public health response to population ageing. *The Lancet, 385*(99968), 658–661.

Cast from clay. (2018). *A new model for think tank communications*. Blog. https://castfromclay.co.uk/blog/2018/8/7/a-new-model-for-think-tank-communications-part-ii. Accessed 8 Dec 2019

European Commission. (2015). *Growing the European silver economy*. http://ec.europa.eu/research/innovation-union/pdf/active-healthy-ageing/silvereco.pdf. Accessed 13 Dec 2019.

Frameworks Institute. (2020). *How do we do it?* https://www.frameworksinstitute.org/sfa-overview.html. Accessed 2 Nov 2019.

Government of New Zealand. (2019). *The well-being budget 2019*. https://treasury.govt.nz/sites/default/files/2019-05/b19-well-being-budget.pdf. Accessed 8 Dec 2019.

Grenier, A., & Guberman, N. (2009). Creating and sustaining disadvantage; the relevance of a social exclusion framework. *Health & Social Care in the Community, 17*(2), 116–124.

HelpAge International. (2016, December). *International glossary* (Unpublished paper).

HelpAge International. (2019a, July). *Ageing and the SDGs, ensuring visibility and inclusion of older people*. London: HelpAge International.

HelpAge International. (2019b, August). *Operational definitions* (Unpublished paper).

HelpAge International. (2019c). *An older world with increasing exposure to disasters*. Infographic.

HelpAge International and AARP. (2018). *Global AgeWatch insights, the right to health, the right to be counted*. London: HelpAge International.

HelpAge International and AARP. (2019). *Tanzania insights, the right to health and access to universal health coverage for older people*. London: HelpAge International.

Inter-Agency and Expert Group on Sustainable Development Goal Indicators. *Final list of proposed Sustainable Development Indicators* (E/CN.3/2016/2/Rev.1). https://sustainabledevelopment.un.org/content/documents/11803Official-List-of-Proposed-SDG-Indicators.pdf. Accessed 8 Dec 2019.

International Labour Organisation. (2017). *World social protection report 2017–19*. Geneva: ILO.

Juergens, F. (2019). *Supporting MANEPO's advocacy for the establishment of a universal social pension in Malawi* (Unpublished paper).

Mihnovits, A. (2020, June). *Official statistics and COVID-19, capturing evidence on older people for response and recovery*. HelpAge International.

Peroni, L., & Timmer, A. (2013). Vulnerable groups: The promise of an emerging concept in European human rights convention law. *International Journal of Constitutional Law, 11*(4), 1056–1085.

Phoenix, C., & Parravani, E. (2019). *Older people's experiences of ageing and ageism in Serbia, Costa Rica, Pakistan and the Gambia*. London: HelpAge International.

Pullinger, J. (2018). *Why we need better data to improve the lives of ageing populations*. https://civilservice.blog.gov.uk/2018/12/13/why-we-need-better-data-to-improve-the-lives-of-ageing-populations/.Blog. Accessed 8 Dec 2019

Republic of Rwanda. (2019). *2019 Rwanda Voluntary National Review (VNR) report*. https://rwandaun.org/site/rwanda-voluntary-national-review-2019/.pdf. Accessed 3 Nov 2019.

Sleap, B. (2019a). *Living, not just surviving*. London: HelpAge International.

Sleap, B. (2019b). *Keeping our dignity*. London: HelpAge International.

Stakeholder Group on Ageing. (2019, September 24–25). *Presentation by Roseline Kihumba on behalf of Stakeholder Group on Ageing to CSO Forum held during SDG Summit* (Unpublished paper).

Straus, S. E., Tetroe, J., & Graham, I. (2009). Defining knowledge translation. *CMAJ, 181*(3–4), 165–168. https://doi.org/10.1503/cmaj.081229.

The SDGs Kenya Forum. (2019). *The second progress report on implementation of SDGs in Kenya, Civil Society Report 2019*. http://planning.go.ke/wp-content/uploads/2019/07/Reformatted-Template.pdf. Accessed 3 Nov 2019.

The Sustainable Development Goals Center for Africa, Sustainable Development Solutions Network. (2019). *2019 Africa SDG Index and Dashboards Report*. https://sdgindex.org/reports/2019-africa-sdg-index-and-dashboards-report/. Accessed 3 Nov 2019.

Tilley, H., Shaxson, L., Young, J., Rea, J., & Ball, L. (2017). *10 things to know about how to influence policy with research*. London: ODI.

United Nations. (2015). *Transforming our world: The 2030 agenda for sustainable development, A/Res/70/1*. https://sustainabledevelopment.un.org/post2015/transformingourworld/publication. Accessed 6 Dec 2019.

United Nations. (2019). *Follow-up to the international year of older persons: Second world assembly on ageing* (Report of the Secretary General to the General Assembly). https://undocs.org/A/74/170. Accessed 3 Nov 2019.

United Nations Department of Economic and Social Affairs (UNDESA). (2019). *World population ageing 2019 highlights*. New York: United Nations.

United Nations, Economic and Social Council. (2018). *Report of the inter-agency and expert group on Sustainable Development Indicators*. Note by the Secretary General to the Statistical Commission. https://unstats.un.org/unsd/statcom/50th-session/documents/2019-2-IAEG-SDG-EE.pdf. Accessed 3 Nov 2019.

United Nations, Economic and Social Council. (2019). *Special edition: progress towards the Sustainable Development Goals* (Report of the Secretary General to the High Level Political forum on sustainable development. E/2019/68). https://unstats.un.org/sdgs/files/report/2019/secretary-general-sdg-report-2019%2D%2DEN.pdf. Accessed 3 Nov 2019.

United Republic of Tanzania. (2019). *Voluntary National Review (VNR) 2019, Empowering people and ensuring inclusiveness and equality*. https://www.nbs.go.tz/index.php/en/sdg/428-voluntary-national-review-vnr-2019-empowering-people-and-ensuring-inclusiveness-and-equality.pdf. Accessed 3 Nov 2019.

UNSD and World Bank. (2 June 2020). The global COVID-19 survey of National Statistical Offices, preview of main results presented at Open virtual meeting of the IAEG-SDG, Covid-19 impacts and resources on data collection, SDG monitoring and on vulnerable groups, 2 June 2020, https://unstats.un.org/sdgs/meetings/virtual-2jun2020/

Viennet, R., & Pont, B. (2017). *Education policy implementation: A literature review and proposed framework* (OECD Education Working Paper No. 162). http://www.oecd.org/official-documents/publicdisplaydocumentpdf. Accessed 8 Dec 2019.

Walsh, K., Scharf, T., & Keating, N. (2017). Social exclusion of older persons: A scoping review and conceptual framework. *European Journal of Ageing, 14*, 81–98. https://doi.org/10.1007/s10433-016.

Chapter 29
The Role of Pension Policies in Preventing Old-Age Exclusion

Jim Ogg

29.1 Introduction

Pension systems are a major component in reducing social exclusion in older-age. The introduction of pensions throughout many countries during the twentieth century was primarily a measure designed to reduce poverty in old-age. Without pensions, few options were available for older people to secure an income, and an absence of income is one of the main determinants of social exclusion in later life (Walsh et al. 2017). Many, if not most of the jobs associated with industrial or agricultural economies of the early twentieth century were manual and demanding and, in the absence of developed retirement systems, most older people worked until they were physically unable to continue. Levels of income in paid employment over the life course were mostly insufficient to enable saving for retirement. In the absence of pensions, intergenerational family transfers (including cohabitation), mainly by children to their ageing parents, were the most common form of ensuring that basic needs in old-age were met.

As state pension systems were introduced and with universal coverage in most industrialised societies, retirement became an institutional period of the life course, defined as an absence of paid work and the receipt of a guaranteed income (Kohli 2007). To be sure, most pensions were well below the level of income workers had received before retirement. For example, although pensions had become almost universal in the United Kingdom (UK) by the 1950s, their level was low compared to previous wages and most retirees did not have enough pension income to participate fully in social life. Writing at the time, Peter Townsend in his study of the family life of older people noted that:

J. Ogg (✉)
Caisse Nationale d'assurance Vieillesse, Paris, France
e-mail: jim.ogg@cnav.fr

K. Walsh et al. (eds.), *Social Exclusion in Later Life*, International Perspectives on Aging 28, https://doi.org/10.1007/978-3-030-51406-8_29

> If the pension had ensured a more comfortable standard of life men might not have had the depressing sense of having become "poor relations" and might have held their heads higher among their children (Townsend 1957, p.147).

Nevertheless, as the value of pensions continued to rise throughout the 1960s and 1970s, the gains in terms of enabling older people to participate fully in the social and civic life of their communities were numerous. Workers were able to look forward to a planned and secure retirement, in the knowledge that they would receive a guaranteed income. Pensions that were calculated on the basis of "defined benefits" became widespread and workers mostly knew in advance the value of their pension since the benefits accrued were linked to earnings and employment careers and the level of future pension was pre-defined and guaranteed. Occupational pensions administered by employers also developed alongside the "first pillar" state pensions. With income security in old-age, residential independence became the norm, as witnessed by the large increase throughout western Europe in the number of older one-person households during the 1960s. Older people relied less and less on their kin for their basic needs. A regular income in old-age also enabled retirees to participate in leisure and cultural activities, thereby reducing significantly the risk of social exclusion. This led to what some commentators have referred to as a "golden age" in the history of pensions. In the UK, the majority of early baby boomers (individuals born in the late 1940s and early 1950s) who began to enter retirement at the beginning of the twenty-first century and who were living in a couple, received total pension incomes at the same or higher level than the incomes they received when they were working (Chandler and Tetlow 2014). In such situations, social exclusion in old-age was significantly reduced and where it did exist, factors other than income were determinant.

As pension systems developed and coverage extended to all workers, specific redistributive elements were also incorporated to protect older people from poverty, either by ensuring a minimum level of pension income for retirees whose contributions would not normally allow an adequate pension, or by providing a basic income to individuals who had never worked. Survivor pensions also became common, whereby the loss of income caused by the death of a spouse with pension rights (usually a man) was compensated by transferring a proportion of the pension to the remaining spouse. These measures were, and still are, important components of pension systems and they are discussed in more detail below.

29.2 The Contribution of Pensions to Income Adequacy

Clearly, pensions have played a major role in the reduction of poverty (Jeffreys 1989), although the accumulation of assets is also an important factor. Recent figures relating to Europe show that from 2008 to 2016, the number of people aged 65 and over at risk of poverty or social exclusion in the European Union (EU) decreased by around 1.9 million (OECD 2018). Moreover, pensions mitigate against material deprivation, defined as "the inability to possess the goods and services and/or engage in activities that are ordinary in the society or that are socially perceived as 'necessities;'" (Fusco et al. 2010, p.7) [see also Ogg and Myck, Chap. 2, Sumil-Laanemaa et al., Chap. 3, and Myck et al., Chap. 24, this volume for a discussion and empirical analysis of material deprivation in later life]. Although it is difficult to quantify the impact that pensions have on reducing exclusion and on living standards in general, one measure is the theoretical replacement rate (TRR), an indicator of the level of pension income after retirement as a percentage of individual earnings at the moment a pension is claimed (or as an average of earnings). Figure 29.1 shows the TRR in a selected number of European and near-neighbour countries. In 2017, on average in the European Union (28 countries), the replacement ratio of pensions was 0.58, illustrating their important role in the provision of adequate incomes in old-age.

This important role that pensions play in providing income in old-age conceals gender differences, more commonly known as the gender pension gap that represents the difference between the average pre-tax income received as a pension by women and compared to men. As far as pensions in the EU 28 are concerned, the gender pension gap ranges from 1.8 to 48.7%, with an average of 37.2% for individuals in the age group 65–79 years (OECD 2018, p.69). Recent trends suggest that "while slight decreases in gender gaps in pensions have been observed in the EU on average since the [global financial] crisis, the gaps remain almost stable in many countries, including in those where it is highest" (OECD 2018, p.70).

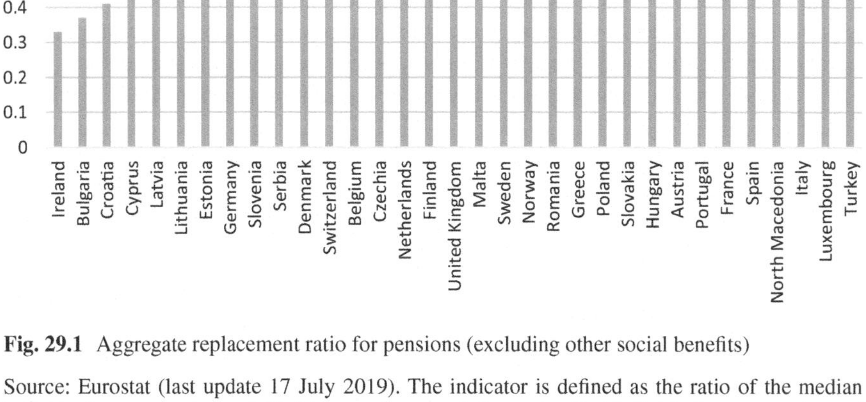

Fig. 29.1 Aggregate replacement ratio for pensions (excluding other social benefits)

Source: Eurostat (last update 17 July 2019). The indicator is defined as the ratio of the median individual gross pensions of 65–74 age category relative to median individual gross earnings of 50–59 age category, excluding other social benefits. The indicator is based on the EU-SILC (statistics on income, social inclusion and living conditions)

A longer life expectancy for women has consequences for income in later life, especially bearing in mind higher rates of poverty among older women compared to men. More than 20% of women aged 65 years and above are at risk of poverty or social exclusion in the EU, compared to 15% of men in the same age group (OECD 2018).

In addition to gender inequalities, other sectors of the population are disadvantaged in terms of access to pensions. International migration and the administrative barriers in harmonising a working career undertaken in two or more countries places specific risks of exclusion on migrant workers. In the EU, mobile citizens are entitled to a pension from each Member State in which they were insured. However, accessibility rules differ between countries as, for example, when a condition of residence is required to obtain a pension. Also, some countries allow access to their pension systems for regular migrants working in sectors such as agricultural work, construction work or social care, whereas in other countries this is not the case. For these workers, who in retirement return to their home country, the "portability" of the rights they have accrued and the ability to access them once in their home country poses substantial risks for exclusion in old-age. Inequalities in access to pensions also exist for individuals who have not been able to fulfil the eligibility requirements for a pension due to career gaps because of disability and poor health. Since income in old-age is mainly provided through pensions, and pensions are dependent on paid work over the life course, disabled individuals who cannot secure full-time paid work over the life course are exposed to specific risks.

Although the contribution that pensions have made to minimising social exclusion is beyond doubt, there have been a number of important systemic changes to the way that pensions are calculated and managed. Central to these changes is the shift away from the public sector and employers' responsibility to ensure adequate pensions, to the individualisation of retirement income responsibility. Through tax incentives, policies have been introduced encouraging individuals to make personal provision for their pensions, mostly through financial markets managed by intermediaries (banks, asset management companies etc.). Ageing populations have particular consequences for pension systems, particularly those which rely upon pay-as-you-go systems, whereby current contributions finance current pension expenditure. Again, shifts towards defined contributions within public first pillar pension systems place the responsibility for accumulating pension rights firmly on the individual. As Krekula and Vickerstaff (2020) note, "this narrative of individual responsibility replaces an earlier sense of moral economy in which the reproduction of labour meant that the young and old had privileged positions in society based on their future and past contributions" (2020, p. 38). Under these circumstances, the very notion of retirement is brought into question (Phillipson 2019) since certain sectors of the population are obliged to continue working to secure an adequate income in old-age. Moreover, changing labour markets and economic crises often undermine the ability of older individuals to find paid work or lead to a reduction in the value of their pensions due to the bad performance of pension funds and investments. In addition, financial crises, past and ongoing, adversely affect women since they are more likely than men to be employed in the temporary, low-skilled and part-time jobs that result from economic downturns. The risks of social exclusion in the face of these transformations are spread unequally throughout society, and many pension systems are grappling with the problem of squaring the circle of sustainability and equity. In the following section, we examine three major challenges that pension systems face if they are to continue to be one of the main mechanisms in preventing exclusion in old-age: financial sustainability; pensions and global finance; and creating stable labour markets.

29.3 Challenges for Pension Systems

29.3.1 Financial Sustainability

Faced with ageing populations and increased life expectancy, structural changes to pension systems have been, and continue to be, necessary in order to ensure their financial sustainability. Three parameters that are common to all pension systems can be adjusted. First, the duration of contributions over the working life that are needed in order to receive a full pension can be increased. Most countries have adopted this measure as well as switching to (or introducing) a defined contribution system whereby the level of contributions and not the final benefit, is pre-defined. Moreover, the amount of pension that is finally paid depends not only on the duration of contributions, but also on the return of investments made by the pension scheme. In this way, building-up a pension can be likened to a savings scheme in which the final amount paid out depends upon how much is paid in and how well or badly the savings have performed in the financial market. Defined contribution pension schemes (whether public, occupational or private), and the increased duration of contributions which is a feature of them, clearly have consequences for economic exclusion in later life. Since it is necessary to work longer in order to secure an adequate pension, many individuals who cannot work through illness, disability or because of caring responsibilities within the family, together with those who cannot find work, are exposed to a heightened risk of entering older-age without an adequate level of income. Protective measures for these vulnerable groups are discussed in the next main section.

The second parameter of adjustment to pension systems which aims to maintain financial sustainability is the raising of the minimum age of pension eligibility. Again, most European countries have adopted this measure (with some, notably Poland, oscillating between increasing and decreasing the minimum state pension age according to the political ideology of governments in office). As with the shift from defined contribution pension schemes, the working life is extended and certain groups are exposed to the risk of economic exclusion.

The third parameter of reform consists of reducing the value of a pension. Although extending the working life and linking pensions to life expectancy also means that the total value of pensions paid out is lower than it would have been in the absence of these reforms, it is also possible to reduce the value of individual pensions. Politically unpopular, most governments avoid this adjustment, although it was one made by the Greek government following the 2008 global financial crisis (Tinio and Lyberaki 2012). An alternative to cutting the total amount of pension paid is to make changes to the indexation of pensions (mostly from wages to prices). For example, in 2017 in Australia, a change in the indexation of pensions to prices instead of average male weekly earnings resulted in lower pensions for 330,000 retirees (Brooke 2020).

29.3.2 Pensions and Global Finance

Coupled with the shift to defined benefit contributions and the individualisation of pension income responsibility through the growth of occupational and private pensions is the increasing role of globalised financial markets in pension systems. Pension systems based on long-term savings schemes invested in financial markets gained world-wide popularity from the 1980s (notably in the case of Chile). In Europe, "several countries, including Sweden and some new Member States such as Bulgaria, Estonia, Croatia, Latvia, Lithuania, Hungary, Poland and Slovakia, have switched part of their public pension schemes into (quasi-) mandatory private funded schemes" (European Commission 2018, p.51). As with any financial investment, significant risks are borne in the management of pension funds and the total value of a pension is determined by the performance of the funds (and how they have been managed). Following the 2008 global financial crisis, the value of pensions was literally wiped out in some countries, notably in Greece but also for some pension funds in the United States of America: "The 2008 economic crisis wreaked havoc on the value of older Americans" individual retirement resources. The value of defined contribution plan balances shrunk as the stock market dropped, equity in housing plummeted, and many had to tap into retirement savings in pre-retirement years to make ends meet" (Street and Ní Léime 2020).

Since the 2008 economic crisis, European occupational pension funds "continue to be negatively affected by the persistent low interest rate environment" (European Insurance and Occupational Pensions Authority 2019, p.34). Many countries have legislated to tighten up investment risk strategies, particularly in relation to supplementary pensions (occupational and private). In 2019, the European Parliament and EU member states reached an agreement on the proposal for a pan-European personal pension product (PEPP), a voluntary scheme for saving for retirement with "strong consumer protection" (European Commission 2019). Within individual countries, protection measures usually take the form of an overseeing regulatory body, as is the case in Ireland since 2018: if a pension fund is in deficit, a financial proposal must be submitted to the Pensions Authority within 6 months.

Hassel and Wiβ (2019) point out that the global financial crisis has led to "a re-assessment of the role of pre-funded private pensions as a complementary, rather than a superior, source of old-age income" (p.1). They suggest that collective occupational schemes administered by social partners may be one solution to counter the trend of treating pension funds in the same way as any investment strategy. Nevertheless, risks will always be a component of pension funds with new and perhaps unforeseen risks on the horizon. A recent article in the Financial Times, for example, stated that "fourteen of the UK's biggest pension funds have been warned by lawyers they risk legal action if they fail to consider the effects of climate change on their portfolios" (Financial Times, 13 August 2018).

Controlling the financial management of pension funds may go some way to protecting the future value of total pension income. However, with the increasing individualisation of pension income responsibility, many governments are placing the onus on individuals to devise and choose their own investment strategies and to be accountable for the gains and losses. The assumption is that given the "right" information, individuals are able to make informed choices regarding the financial products on offer with regard to a future pension. However, this assumption is problematic. Kaifala et al. (2019) question the way in which financial experts and accountants treat the key dimensions of pensions, such as their predictability and stability and the way in which information is communicated to clients. Also, the high degree of financial literacy needed to make informed investment choices for future pension income excludes large sectors of the population who do not have such skills.

29.3.3 Creating Stable Labour Markets

Pensions are built up through paid work, but in recent years labour markets have been characterised by an increase in precarious and low-paid jobs that fail to allow the work-force to build up sufficient contributions for their pensions. For example, "during the financial crisis of 2008–2013, Finland's proportion of precarious work increased to 13%, surpassing 1990s recession levels" (Salonen et al. 2020). The rise in short-term contracts and part-time jobs affects particularly young adults who enter the labour market for the first time and older adults who seek to remain in it. Moreover, many, if not most, of the jobs that are insecure are low-paid and entail low-quality work. Working conditions are often harsh and older workers commonly lack skills that would enable them to diversify or are quite simply physically not able to undertake the jobs on offer. Improving the quality of working conditions is therefore an important component of safeguarding adequate pension income.

Retaining older workers in the labour force also requires significant investment in training and the acquisition of new skills. Older workers will need to keep up with technology advances, introduced into their workplace, especially as human labour is replaced by automation. Although there are examples of good practice in the training of older workers, ageism means that they receive less training than younger workers (Krekula 2018) and they are often excluded from new technology training.

29.4 Protective Measures Against Exclusion in Pension Systems

The challenges to pension systems described above mean that it will be crucial in the coming years to ensure that "first pillar" pension schemes retain a redistributive element that protects the most vulnerable sectors of society in the event of not being able to build up sufficient sources of income in old-age. In some countries, a minimum guaranteed pension exists for individuals with no or low financial resources although their value can differ substantially from one country to another. For example, in France, the *Allocation de solidarité aux personnes âgées* (ASPA) is paid by the state National Pension Fund (€868.20 per month in 2019) to individuals aged 65 years and above whose contributions are low and who would normally have received a pension lower than the ASPA rate. A "social pension also exists in Bulgaria for people aged 70 years and above when the annual income of a member of their household is less than the guaranteed minimum income established in the country in the previous 12 months…this social monthly pension is 120.98лв (€62), one-third of the amount that is set as the poverty line (314 лв or €160 for 2017)" (Trifonova and Lillova 2020).

"Top-up" pensions are also important where individuals have had long careers and made full contributions to the pension system, but on account of their low wages would normally receive a low pension. For example, in Austria, although there is no minimum pension, retirees with low earnings-related benefits receive a means-tested top-up (*Ausgleichszulage*) which in 2017 amounted to €889.84 per month for a single-person household (Hass et al. 2020).

In many countries, survivor pensions are important in maintaining incomes. Survivor pensions were designed to protect spouses who risked a large fall in income when their husband/wife died. Given the typically greater life expectancy of women over men, the beneficiaries of survivor pensions are mostly women, and this source of income is especially important where no or limited pension rights have been built up. However, in most countries survivor pensions were paid only in the case of marriage or registered partnerships, with common-law spouses being excluded. In some countries, such as Finland, survivor pensions were also designed to protect under-age children (who lived with the surviving spouse). With changing family configurations, many survivor pensions are being reformed, and in some countries there is considerable debate over the need to abolish them given that many women have acquired their own pension rights and therefore a survivor pension is not needed. Abolishing survivor pensions outright would undoubtedly place some women at risk of not receiving an adequate income and it will be important for future policy to make pensions more inclusive and adapted to societal transformations.

Pension systems will need to take into account workers in hazardous jobs for whom it is unreasonable to suppose that they should extend their working life in order to secure adequate pension income. Measures are in place in some countries. For example, in Austria, workers in physically demanding jobs for at least 10 of the 20 years immediately preceding the legal retirement age ("heavy labour pension") can retire early (OECD 2017). In France, a personal account aimed at preventing the impact of harsh working conditions was introduced in 2016. Since October 2017, the definition of annual thresholds identifies six occupational risk factors. The account allows employees exposed beyond the thresholds to gain points, which can be used to fund either training opportunities to access less arduous jobs, or a reduction in working hours with wage-loss compensation or retiring earlier with a maximum of 2 years earlier than the legal age of retirement. These measures contribute to safeguarding adequate pension income and reducing exclusion in old-age.

29.5 Conclusion

Pension systems play a crucial role in preventing social exclusion in later life. As countries address current demographic and economic challenges, it will become increasingly important to ensure that all sectors of society are protected against economic exclusion in old-age. This means addressing issues such as the extended working life and the consequences for individuals excluded from paid work, tackling gender pay gaps throughout a working career, increasing the "portability" of accrued pension rights between countries for migrant workers, and greater recognition of the value of unpaid work through measures that give access to pensions. Future generations of retirees are likely to have more diverse profiles than current generations, with important sectors of the population who will have accumulated periods of inactivity and low pay. The increasing deinstitutionalisation of the life course and the continued spectre of neo-liberal policies based on individual responsibility for the provision of income in older-age pose specific risks to the sustainability of pension systems hitherto built on the premises of intergenerational solidarity and equity. Redistributive measures will continue to be necessary, either being built-in to pension systems or aligned with them. These can be provided by fiscal reforms and the provision of universal basic pensions indexed to the purchasing power of working populations. Given these measures, the risk of economic exclusion in old-age can be significantly reduced, allowing individuals and their families to fully participate in all domains of social life.

Editors' Postscript

Please note, like other contributions to this book, this chapter was written before the COVID-19 pandemic of 2020. The book's introductory chapter (Chap. 1) and conclusion (Chap. 34) consider some of the key ways in which the pandemic relates to issues concerning social exclusion and ageing.

References

Brooke, E. (2020). Australia. In A. Ní Léime, J. Ogg, D. Street, C. Krekula, M. Rašticová, M. Bédiová, & I. Madero-Cabib (Eds.), *Extended working life policies: International gender and health perspectives* (pp. 129–139). New York: Springer.

Chandler, D., & Tetlow, G. (2014). *Retirement in the 21st century* (IFS report R98). London: Institute of Fiscal Studies.

European Commission. (2018). *The 2018 ageing report. Economic & budgetary projections for the 28 EU Member States (2016–2070)*. Brussels: European Commission.

European Commission. (2019). *Press release: Capital Markets Union: Commission welcomes political agreement on new rules to help consumers save for retirement*. https://europa.eu/rapid/press-release_IP-19-1108_en.htm. Accessed 1 Aug 2019.

European Insurance and Occupational Pensions Authority. (2019). *Financial stability* (Report June 2019). Luxembourg: Publications Office of the European Union.

Fusco, A., Guio, A.-C., & Marlier, E. (2010). *Income poverty and material deprivation in European countries, theme: Population and social conditions*. Collection: Methodologies and working papers, European Union, 2010, Cat. No. KS-RA-10-030-EN-N.

Haas, B., Gstrein, M., & Bildsteiner, R. (2020). Austria. In A. Ní Léime, J. Ogg, D. Street, C. Krekula, M. Rašticová, M. Bédiová, & I. Madero-Cabib (Eds.), *Extended working life policies: International gender and health perspectives* (pp. 141–152). New York: Springer.

Hassel, A., & Wiβ, T. (2019). The political economy of pension financialisation: Public policy responses to the crisis. *Journal of European Public Policy, 26*, SI. https://doi.org/10.1080/13501763.2019.1575455.

Jeffreys, M. (Ed.). (1989). *Growing old in the twentieth century*. London: Routledge.

Kaifala, G.B., Paisey, C., & Paisey, N. J. (2019). The UK pensions landscape – A critique of the role of accountants and accounting technologies in the treatment of social and societal risks. Critical Perspectives on Accounting. Available online: https://doi.org/10.1016/j.cpa.2019.06.005. Accessed 4 July 2019.

Kohli, M. (2007). The institutionalization of the life course: Looking back to look ahead. *Research in Human Development, 4*(3–4), 253–271.

Krekula, C. (2018). Time, precarisation and age normality: On internal job mobility among men in manual work. *Ageing & Society, 39*, 2290–2307. https://doi.org/10.1017/S0144686X1800137X.

Krekula, C., & Vickerstaff, S. (2020). The 'older worker' and the 'ideal worker': A critical examination of concepts and categorisations in the rhetoric of extending working lives. In A. Ní Léime, J. Ogg, D. Street, C. Krekula, M. Rašticová, M. Bédiová, & I. Madero-Cabib (Eds.), *Extended working life policies: International gender and health perspectives* (pp. 29–47). New York: Springer.

OECD. (2017). *Key policies to promote longer working lives. Various countries*. https://www.oecd.org/els/emp_Key%20policies_Final.pdf. Accessed 3 July 2019.

OECD. (2018). *Pensions at a glance 2017. OECD and G20 indicators*. Paris: OECD Publishing. https://doi.org/10.1787/pension_glance-2017-en. Accessed 4 Mar 2019.

Phillipson, C. (2019). 'Fuller' or 'extended' working lives? Critical perspectives on changing transitions from work to retirement. *Ageing & Society, 39*(3), 629–665.

Salonen, L., Kähäri, A., & Pietilä, I. (2020). Finland. In A. Ní Léime, J. Ogg, D. Street, C. Krekula, M. Rašticová, M. Bédiová, & I. Madero-Cabib (Eds.), *Extended working life policies: International gender and health perspectives* (pp. 251–260). New York: Springer.

Street, D., & Ní Léime, Á. (2020). Problems and prospects for current policies to extend working lives. In A. Ní Léime, J. Ogg, D. Street, C. Krekula, M. Rašticová, M. Bédiová, & I. Madero-Cabib (Eds.), *Extended working life policies: International gender and health perspectives* (pp. 85–113). New York: Springer.

Tinio, P., & Lyberaki, A. (2012). Labour and pensions in the Greek crisis: The microfoundations of disaster cover. *Südosteuropa. Zeitschrift für Politik und Gesellschaft., 3*, 363–386.

Townsend, P. (1957). *The family life of old people*. London: Routledge/Kegan & Paul.

Trifonova, T., & Lillova, K. (2020). Bulgaria. In A. Ní Léime, J. Ogg, D. Street, C. Krekula, M. Rašticová, M. Bédiová, & I. Madero-Cabib (Eds.), *Extended working life policies: International gender and health perspectives* (pp. 173–182). New York: Springer.

Walsh, K., Scharf, T., & Keating, N. (2017). Social exclusion of older persons: A scoping review and conceptual framework. *European Journal of Ageing, 14*, 81–98. https://doi.org/10.1007/s10433-016.

Chapter 30
Social Policy for Older People in the Post-Soviet Space: How Do Pension Systems and Social Services Influence Social Exclusion?

Irina Grigoryeva, Oksana Parfenova, and Alexandra Dmitrieva

30.1 Introduction

Various approaches currently exist to conceptualising and measuring social exclusion (Burchardt and Le Grand 2002; Walsh et al. 2017). By expanding the concept of poverty and material limitations, researchers have shown that exclusion can be defined not only as a lack of financial opportunities, but also as a sum total of various barriers (in education, access to healthcare, labour market participation etc.) that jeopardise an individual's or a group's social and systemic integration (Sen 1999). Exclusion has begun to be interpreted as not only material, but also symbolic limitations, a disruption of social and symbolic connections (Silver 1994). The vertical class stratification has been replaced by a horizontal differentiation that distinguishes insiders from outsiders (Abrahamson 2001). In this sense, both individuals and specific groups of people may experience forms of social exclusion (Levitas et al. 2007). The social status of older people, particularly in the post-Soviet space, is characterised by multiple structural barriers that prevent them from enjoying an active lifestyle. Some of these barriers are hard to overcome, as they have to do with older people's state of health. Older people can become marginalised not only through financial insecurity, but also through loss of social contacts linked to the workplace and a reduced ability to socialise with friends and family. The latter is of growing relevance as a result of strong family nuclearisation (Eliseeva and Kletsin 2010).

I. Grigoryeva (✉)
University of St. Petersburg, St. Petersburg, Russia
e-mail: soc28@yandex.ru

O. Parfenova
Sociological Institute of FCTAS RAS, St. Petersburg, Russia

A. Dmitrieva
Support, Research and Development Center (SRDC), Kyiv, Ukraine

K. Walsh et al. (eds.), *Social Exclusion in Later Life*, International Perspectives on Aging 28, https://doi.org/10.1007/978-3-030-51406-8_30

Evidence from European Union (EU) member states suggests that older adults experience less social exclusion in countries with greater levels of social protection, with income and health conditions having more impact on social exclusion than age and gender (Jehoel-Gijsbers and Vrooman 2008). A recent scoping review identified six key domains relating to social exclusion of older people: neighbourhood and community; services, amenities and mobility; social relations; material and financial resources; socio-cultural aspects; and civic participation (Walsh et al. 2017). In our analysis, we consider policies relating to pensions and social services, which belong to the material and financial resources and services, amenities and mobility domains, respectively.

Against this background, post-Soviet countries illustrate the complexity of challenges relating to social exclusion, as later life in these countries is marked by relatively poor health, low life expectancies, and reduced quality of life. Using the examples of Russia and Ukraine, this chapter examines characteristics of the two most important spheres of social welfare, pension provision and social services, and considers how these are changing. Using the examples of Russia and Ukraine, we pose the question: how do modern pension reforms and the structure of social services in the post-Soviet space affect the social exclusion of older people? Russia and Ukraine were chosen because they illustrate important policy trends, given their ageing populations, both countries have rather lagged behind other post-Soviet states in introducing vital pension reforms and in reforming social services for older people. Moreover, pension reforms in both countries began almost simultaneously – in 2018 in Ukraine and 2019 in Russia – and continue to progress at the time of writing.

Starting from the 1990s, falling living standards could be observed across the entire post-Soviet space due to inflation and cuts in pension benefits. Researchers who analyse the overhaul of Russian social policies in the new market environment consider post-Soviet bureaucracy, unable to adapt to the new market conditions, to be the main obstacle to reform (Cook 2007; Grigoryeva 2017). Examining the transformation of the post-Communist "legacy" into Russian social policies, Cook (2007) concluded that by 2007 the sphere of social security in Russia manifested a relatively low level of social security and excluded a significant portion of the population from basic services and social insurance and service provision. One can counter her argument by pointing out that, at the time, everyone was and still is covered by compulsory medical insurance and universal pension insurance or provision. Persons falling short of the length of service required for an occupational pension receive a social pension. Contemporary studies into Russian state-operated services for older people show, however, that there is now even more bureaucracy in the sphere of social services, and that has become a problem not only for older service users but also for service providers (Parfenova 2018; Grigoryeva et al. 2019a, b; also see Széman et al. this volume).

In considering our research question in the sections that follow, we draw on an analysis of legislation relating to pension and social services reforms in Russia and Ukraine, publicly available statistical data, and evidence from research conducted in both countries.

30.2 The Russian Case

The need to reform the pension system, modify its parameters, and give more careful consideration to individual insurance rights (unaccounted for due to closure of numerous companies and their employees having no documentation to prove their length of service), has been discussed in Russia since the mid-1990s. A series of laws have been passed to that effect, including, for example, the law *On Individual (Personalised) Accounting in the Compulsory Pension Insurance System,* and all citizens now receive an individual social security card (FL 27, 1996). This has, however, proved to be a mere formality. The new law had no effect on pension payments, since these are calculated based not on the data thus accounted for, but on a special averaging formula. In 2001, basic laws on pension provision (FL 166, 2001) and pension insurance (FL 167, 2001) were adopted that made provisions for a three-pillar pension consisting of old-age security, insurance payments, and personal savings. However, due to companies constantly being in tax arrears and the Pension Fund of the Russian Federation growing ever more dependent on transfers from the state budget, actual pension payments failed to exceed the minimum wage and did not keep pace with inflation.

Also noteworthy is the falling average life expectancy across the post-Soviet space, especially among men. By the mid-2010s, this tendency had considerably slowed down, but average male life expectancy has not yet reached 70 years, as was the case during the Soviet era. It was exactly this relatively short average lifespan and, especially, the low healthy life expectancy that constituted the principal argument against increasing retirement ages. For men, the relatively short post-retirement survival period has persisted, and the gender gap has remained static. In comparison with Russia's nearest neighbours, such as Finland, and other post-Soviet states, Russia has the shortest length of life (including healthy life expectancy) among both men and women (Table 30.1).

The requirement for pension reform was nevertheless constantly felt and brought up in Russia, as well as in the Ukraine. The government of the Russian Federation announced the launch of the pension reform on 14th June 2018. Two days later, a draft of the federal law *On Amendments to Certain Legal Acts of the Russian Federation Regarding the Granting and Payment of Pensions* was introduced for

Table 30.1 Life expectancy and healthy life expectancy

Country	Average life expectancy at birth (years)		Average healthy life expectancy at birth (years)	
	Men	Women	Men	Women
Russia	66.4	77.2	59.1	67.5
Ukraine	67.6	77.1	60.3	67.6
Finland	78.7	84.2	69.8	73.5
Estonia	73.1	82.1	64.6	71.4
Armenia	71.2	78.1	63.6	68.7

(Source: World Health Organization, 2016)
http://apps.who.int/gho/data/view.main.SDG2016LEXv?lang=en

consideration into the State Duma (Parliament). The main feature of the reform was that retirement age would increase gradually, over a 10-year period (*i.e.* by 2028), to 60 years for women and 65 years for men. The length of pensionable service required to receive an occupational pension would increase to 15 years as early as 2025.

In Russia, prior to the reform, social pensions were available to women from age 55 and to men from age 60 (FL 166, 2001). One of the latest versions of this regularly updated law instantaneously raised the age of retirement to 60 years for women and 65 years for men. This immediately produced a group of around three million people who were to receive no pension whatsoever. The only income transfers they are entitled to are social welfare payments. The most recent amendment of the same law will see these age norms increase by five additional years, to 65 and 70 years respectively for women and men (FL 350, 2018).

In this case, changes will not be implemented immediately but will follow a stipulated timeline from 2019 to 2023. Notably, retirement age for social pension recipients is planned to increase more rapidly than in the case of occupational pensions. The latter are governed by an act that is largely incomprehensible to ordinary citizens concerning the length of pensionable service; according to this act, in 2008 one needed no less than 5 years of service to qualify for an occupational pension. Subsequently, the state increased the required length of service, so that in 2019 an applicant needs to show at least 9 years of employment, and by 2025 the requirement will increase to at least 15 years of employment. However, the difference between an old-age pension with minimal length of pensionable service and that with, say, 30 years of service is insignificant. The average monthly occupational pension awarded on 1st January 2019 amounts to 14,102 RUB (€196), whereas a social pension equals 9904 RUB (€137) (Federal State Statistics Service 2019). Such a negligible difference discourages people from contributing to the national pension scheme or to other social insurance funds. Instead, people frequently declare a fictitious minimum wage, so the employer would pay only minimal social contributions.

Research on employment in retirement in contemporary Russia suggests that many people continue to work after reaching statutory retirement age. They often do so not so much for the extra income as for the desire to remain included in an active social life. Moreover, while older people remain capable of continuing their education, they are limited by common prejudices and the inadequacy of the state's social policies (Rogozin 2012; Grigoryeva et al. 2019a, b). Studies of older people's labour potential in Russia suggest that the situation regarding post-retirement employment will improve once people with sufficient educational resources and the skills necessary to work with new technologies start to retire (Smolkin 2014). However, it is worth noting that different groups of pensioners have different motivations for continuing to work. While some people do not want to retire, others continue to be employed in informal ways for many years.

Along with the pension system transformation, the development of social services for older people took off at the end of the Soviet period. A system of social work and social services, as we currently understand them, began to evolve in Russia in the early 1990s. Development took place in three directions simultaneously: as a system of professional training; conceptualisation of emerging practices and adaptation of theoretical approaches in the Russian context; and a system of social services (social practices) for the population. At present, after the Pension Fund of the Russian Federation, the most notable actor in the sphere of social support is a network of state-operated specialised centres and branches of home care services for older people and persons with disabilities. Home-based care grew rapidly in Russia from late 1980s and early 1990s and by 2017 over one million citizens were being supported by such centres and branches [also see Széman et al. this volume]. This is over five times the number of older people receiving social and socio-medical care in state-operated nursing homes. In 2016, there were 253,382 people living in nursing homes across Russia (Rosstat 2018).

In 2015, a new federal law on social services was passed (Federal Law 442). Transformations that took place in the sphere of social services are best considered in the context of a neoliberal turn. Research suggests that, in practice, liberalisation is limited to a significant increase in service fees, some relaxation of the rules regarding access to services (people can receive services wherever they live rather than only at their registered domicile), and involvement in social services of non-governmental and commercial organisations (Parfenova 2018). Social workers receive higher wages, offset by an increased workload and staff cuts. Paradoxically, along with fee increases and an expanded list of services provided, new regulations also rigidly limit the amount of time allotted for service provision and make it impossible to flexibly modify the number and type of services a client requires. All of this leads to constant manoeuvering both by service recipients and providers forced to replace certain services with others and, consequently, to mutual discontent. The passing of FL 442 did not make the situation for clients cared for at home any better; to the contrary, they were aggravated by increased fees and additional bureaucracy. Due to lack of information or by force of habit in a situation when alternative arrangements are available through non-governmental organisations, older people tend to prefer a governmental service. While experts from state-operated social service centres give the situation a reflexive and critical assessment, their opinions and wishes are not taken into account by the relevant authorities. In the regions (especially in rural areas), NGOs and commercial organisations are virtually non-existent (Parfenova 2018). Apparently, the more functional and flexible services offered by NGOs and commercial organisations lose out to the rather rigid and limited, but “reliable and familiar” state services, the preservation of which is in the interest of all levels of the existing system of social services. Older adults themselves most likely lack information and stick to the familiar format of service. On the whole, in rural areas one can observe an increasing role of informal relations in the sphere of adult social care [see Széman et al. this volume for a more in-depth discussion of the home care provisions in Russia].

Research on social exclusion in the Russian context distinguishes seven parameters of social exclusion: work; health; education and culture; relationships; connections; autonomy; and housing (Tikhonova 2004). When applied to older people with restricted mobility in contemporary Russia, these parameters acquire a specific meaning. Our inquiry into the clients of state-operated social services highlights a number of key points. The category of "work" is practically irrelevant for older people due to poor health. Those who receive home-based social services from the state are, by and large, unfit for work, with some having ceased employment upon retirement. In relation to "health", the situation is also idiosyncratic. In theory, older people have access to medical services. Moreover, they frequently enjoy a certain number of privileges relating to health care. However, older people's state of health is typically so poor that even going to a doctor is often problematic. Physical limitations due to poor health have a visible impact on older adults' lifestyles, with recipients of home-based social services either rarely or never leaving their homes. Things are different for "mobile" service users whose health condition does not prevent them from benefitting from integration measures offered by social services centres. The category of "education and culture" in this case may be seen as elusive. Home-based clients of social services cannot, in fact, satisfy their current needs for education and culture due to poor health, whereas clients from the mobile group, capable of attending excursions and classes, have opportunities for social integration. The category of "connections" is presently hard to assess, while the category "relationships", as our study shows, also draws a distinction between mobile and less mobile older people (Parfenova 2017). In the absence of physical limitations, people who are mobile have more opportunities for integration in communities, both through state-operated social centres and on their own. Disabled service users, nevertheless, get a chance to expand their communicative space through contact with a social worker. The category "autonomy" pre-supposes physical fitness as the major prerequisite for active participation in social life. Thus this parameter is only applicable to mobile service users. In relation to the final category, housing, most clients are provided with accommodation, so no special practices of exclusion are to be found here. Rather, the opposite is true: home-based services are not infrequently required by older people living alone in a place of their own (Parfenova 2017).

30.3 The Ukranian Case

Turning to the case of policy relating to social exclusion of older people in Ukraine, a useful starting point is that expenditure attributed to people of pensionable age represents over 50% of the total Ukrainian social security budget. This is due to the ageing population and a relatively low retirement age, leading to a greater number of persons above the cut-off age, as well as a considerable array of privileges granted to older people (for example, all pensioners have a right to free travel on municipal and peri-urban public transit).

Over the long term, issues associated with the stability and efficacy of the Ukrainian pension system are related to demographic trends, in particular to low fertility and the progressive ageing of the country's population. By 2050, the ratio of persons over 65 years of age to those aged 15–64 is forecast to increase to 38%, and that between pensioners and those paying pension contributions, to 132%

(Social Care 2009). Throughout the post-Soviet period, informal (unregulated) employment on a large scale has characterised the Ukrainian economy, leading to practices of income under-declaration and tax evasion. Even when labour relations were properly formalised, a significant portion of income remained undeclared (in the form of cash payments). Thus, the shortage of funds in the Pension Fund has as much to do with population ageing as with widespread unregulated employment.

Pension reform in Ukraine was introduced in 2018. To this effect, on 3rd October 2017 the Supreme Rada (parliament) adopted the Law of Ukraine №2148-VIII, and, after, The Law No 2449-VIII. The reform introduced gradual changes to a number of pension system parameters over the subsequent 10 years (*i.e.* until 2027). At the core of these changes is the length of pensionable service, which should be 35 years for retirement at age 60. Thus, the Ukrainian pension reform focuses on "legalising" pensionable service, that is, returning labour market and employment to the situation that allows for statutory pension insurance and pension calculation based on length of pensionable service and salary. Immediately, starting from 2018, previously awarded pensions were recalculated based on the average salary in the 3 years preceding retirement (from 2014 to 2016). They currently amount to 3764 UAH (approximately €120) monthly. However, the minimum pension is very small, amounting to only 1564 UAH (approximately €50 monthly). As of 2019, pensions will be calculated based on the average salary in the last 3 years of employment and the cost of 1 year of pensionable service equivalent to 1%. Prior to the reform, the coefficient was equal to 1.35%. In fact, the regulation that the statutory pension is to be calculated based on the average salary of the 3 years preceding retirement is similar to the calculation used during the Soviet period, except that at this earlier time it was the final 2 years of service that calculations were based on. This condition obviously encourages people to access regularised employment, with a reported salary, at least in the last few years before reaching retirement age.

While the statutory age of retirement has formally remained the same, at 60 years for both men and women, in practice requirements for pensionable service have become more stringent. From 2018 onwards, only those Ukrainians are qualified to retire at 60 who have worked and paid pensionable contributions for 25 years and more. Every year, requirements regarding the length of pensionable service will increase by 12 months per year. Thus by 2028, one would need 35 years of pensionable service in order to retire at age 60. In contemporary society, where education and training take up a significant portion of one's life, this will not be straightforward. People falling short of 35 years of pensionable service will only be able to retire at 63 or even 65 years of age. Should someone have under 15 years of pensionable service by the age of 65, they will receive no pension at all. Instead, they will be entitled to receive means-tested social assistance payments, the size of which will be based on the older person's household income.

The Ukrainian pension reform has made provisions for temporary social assistance to citizens in the period between 1st January 2018 and 31st December 2020. It is granted to persons unfit to work who have reached retirement age and have at least 15 years of pensionable service, but no right to an occupational pension. Financial assistance will be provided until the persons who have become unfit to work have reached the age of entitlement to old-age income transfers, equivalent to a minimum wage. Academy member E.M. Libanova, one of the authors of the reform, believes that these 3 years will give people time to acquire all proof of earlier employment not formalised at the time or to have worked the requisite length of time needed to increase their pensionable service and the size of pension, respectively (Libanova 2017). Citing E.M. Libanova, *Novosti Ukrainy* note that "*for a number of years, people were reluctant to receive an officially reported salary*". There are still a lot of people in Ukraine who wish to subsist on social assistance alone:

"Recently at an employers meeting in Ivano-Frankivsk, someone stated that he would be willing to pay up to 15,000 UAH, but his employees requested that he pay them less, albeit under the table. That is, a person wishes to receive a salary, but also not to give up a state subsidy of 3,000 UAH, and this government money means more to them than the same 3,000 UAH they could have earned officially" (Maksimovich 2018).

Social services in the Ukraine were formalised through normative acts somewhat later than in Russia, namely in 2003 in a law entitled *On Social Services* (The Law of Ukraine 2003). For instance, Article 5 of this law makes provisions for two forms of social care: financial assistance and social services. Part 4 of Article 5 of the law defines such social services as social welfare facilities, psychological, socio-pedagogical, socio-medical, socio-economic, legal, advisory services, as well as help with employment and other pratices. This classification is similar to its Russian counterpart. It remains uncertain and incomprehensible precisely which services are included in the "material service". As in Russia, the concepts of service, support, help, protection and such, lack clear definitions and are closely related and thus often overlap. However, in Ukraine, "non-state-operated providers of social services, such as charities and religious organizations, as well as natural persons whose activities have to do with providing social services have become widespread" earlier than in Russia (Gorova 2012, p.446).

30.4 Conclusion

Responding to our principal question of how, using the examples of Russia and Ukraine, recent pension reforms and the structure of social services in the post-Soviet space affect the social exclusion of older people is far from straightforward. In theory, pension reforms in both countries ought to have extended the period of paid employment and increased social inclusion of older adults. However, in practice. The reforms have reduced older people's real incomes. While older people were once able to receive a salary alongside their pension on reaching statutory retirement age, they now have to wait for this opportunity for a few more years. The group at greatest risk of social exclusion in terms of their material circumstances are those older adults who live alone and are no longer able to work due to poor health or a lack of suitable employment, especially in rural areas. In these circumstances, older people have limited opportunities to receive help and support from other sources. Low income, with an average pension equalling 14,151 RUB, (approximately €196 monthly; Russian Pension Foundation 2019), restricted mobility, and a narrow choice of care providers make such individuals most vulnerable to risks of exclusion.

In relation to pension provisions, fair accounting and assessment of pensionable service should be prioritised by policymakers. Moreover, peculiarities typical of older people in post-Soviet nations hinder both pension reform and modernisation of social services. The current cohort of older adults was the first to see itself as "the lost generation". They consider themselves to have been victims of rapid socio-economic change. These people intended to retire according to "Soviet" rules and to receive a decent pension, in spite of the many years that have passed since the fall of the USSR. However, in reality, they did not receive a decent pension and came to realise that they may never again have secure employment comparable to that which they had prior to retirement. At only 60–65 years of age, these pensioners have not yet lost much in terms of qualifications and fitness to work. In practice, employment services offer older people only those vacancies that require few or no qualifications. As a result, in post-Soviet countries, such as Russia and Ukraine, the social elevator only works in one direction in later life – downwards.

Thus, low income combines with chronic illnesses and difficulty accessing quality medical services, especially in remote rural areas, as well as a very basic form of social care offered by monopolistic state-operated service providers. In our view, the combination of these factors serves as the key factor influencing the social exclusion of older people in the post-Soviet space. With pensions and social services representing sub dimensions of exclusion from material and financial resources and from services, amenities and mobility (Walsh et al. 2017), we assume that exclusion in these areas also shapes exclusion in other domains. However, this requires further research and conceptual development. As for modern state policy in Russia and Ukraine, we can identify a need for state policies to focus more strategically on preventing illness, increasing healthy life expectancy, and promoting the practice of self-care in order to reduce risks of social exclusion in older-age.

Editors' Postscript

Please note, like other contributions to this book, this chapter was written before the COVID-19 pandemic of 2020. The book's introductory chapter (Chap. 1) and conclusion (Chap. 34) consider some of the key ways in which the pandemic relates to issues concerning social exclusion and ageing.

Acknowledgments The research for the introduction and sections on Russia, conducted by I. A. Grigoryeva, was supported by the Russian Science Foundation (project №19-18-00246 "Challenges of the transformation of Welfare State in Russia: institutional changes, social investment, digitalization of social services").

References

Abrahamson, P. (2001). Social exclusion and poverty [Abrahamson P. Social'naja jekskljuzija i bednost']. *Obshhestvennye nauki i sovremennost' – Social Sciences and Modernity*, (2), 158–166.

Burchardt, T., & Le Grand, J. (2002). Degrees of exclusion: Developing a dynamic, multidimensional. In J. Hills, J. Le Grand, & D. Pichaud, *Understanding social exclusion* (pp. 30–43). New York: Oxford University Press.

Cook, L. J. (2007). *Postcommunist welfare states. Reform politics in Russia and Eastern Europe*. Ithaca: Cornell University Press.

Eliseeva, I., & Kletsin, A.A. (2010). Urban family in Russia: Current trends. *Petersburg Sociology Today* [Peterburgskaya sotsiologiya segodnya], (2): 127–146. (in Russian).

Federal State Statistics Service (Rosstat). (2019). https://www.gks.ru/storage/mediabank/doc3-1-1.htm. Accessed 22 Sept 2019.

Gorova, A. V. (2012). Nederzhavnyy sektor nadannya sotsial'nykh posluh: suchasnyy stan ta perspektyvy rozvytku. In S. V. Kivalov (Ed.), *Aktual'ni problemy derzhavy i prava: Zbirnyk naukovykh prats'* (Vol. 63, pp. 445–450). Odesa: Yurydychna literatura. (In Ukrainian).

Grigoryeva, I. A. (2017). One hundred years of social policy in Russia. *The Journal of Social Policy Studies, 15*(4), 495–496.

Grigoryeva, I. A., Sizova, I. L., & Moskvina, A. Y. (2019a). Social services for the elderly: Implementation of the Federal Law No. 442 and future prospects. *Monitoring of Public Opinion: Economic and Social Changes, 4*, 125–144. https://doi.org/10.14515/monitoring.2019.4.09.

Grigoryeva, I., Vidiasova, L., Dmitrieva, A., & Sergeyeva, O. (2019b). *Elderly population in Modern Russia: Between work, education and health*. Springer.

Jehoel-Gijsbers, G., & Vrooman C. (2008). *Social exclusion of the elderly: A comparative study of EU Member* (ENEPRI Research Report No. 57). Available at SSRN: https://ssrn.com/abstract=2027886. Accessed 22 Sept 2019.

Levitas, R., Pantazis, C., Fahmy, E., Gordon, D., Lloyd, E., & Patsios, D. (2007). *The Multi-dimensional analysis of social exclusion*. Bethesda: Bristol Institute for Public Affairs, University of Bristol.

Libanova, E. M. (2017). Ministerial conference on ageing: A sustainable society for all ages: Realizing the potential of living longer. *UNECE conference* (pp. 21–22). Lisbon. http://www.unece.org/pau/ageing/ministerial_conference_2017.html. Accessed 10 Aug 2019.

Maksimovich, M. (2018). *Sociologist: Ukrainians are used to relying only on the state*. News of Ukraine. https://replyua.net/news/106356-sociolog-ukraincy-privykli-polagatsya-tolko-na-gosudarstvo.html. Accessed 20 Sept 2019.

Parfenova, O. (2017). *Care for the old people in state social services*. PhD dissertation. https://search.rsl.ru/ru/record/01006654185. Accessed 22 Sept 2019 (in Russian).

Parfenova, O. (2018). Transformation of social services for the elderly in the regional context of modern Russia. *The Journal of Sociology and Social Anthropology [Zhurnal sotsiologii i sotsialnoy antropologii], 21*(2), 165–186. https://doi.org/10.31119/jssa.2018.21.2.6. (in Russian).

Rogozin, D. M. (2012). The liberalization of aging, or labor, knowledge and health at an older age. *Sociological Journal, 4*, 62–93. (in Russian).

Rossat. (2018). http://www.gks.ru/wps/wcm/connect/rosstat_main/rosstat/ru/statistics/population/generation/#

Russian Pension Foundation. (2019). https://pfrp.ru/faq/srednyaya-pensiya-v-rossii.html. Accessed 10 Aug 2019.

Scharf, T., & Keating, N. (Eds.) (2012). Social exclusion in later life: A global challenge. Bristol: The Policy Press.

Sen, A. (1999). *Development as freedom* (1st ed.). New York: Oxford University Press.

Silver, H. (1994). Social exclusion and social solidarity: Three paradigms. *International Labour Review, 133*(5–6), 531–578.

Smolkin, A. A. (2014). The labor potential of the elderly. *Sociological Studies, 5*, 97–103. (in Russian).
Social Care and Social Inclusion in Ukraine. (2009). *Ukrainian center for social reforms Kiev*. http://www.ucsr.kiev.ua/public_en.html. Accessed 22 Sept 2019.
Tikhonova, N. (2004). Social exclusion in Russia. In N. Manning & N. Tikhonova (Eds.), *Poverty and social exclusion in the New Russia* (pp. 109–149). London: Ashgate.
Walsh, K., Scharf, T., & Keating, N. (2017). Social exclusion of older persons: A scoping review and conceptual framework. *European Journal of Ageing, 14*(1), 81–98.
World Health Organization. (2016). Life expectancy and Healthy life expectancy. Data by country. https://apps.who.int/gho/data/view.main.SDG2016LEXv?lang=en. Accessed 3 December, 2020.

Legal Acts

Federal Law N 166-FL on December 15, 2001 'On State Pension Provision in the Russian Federation'.
Federal Law N 167-FL on December 15, 2001 "On Compulsory Pension Insurance in the Russian Federation".
Federal Law N 350-FL on October 3, 2018, 'On Amendments to Certain Legislative Acts of the Russian Federation on the Purpose and Issues of Pensions'.
Federal Law N 422-FL on December 28, 2013 'About Bases of Social Services Of Citizens in the Russian Federation'.
Federal Law of Russia N 27-FL on April 1, 1996 'On individual (personified) accounting in the system of compulsory pension insurance'.
The Law of Ukraine №2148-VIII, 03 October 2017. On Amendments to Some Legislative Acts of the Ukraine Regarding Pension Increases. he Law of Ukraine No. 966-IV on June 19, 2003 'On Social Services'.
The Law of Ukraine. No. 2449-VIII on June 7, 2018. 'On introducing an amendment to the relevant legislative acts of Ukraine on pension'.

Chapter 31
How Can Urban Design and Architecture Support Spatial Inclusion for Nursing Home Residents?

John Andersen, Annette Bilfeldt, Marianne Mahler, and Lone Sigbrand

31.1 Introduction: Key Concepts of Spatial and Community Exclusion Related to Urban Design and Planning Traditions

Older persons who experience difficulties related to risks of deteriorating health and lack of mobility (Walker 2010) may face challenges in gaining access to the social life of their residential neighbourhoods. The concept of *ageing in place* thematises the considerable importance to older people's quality of life that is associated with continued participation in the life in their local area and in the maintenance of connections with neighbourhoods and communities. People may have lived in the same place for their entire lives and may often prefer to remain within the community with which they are most familiar (Wiles 2005; Philips et al. 2010). Ageing in place implies that ageing happens in a specific spatial environment – the familiar environment of one's own home, community and neighbourhood – rather than in an unfamiliar, institutional environment (Moulaert et al. 2018).

While the overwhelming majority of older people in Europe live in domestic settings, it is important not to overlook the role played by institutional settings as places where people may spend their later lives. In this context, nursing home residents should have the possibility to be part of the social life of the cities, communities or neighbourhoods in which they live. Whether or not the nursing home is

J. Andersen (✉)
Department of People and Technology (IMT), Roskilde Universitet, Roskilde, Denmark
e-mail: johna@ruc.dk

A. Bilfeldt
University of Greenland, Nuuk, Greenland

M. Mahler
University of Copenhagen, Copenhagen, Denmark

L. Sigbrand
Department of the Built Environment, Aalborg University, Aalborg, Denmark

K. Walsh et al. (eds.), *Social Exclusion in Later Life*, International Perspectives on Aging 28, https://doi.org/10.1007/978-3-030-51406-8_31

situated in the same area that the resident has lived in for years, remaining or becoming part of a neighbourhood and local community when moving to a nursing home is of great importance for individuals' quality of life [also see Villar et al. this volume]. The concept of ageing in place can, therefore, also have meaning for people who move into a nursing home, providing an opportunity to improve their quality of life in an institutional setting in a new neighbourhood. In such situations, the idea of ageing in place can be expanded to encompass the notion of *ageing in a new place* or of *ageing in a new local area.*

Against this background, architecture and urban planning policy can play a crucial role for the social inclusion of older persons who reside in nursing homes, not least by ensuring that residents are able to access to their surroundings.

31.2 The Human Dimension of Urban Design and Planning

The importance of the human and social dimensions of city planning and development – how urban structures affect community life and social interaction and "liveability" in neighbourhoods – has a long history in urban planning policy and urban movements. This encompasses the iconic work of Jane Jacobs (1961/69), advocacy and empowerment planning in the 1960s (Davidoff 1965), and the work of contemporary communicative and social justice planning theorists like Patsy Healy (2003) and Peter Marcuse (2011). Jan Gehl, the Danish architect, developed the concept of "life between buildings" in order to embrace the entire spectrum of activities that combine communal spaces in cities and residential areas in meaningful and attractive ways (Gehl 1971). Gehl underpinned the idea that social activities in an urban design perspective could be characterised as encompassing "all activities that depend on the presence of others in public spaces" (Gehl 1971 p.10). According to Gehl, social activities occur spontaneously as a direct consequence of people moving about and being in the same spaces:

> 'Social activities include children at play, greetings and conversations, communal activities of various kinds, and finally – as the most widespread social activity – passive contacts, that is simply seeing and hearing other people'. (Gehl 1971, p.10; see also Carmona and Tiesdell 2007).

With this definition of social activities, Gehl points out the fundamental importance of urban planning in framing the possibility for social life activities to take place.

Ray Oldenburg (1999), the American sociologist, argues in his book *The Great Good Place* that "third places" – informal public gathering places, where people can gather outside work and home in inclusively sociable places – are essential for a functioning civil society, democracy and civic engagement. Meeting places, where the concerns of work and home are put aside and people gather simply for the pleasure of good company and lively conversation, are the heart of a community's social vitality and the grassroots of democracy. He emphasises the importance of places where individuals feel at home and comfortable and where they may come and go as they please. Oldenburg pointed out that without neutral ground in the neighbourhoods where people live, association outside the home will be impoverished:

> 'Neighbours will never associate, if there is no place for them to do so. The third place may be a solution in reframing the way interpersonal interaction is approached on an individual level'. (Oldenburg 1999, p.88).

In urban planning, architecture and design, we often find that framing possibilities for older people to gain access to urban space is absent from the agenda. But social life in a third-place perspective is important for older residents of nursing home. Access to association on neutral ground in the neighbourhood outside the institution can be very important for nursing home residents whose everyday life is institutionalised. The importance of access to a social life does not disappear as one gets older, even though the need may change character with increasing age. As a researcher on ageing, Sari Rissanen (2013) established that access to a social life is just as important for older persons' quality of life as good physical health. This applies regardless of whether people live in their own domestic home or in a nursing home (Rissanen 2013).

Despite the fact that urban planning debates engage with the need to respond to demographic change, the focus is primarily on where to place older persons and less on enabling older persons, as citizens with the right to a social life, to participate in practice in city life in their neighbourhood and in the local community. Buffel et al. (2019) emphasise:

> 'the need for a stronger embedding of the age-friendly mission in a **citizenship-** and **rights-based** narrative of ageing, one that is centred on values of equality, community empowerment and spatial justice'. (p.288).

In general, this type of approach may be especially challenging for nursing home residents.

31.3 Social Inclusion in Indoor and Outdoor Environments in a Capability Perspective

The capability approach, a moral-philosophical theoretical framework concerning well-being, development and justice, has been pioneered by the economist-philosopher Amartya Sen and further developed by the philosopher Martha Nussbaum. The concept entails two core normative claims: first, the claim that the freedom to achieve well-being is primarily of moral importance; and second, that the freedom to achieve well-being is to be understood in terms of people's capabilities, which refers to individuals' real opportunities to do and be what they have reason to value (The Stanford Encyclopedia of Philosophy 2016). In Nussbaum's perspective, the key focus is on the freedom to achieve well-being as a matter of what people are able to do and to be, and thus the kind of life they are able to live in practice:

> 'What is each person able to do and to be? It is focused on choice or freedom, holding that what the crucial good societies should be promoting for their people is a set of opportunities, or substantial freedoms, which people may or may not exercise in action: the choice is theirs'. (Nussbaum 2011, p.18).

The capability concept contains the central values of the WHO Healthy Ageing definition, which includes participation, justice, autonomy and safety (Hörder 2016). In this perspective there is a political obligation to frame capability for everybody (Nussbaum 2011), with respect for the notion that everyone should have the human freedom to live a life they have reason to value (Sen 1982). With reference to the potential vulnerability of some older persons (Katz 2010), a core feature of the capability perspective is not to normalise social exclusion of older individuals, but to provide a basis for their social inclusion in the way they value being included, however vulnerable they might be (Wiles and Jayansinha 2013).

Against this background, an important question concerns how nursing home architecture can make it possible for residents living in a nursing home to participate in urban life and be part of the social activities that they value.

31.4 The Historical Context

Often called "old people's homes", in earlier times, nursing homes were typically placed in quiet areas removed from city life, where the residents often had only a small bedroom and a shared bathroom and ate their meals in a communal dining hall. Compared to the general housing standard in Denmark, this nursing home standard gradually came to be seen in the policy and planning discourse of the 1980s as out-dated. In accordance with legislation introduced in 1987 (the Social Housing Act [*Almenboligloven* 2019]), most nursing homes in Denmark are now organised as general social housing for older persons with associated care and service functions. This means that (unlike in former "old people's homes") residents have individual leases and pay rent and other expenses for their own homes and shared facilities. They also have democratic rights regarding the running of the nursing home. Besides having their own individual homes, with a bedroom, small living room, kitchenette and bathroom, residents share dining and living facilities and have access to public facilities like cafés, physical training gyms, music activities and such together with other, mostly older people, living in the same residential neighbourhood. Depending on their abilities, both residents in the nursing home and residents in the surrounding residential areas have the option of meeting, interacting and enjoying social activities together.

Compared to the former institutionalised nursing homes, modern nursing homes are similar to ordinary housing, with private and common facilities but with additional care for residents in need.

31.5 New Knowledge About How to Protect Vulnerable Residents Through Nursing Home Design

Recent reviews of relevant national and international research compiled in a national guideline for Danish nursing homes show that design of the physical environment is of great importance for older persons' well-being and quality of life. It is important to be able to stay connected to the local area you live in and to continue to feel part of a community. The guidelines of the Department of the Built Environment (the former Danish National Building Research Institute) (Sigbrand et al. 2019) argue that a nursing home should provide easy access to the surrounding local society, both for residents and their visiting relatives.

Compared to the situation in the 1980s and 1990s, the profile of nursing home residents has changed significantly. Today, since the majority of nursing home residents can be classified as "frail", they are mainly dependent on living in a supportive environment (The Ministry of Health 2017). Under these circumstances, it is expected that nursing homes should have a homely atmosphere, good access to daylight, and close contact to nature, both visually and directly in a secure outdoor area. If these elements exist in a nursing home, the quality of life of residents, judged to be vulnerable, may improve and medication be reduced or avoided altogether (Sigbrand et al. 2019; Siren et al. 2019).

31.6 Four Nursing Home Concepts and Spatial Inclusion

Based on pioneering examples of nursing home planning principles that aim to integrate the surrounding local community and to facilitate social inclusion of nursing home residents, we now proceed to present four distinct contemporary cases from The Netherlands and Denmark. The criteria for the case selection draw on principles of "strategic exemplarity" (Flyvbjerg and Sampson 2001). In this sense, the aim is to illustrate how new trends in architecture and urban policy can support nursing home residents to become part of local city and social life. The cases have been chosen with reference to innovation of existing approaches in the field or a "best case" criterion, *i.e.* projects that demonstrate *political and public* awareness (*e.g.* at local government level) and innovative *professional* commitment and visibility (by architects, planners and nursing home professionals) to overcome or reduce the risks of social exclusion faced by nursing home residents.

The first case is the *Closed Village*: the de Davidoff nursing home in Amsterdam (https://hogeweyk.dementiavillage.com/). This project was completed in 2009 and is designed as a closed village for older people living with severe forms of dementia. The Hogeweyk project consists of 23 houses and is home to 152 residents. In spite of their cognitive impairment, residents are enabled to live a normal life with *freedom in safety*. All buildings are closed to the surrounding neighbourhood, and only one gate opens to the outside world. This ensures that residents can safely roam freely in the streets and park without getting lost. A restaurant, theatre, supermarket, hair salon and different activity rooms can be used by residents and visiting relatives. The nursing home is situated in a residential area and residents from the local neighbourhood are invited inside to use the different facilities and to stroll in the streets and park. In this way, residents can remain connected to society outside the nursing home.

The second case is the *Intergenerational Neighbourhood*: the planned nursing home Ingeborggaarden (https://www.frederiksberg.dk/sites/default/files/meetings-appendices/53F4AEA9-BC1D-40E0-91B7-F6F8669BA271/2535700-2694951-1.PDF) is located in Frederiksberg Municipality in the Copenhagen Region. The political context here was that the City Council was inspired by the WHO programme, Global Age-Friendly Cities (WHO 2018). A local left-wing politician, Thyge Enevoldsen, had placed the political focus for more than 20 years on the importance of framing rights and quality of life for Frederiksberg's nursing home residents. It is a nursing home that is planned to have a close relationship with the neighbourhood *i.e.* with the local football club through common areas, both inside and outside the building, that frame intergenerational meeting places and meetings between younger and older community residents. Nursing home residents have the possibility to watch the young football players, meet them in the cafés, interact with them and maybe even help them with homework. The nursing home is about to be constructed in an urban residential area and is expected to be completed in 2023. It will accommodate approximately 200 residents with either cognitive impairment or physical disabilities, living in housing groups comprising 10–13 individual homes with shared living rooms, dining rooms and balconies. The overall approach of the nursing home is openness towards the neighbourhood, with communal facilities on the ground floor and a city park. The plan is to take care of the special needs of residents with severe dementia in a common, sheltered day centre connected to *a secret garden*, located at the heart of the building away from noisy activities. The plan also envisages that, depending on their wishes and needs, all residents will be able to follow and participate in activities connected to the local football club and wider neighbourhood.

The third case is New Soelund (http://www.detnyesoelund.dk/) in Copenhagen, which we call *Age-Friendly Urbanism*: The Danish social housing association, KAB, is building a new nursing home close to one of the city's most attractive and lively neighbourhoods, Noerrebro. New Soelund will replace an existing, outdated nursing home in a central, densely-populated residential area. It will become the largest nursing home in Copenhagen, with 360 residents living on a daily basis in smaller housing groups of 8–12 people who share dining and living areas, co-housing for 20 senior citizens, 150 housing units for young people, a day-care centre for approximately 75 children, and roof gardens for school pupils from the surrounding neighbourhood. Moreover, New Soelund will provide the neighbourhood with small shops and other facilities. New Soelund is expected to be ready to welcome its first residents in late 2022. This particular case provides an example of how municipalities and non-profit social housing associations have started to work with the idea of age-friendly urbanism in order to facilitate generational integration and avoid spatial exclusion of nursing home residents from the local neighbourhood. The nursing home is placed on a relatively quiet site close to one of the lakes in Copenhagen, where there are pedestrian and cycle paths, so that pedestrians and cyclists pass by during the daytime and evening hours. A *town square for generations,* with benches and cafés, makes New Soelund attractive for people who pass by to take a break, thereby enabling contact between residents and non-residents. At the same time, the aim is to use the nursing home as an urban frame for social activities, and to provide a context within which residents can experience urban life, fresh air, and contact with passers-by and also with young people on their way to and from school.

The final case is Dagmarsminde in Graested, which we call *the Caring Countryside Oasis,* was opened in 2016 in the countryside north of Copenhagen (http://dagmarsminde.dk/). Dagmarsminde is a small nursing home with 10 separate units for 11 residents, all with severe dementia. The residents have their own individual bedrooms and bathrooms. They live in a very homely environment, sharing living and dining areas, a conservatory, library and a wellness and sensory room. The building is surrounded by a large fenced garden with a henhouse, rabbits and an enclosure with goats, which is situated next to fields and a forest. The building is a remodelled carpentry workshop. The nursing home is described as *a caring oasis,* and, compared to other large nursing homes, Dagmarsminde could be regarded as a pioneer case when it comes to the scale of the nursing home and the approach to the care of residents. Close contact to nature and animals, access to daylight, and a high degree of homeliness are central elements of the care provided, which focuses on supporting residents' well-being and quality of life with less medication. Depending on the abilities and needs of individual residents, care staff take trips, for example to the beach or forest. Family members are an important part of daily life and activities even though there is a fairly long distance to a city, and young children in the neighbourhood or grandchildren come to do their homework at the dining table, as they do in an ordinary home. By taking tours and inviting people in to take part in their daily life, residents maintain their connections with the social life of the community beyond the nursing home.

Residents with severe dementia are often sensitive to excessive stimulation, whether from being surrounded by many people or by engaging with the noisy and hectic activity of city life. However, visual contact, such as seeing and hearing other people is important: "Enjoying a view, listening to music, or simply watching other people's activities, visitors or staff, can be engaging activities" (Scheel Thomasen 2013 p.112). Close contact with nature, broadly understood, is another important factor for such residents with such sensitivities in order that they can feel at ease and comfortable. Easy access to nature is important in providing sensory stimulation (Clancy 2016) and is the focus of the Dagmarsminde nursing home.

31.7 Discussion

Drawing the threads of this chapter together, it is evidently important to focus on capability when creating opportunity structures through planning and designing nursing homes for the future, both with regards to residents with and without dementia. However, there is not only one simple response to the question about how architecture and urban policy approaches can frame spatial inclusion for nursing home residents. The four illustrative cases highlight different approaches to creating possibilities for facilitating social inclusion of older nursing home residents in the surrounding neighbourhood and local society.

For Dagmarsminde, the radical answer was to "go back to nature" and to locate the nursing home with easy access to nature and to use actively the natural facilities in the daily practices of care work and social activities. Dagmarsminde, from a capability perspective, functions well by supporting life quality in such a way that the residents have opportunities to participate in social activities according to their own individual conditions, without being obliged to engage in activities that may cause them undue stress.

As for the Hogeweyk project, the scheme has aimed to provide opportunities for the residents with severe dementia to roam safely and freely in a "city-like" environment within the area of the nursing home. From a capability perspective, the result is that residents can join a "city-like" social practice in a safe way, but without accessing the surrounding neighbourhood. De Hoogeweyk provides a quiet city area for the local neighbourhood, with non-residents invited inside to use the different facilities alongside residents and to stroll in the streets and park, offering an alternative to the noisy city-life outside.

From Ray Oldenburg's "third-place perspective", both Ingeborggaarden and New Soelund are planned in ways that contribute to age-friendly urbanism with emphasis on informal public gathering places, where people can congregate outside work and home in inclusive, sociable places. These housing schemes can frame the social life of residents by providing opportunities on a daily basis to connect with citizens outside the nursing home.

The Ingeborggaarden nursing home, situated in a quiet part of Frederiksberg Municipality, aims to foster intergenerational interaction in everyday life and to avoid age segregation. It combines indoor facilities for residents, including providing possibilities for peacefulness for residents with severe dementia in the "secret garden", with age-friendly outdoor surroundings and facilities, in order to share facilities with the local community for residents who want to be part of social life in the neighbourhood. Ingeborggaarden is a key part of the municipality's plan to be "the city of generations". Communal areas and facilities like a café are connected to the nursing home. The scheme offers the younger generation of football players the possibility to have daily contact with the older generation. Informal conversations and help with homework can support and sustain important relationships between generations.

With New Soelund positioned in an attractive location, close to the city of Copenhagen's lakes and its well-used pedestrian and cycle paths, residents will have direct access to a vibrant metropolitan life. The residents will become an integrated part of the urban neighbourhood with opportunities for direct contact with younger generations in the shared areas. New Soelund represents an innovative contribution to urban social life by inviting local residents, bypassing pedestrians and cyclists, to use the place in front of the nursing home together with the nursing home residents. That said, there are also challenges associated with this development. In particular, the residents who formerly lived in the old Soelund were moved away long before the building process started. Former residents felt it was unjust that they had to leave their home by the lakes. Since they and their neighbours felt that their views were not taken into account in the planning process, it will be important to follow and evaluate the development and impact of the nursing home in the years to come.

With regard to the capability perspective, it is important to investigate whether residents of Ingeborggaarden will indeed become part of the social life of the neighbourhood that surrounds the nursing home in the way that they and their relatives value. It is not clear whether residents will be able to gain access to the surrounding green area if they want to or whether they will be able to navigate the physical environment with a walker or wheelchair, so that the nursing home component of the intergenerational city life will come to fruition as planned. It also remains unclear how social contact between the football players and residents and their relatives will occur.

31.8 Conclusion

The four examples we have described are valuable examples of innovation in nursing home planning and design principles. The cases support, in different ways, the residents' capability to be part of social activities in city life in the way they value – showing respect for individualism and regarding residents as a heterogeneous group with different needs, values and capabilities. From a capability perspective, it is inevitable that residents, relatives, care-workers and neighbours should in future be empowered as important stakeholders in the evaluation as well as in the planning of new nursing homes. This can open up new knowledge about the connection between nursing home locations, design and improved spatial inclusion of nursing home residents (Rissanen 2013, McDonald et al. 2019). In particular, it is important not to forget that nursing home residents, including those who are experiencing cognitive decline, are able to express their wishes and values, if asked.

Editors' Postscript

Please note, like other contributions to this book, this chapter was written before the COVID-19 pandemic of 2020. The book's introductory chapter (Chap. 1) and conclusion (Chap. 34) consider some of the key ways in which the pandemic relates to issues concerning social exclusion and ageing.

References

Almenboligloven. (2019). https://www.retsinformation.dk/pdfPrint.aspx?id=206725

Barry, B. (2002). Social exclusion, social isolation and the distribution of income. In J. Hills, J. Le Grand, & D. Piachaud (Eds.), *Understanding social exclusion* (pp. 13–29). Oxford: Oxford University Press.

Buffel, T., Handler, S., & Philipson, C. (2019). Age-friendly cities and communities: a manifesto for change. In T. Buffel, S. Handler, & C. Philipson (Eds.), *Age-friendly cities and communities: A global perspective*. Bristol: Policy Press.

Carmona, M., & Tiesdell, S. (2007). *Urban design reader*. New York: Architectural Press/ Routledge.

Clancy, A. (2016). Steder rommer elementene. Det nordlige mennesket og stedets betydning for helse og velbefinnende. In Stenbock-Hult, B. & Sarvimäki, A. (Eds.), *Healthy ageing. Nordiske perspektiv på äldres hälsa och främjande av äldres hälsa* (Arcada Working Papers 2/2016).

Dagmarsminde. http://dagmarsminde.dk/. Accessed 30 Mar 2020.

Davidoff, P. (1965). Advocacy and pluralism in planning. *Journal of the American Institute of Planners, 31*(4), 331–338.

De Hogeweyk.: https://hogeweyk.dementiavillage.com/en/kenniscentrum/

Flyvbjerg, B., & Sampson, S. (2001). *Making social science matter- why social inquiry fails and how it can succeed again*. Cambridge: Cambridge University Press.

Gehl, J. (1971). *Life between buildings: Using public space*. Skive: Arkitektens Forlag.

Healy, P. (2003). Collaborative planning in perspective. *Planning Theory, 2*(2), 101–123. Sage Publications.

Hörder, H. (2016). En kapabilitietsansats till Healthy Ageing. In B. Stenbock-Hult & A. Sarvimäki (Eds.), *Healthy Ageing. Nordiske perspektiv på äldres hälsa och främjande av äldres hälsa* (Arcada Working Papers 2/2016).

Ingeborggården. https://www.frederiksberg.dk/sites/default/files/meetings-appendices/53F4AEA9-BC1D-40E0-91B7-F6F8669BA271/2535700-2694951-1.PDF. Accessed 30 Mar 2020.

Jacobs, J. (1961). *The death and life of great American cities*. London: Jonathan Cape.

Katz, S. (2010). Sociocultural perspectives on ageing bodies. In D. Dannefer & C. Phillipson (Eds.), *The Sage handbook of social gerontology* (pp. 357–366). Los Angeles/London/New Delhi/Singapore/Washington: Sage.

Macleod, C., et al. (2017). Re-thinking social exclusion in later life: A case for a new framework for measurement. *Ageing & Society, 39*, 74. Cambridge University Press.

Marcuse, P. (2011). *The three Historic currents of City Planning*. In G. Bridge & S. Watson (Eds.), *The new Blackwell companion to the city*. Oxford: Blackwell Publishing.

McDonald, B., Scharf, T., & Walsh, K. (2019). Creating an age-friendly county in Ireland: Stakeholders' perspectives on implementation. In T. Buffel, S. Handler, & C. Philipson (Eds.), *Age-friendly cities and communities a global perspective*. Bristol: Policy Press.

Ministry of Health (Sundheds- og Aeldreministeriet). (2016) *National undersøgelse af forholdene på plejecentre*. https://sum.dk/~/media/Filer%20-%20Publikationer_i_pdf/2016/National-undersoegelse-af-forholdene-paa-plejec/Undersoegelse-af-forholdene-paa-plejecentre.pdf

The Ministry of Health (Sundheds- og Aeldreministeriet). (2017): *Plejecentre*.https://www.sum.dk/Aeldre/Boliger-til-aeldre/Plejecentre.aspx

Moulaert, T., Wanka A., & Drilling M. (2018). The social production of age, space and exclusion. *Social Studies* 1.

Nussbaum, M. (2011). The human development approach. In M. Nussbaum (Ed.), *Creating capabilities*. Cambridge, MA: Belknap Press of Harvard.

Oldenburg, R. (1999). The Character of Third Places. In R. Oldenburg (Ed.), *The Great Good Place: Cafés, coffee shops, bookstores, bars, hair salons and the other great hangouts at the heart of a community* (2nd ed., pp. 2–42). New York: Marlowe & Company. (First edition published in 1989).

Philips, J., Ajrouch, K.J., & Hillcoat-Nalletamby, S. (2010). *Key concepts in social gerontology* (Sage Key Concepts). London: Sage.

Rissanen, S. (2013). Wellbeing and environment, concepts in the elderly care home context. In A. Hujala, S. Rissanen, & S. Vihma (Eds.), *Designing wellbeing in elderly care homes* (Aalto University publication series Crossover 2.13) (pp. 20–35).

Scheel Thomasen, L. (2013). A good old age? Life as a nursing home resident in Denmark. In A. Hujala, S. Rissanen, & S. Vihma (Eds.), *Designing wellbeing in elderly care homes* (Aalto University, Crossover, 2.13) (pp. 102–114).

Sen, A. (1982). *Choice, welfare and measurement*. Oxford: Basil Blackwell.

Sigbrand, L., Bredmose, A., Jensen, P. H., Kirkeby, I. M., Lygum, V. L., & Mathiasen, N. (2019). *Plejeboliger for personer med demens – detaljer og eksempler* (Nursing homes for people with dementia– Details and examples) Institute of the Built Environment (The Danish building research institute), Aalborg University, Copenhagen.

Siren, A., Grønfeldt, S. T., Andreasen, A. G., & Bukhave, F. S. (2019). *Sociale mursten: En forskningskortlægning af fysiske rammers betydning i velfærdsindsatser*. Copenhagen: VIVE–Viden til Velfærd Det Nationale Forsknings- og Analysecenter for Velfærd.

Soelund. http://www.detnyesoelund.dk/. Accessed 30 Mar 2020.

The Stanford Encyclopedia of Philosophy. (2016) Plato. Stanford.edu.

Vidovićová, L., & Tournier, L. (2020). Community and spatial aspects of exclusion in later life. In K. Walsh & T. Scharf (Eds.), *Reducing old-age exclusion: Collaborations in research and policy* (ROSEnet briefing paper series: No. 2. CA 15122). ISBN: 978-1-908358-72-1.

Walker, A. (2010). Ageing and quality of life in Europe. In D. Dannefer & C. Phillipson (Eds.), *The Sage Handbook of Social Gerontology*. London: Sage.

Wiles, J. (2005). Conceptualizing place in the care of older people: The contribution of geographical gerontology. *International Journal of Older People Nursing* in association with *Journal of Clinical Nursing*, *14*, 100–108.

Wiles, J., & Jayansinha, R. (2013). *Care for place: The contributions older people make to their communities*. *Journal of Aging Studies*, *27*, 93–101. Elsevier.

World Health Organization. (2018). *What is healthy Ageing?*. www.who.int/ageing/healthy-ageing/en/. Accessed 10 Oct 2019.

Chapter 32
Old-Age Digital Exclusion as a Policy Challenge in Estonia and Finland

Anu Leppiman, Iivi Riivits-Arkonsuo, and Anneli Pohjola

32.1 Introduction

Conceptualisations of social exclusion increasingly recognise the significance of digital forms of exclusion. As a consequence, responding to the digital divide has become a key social and policy challenge in contemporary society (Helsper 2012; Martin et al. 2016). The coincidence of increasing longevity and widespread digitalisation characterise all European Union member states, including countries such as Estonia and Finland. This requires effective strategies in both the economic and social spheres (Batut 2016). This chapter aims to explore the challenges posed by digitalisation for ageing populations, the concerns experienced by older people when accessing digital services, and the key elements of digital solutions that are designed to answer older people's needs. We consider these issues in the specific context of Estonia and Finland, as countries that are close to one another as states and nations. At almost all levels and sectors of society, the relations between the two countries are intense. Estonia, like Russia and the Ukraine included elsewhere in this section of the book, is a post-socialist state with a welfare model that differs from Finland. The social structure in Estonia emphasises the principles of individual self-responsibility and self-regulation as well as a government that seeks to avoid interference in individuals' affairs (Leppiman and Tulva 2005). While Estonia has adopted a liberal model, with the hallmarks of a US-style welfare system based on neoliberal and monetarist economic thinking, Finland is typically characterised as having a Nordic welfare state regime. However, in recent times market-liberal thinking has increasingly penetrated the public sector and this trend seems to be

A. Leppiman (✉) · I. Riivits-Arkonsuo
Tallinn University of Technology, Tallinn, Estonia
e-mail: anu.leppiman@taltech.ee

A. Pohjola
University of Lapland, Rovaniemi, Finland

K. Walsh et al. (eds.), *Social Exclusion in Later Life*, International Perspectives on Aging 28, https://doi.org/10.1007/978-3-030-51406-8_32

continuing in Finland, giving rise to problems in linking the market economy and public sector activities (Koskiaho and Saarinen 2019).

As in other nations, the populations of Finland and Estonia are ageing rapidly, with increasing life expectancy contributing to a growth in the numbers and proportions of older people. In Finland, the age groups born after the Second World War are disproportionately large, and Finland is characterised by its high numbers of older people. Over one-fifth of Finland's population (5.5 million) is over 65 years (1.2 million/22%), and an increasing proportion are over 75 years (Statistics Finland 2019). In Estonia, the birth rate after the Second World War was more modest. However, nearly one-fifth (19.6%) of the Estonian population (1.3 million) is over 65 years of age (Statistics Estonia 2019). At the same time, in both countries, the younger age groups are shrinking as a result of low birth rates.

In Estonia and Finland, the use of technology and digital services has become widespread in the public and private sectors. These countries are building a digital society and digitising public services both nationally and across borders. Estonia's and Finland's data exchange layers are connected to one another, enabling cross-border data exchange (Nordic Institute for Interoperability Solutions 2019). However, population ageing poses a fundamental challenge in relation to digitalisation. The rapid growth of Information and Communication Technologies (ICT) facilitates people's lives and offers a variety of digital services. People who have the necessary skills and motivation to use ICTs can benefit considerably from inclusion within a digital society. Digitalisation enables people to learn and to be proactive, especially when they are older and their mobility is reduced. It can help to avoid segregation and facilitate knowledge transfer (Batut 2016). Delivery of digital services influences positively the life of older people, improves quality of life and increases independence (Czaja 2017; Siegel and Dorner 2017). Nevertheless, digital technologies can also have their drawbacks. Not all people have equal access to digital services, resulting in widespread exclusion and the emergence of a digital divide between different user groups (Ihm and Hsieh 2015; see also Poli et al. this volume for a related analysis of old-age digital health exclusion).

In particular, older adults who are economically, socio-culturally, or physically disadvantaged are at risk of being marginalised (Grundy 2006; Yu et al. 2016). For them, digital exclusion, access to information and difficulties in accessing online services can cause problems, uncertainty and insecurity. Drawing on the conceptual model of social exclusion in later life developed by Walsh et al. (2017), where digital exclusion is a feature of the services, amenities and mobility domain, poor accessibility and usability of digital technologies can create barriers for some older people, resulting in their exclusion from the opportunities presented by digitalisation (Yu et al. 2016; Niemi 2017).

Public policy can play a major role in reducing digital exclusion among older people, depending on what kind of values and whose needs are placed at the centre of the policy-making process. It is important for policy to address the risk of exclusion faced by older people who are unable to use the Internet or access e-services when using services and participating in civic activities. Moreover, both the availability and quality of digital services designed for older people are highly dependent on policy decisions.

32.1.1 Multiple Causes of Digital Exclusion

Older people are a heterogeneous group with different capacities and abilities to act. While they are not a separate category to consider, it is necessary to identify the spectrum among them and ongoing changes in their life situations. Older people are characterised by differences in their economic, educational, social and societal roles. It is not only important to take into account the contextual factors of their lives, but also the human and social capital at their disposal (Niemi 2017).

Old-age exclusion involves interchanges between multilevel risk factors, processes and outcomes (Walsh et al. 2017), with digital exclusion representing a key form of exclusion in later life. Older-age is typically associated with a reduced likelihood of using online services (Freese et al. 2006; Sourbati 2007) and older people tend to be on the wrong side of the digital divide (Olphert and Damodaran 2013; Friemel 2016). Digital exclusion can have multiple causes, related to a lack of the fundamental requirements for the democratisation of technology: hardware access (affordability, availability of energy networks), access to the Internet (affordability, availability of infrastructure to connect to a network), and mastery of technology (Castilla et al. 2018). Moreover, commonly identified reasons for old-age digital disengagement include disability, complexity of the technology, social isolation, lower income, and lower education (Olphert and Damodaran 2013; Friemel 2016). Older adults are more likely to be late rather than early adopters of technologies (Chen and Chan 2014). In addition to socio-demographic factors, psychological factors contribute strongly to the digital divide affecting the older population. Older people who feel younger than their chronological age, experience less technology anxiety, feel more confident in using technology, and are more adventurous are more likely to be active participants in a digital society (Peral-Peral et al. 2015).

New technologies have emerged with the rapid expansion of the Internet into modern life. In this regard, older people are more susceptible to certain fears than younger, so-called "digital natives". Older adults are more susceptible to technology anxiety, such as: a concern that technology will be complicated to use; it will intrude into their private life; they may be a victim of fraud if they make online payments; technology is dangerous (Batut 2016).

As suggested by Michael Cahill (1994), digital exclusion is associated with the emergence of new forms of poverty that became social policy challenges even before the ICT revolution. According to Cahill, the new forms of poverty produced by the era are, for example, information and communication poverty and service poverty. Older people are required to stay abreast of the ever-growing knowledge, interpretation, media literacy and digital skills of services, communication with multiple actors, and the maintenance of social relationships. Otherwise, they are in danger of being excluded from access to information and services and are outside of channels which they could influence. The new forms of poverty described by Cahill (1994) are intertwined with the demands of the digital world.

32.1.2 Digitalisation as a Process of Social Change

Digitalisation of society is advancing at a faster pace than people are able to embrace the new technological applications. Hardware, software and operating systems are constantly evolving, and new learning is required all the time. The ability to get used to continuous and consistent change and up-dates in ICT equipment and software presents challenges for younger people as well as older people. The more information technology facilitates everyday life, the higher is our dependence on it (Leppiman 2010). The Internet user penetration rate continues to grow year on year. By 2024, it is predicted that there will be an internet usage rate of 97.5% in Finland (Statista 2018). In Estonia, the objective is to increase the percentage of Internet users among the entire population by 2020, from the current figure of 88–95% (Chancellor of Justice 2019).

Digitalisation has not only become a part of society, but is itself constantly and profoundly changing social development. Indeed, digitalisation is an important and fast-paced process of social change that affects the daily lives of all age groups. It aims at streamlining people's lives, disseminating information, facilitating transactions, delivering services, and increasing inclusiveness, social relationships and networking. It should be about new opportunities created by digitalisation. From a human point of view, the key is how technology can be developed so that it contributes to the smooth running and well-being of people.

According to Finnish statistics, 74% of 65–75 year-olds have used the Internet and 21% have accessed some type of digital service. The corresponding figures for the older-age group (75–89 years) are 31% and 8% respectively, leaving a significant majority of older adults excluded from digital activities. By comparison, almost all people of working age (16–64 years) use the Internet (Statistics Finland 2016). In Estonia, there is also evidence of a digital divide between people aged 15–60 years (internet usage rate: 96%) and older-age groups. A representative national survey showed that 62% of people aged 60–74 years use the Internet compared to only 25% of people over 75 years (Turu-uuringute AS 2019).

The age-related differences in the use of digital technology are significantly influenced by the lack of previous experiences and the alienation of operating logic for hardware, software and network services (Päykkönen 2017). Older-age groups have become socialised in the technology of each era in their generational history and encountered a breakthrough in information technology relatively late in their life course. Furthermore, they have often been out of the labour market for a long time, and do not have either user experience or IT supporting structures. Individual life histories differ concerning the use of technology (Niemi 2017; Koskiaho and Saarinen 2019).

The goals of digitalisation often reflect the long-term future of society, but are expected to be realised in practice in today's society. However, reality does not necessarily come with the kind of comprehensive and rapid digital transformation that we are expecting. In Finland, for example, it is estimated that half a million citizens experience a range of barriers to using e-services (Kestilä and Karvonen 2019). For older people, it is estimated that as many as one million are resistant to adopting digital services (VM 2017) and more than half a million do not use the Internet at all (Statistics Finland 2016). The figures indicate a significant problem of structural exclusion, even though the use of digital applications and the digital inclusion of the ageing population is constantly expanding. However, at the same time, the diversity, incompatibility and complexity of digital applications is also increasing (Pohjola 2017).

32.1.3 Digital Services: Seeking Simplification and Efficiency

While ICT has reduced and improved operations in commercial businesses, digitalisation also reduces the number of touchpoints and limits interaction time between providers and customers (Kukk and Leppiman 2019). All organisations are looking for ways to manage and allocate their funding in the most efficient way. Service providers, when faced by the high costs of maintaining traditional services, will strive in their business processes for the simplification and efficiency that digitalisation enables. One of the most characteristic examples of digitalisation is reflected in the shift towards digital banking. For the past two decades, commercial banks have been closing physical branches. Customers increasingly need to use online channels to stay in touch with their banks, transfer money, check balances, and pay bills. Digital solutions are available to everyone faster than ever before, regardless of time and location. Lack of digital devices, such as personal computers, tablets or smartphones, or lack of skills needed for using them, places part of the population in an unequal position. Older people are expected to use personal computers and smartphones, even though the usage of such devices is much lower among older compared to younger age groups.

In Estonia, the healthcare system has been revolutionised by innovative e-solutions. Patients can view their personal medical data in the Patient Portal, see prescribed medicines and prescriptions' validity and schedule a doctor's appointment. People can also view their pension and social welfare entitlements online. Likewise, in Finland, social services, healthcare services and functionalities are highly digitalised, with a range of e-health services available for citizens (Vehko et al. 2019).

A prerequisite for making the most of these opportunities is internet access and the ability to access digital services. People who lack access are left without corresponding information. It is already taken for granted that welfare information and services are increasingly produced digitally. At the same time, face-to-face services are being minimised for cost reasons and traditional local services are being reduced. When digitalising services, the automatic assumption is that everyone is able and willing to use electronic services instead of having a personal meeting. Along with financial savings, the idea is that almost everyone uses the Internet. However, such assumptions do not specify the scale, level or quality of internet use, for example, among people in different stages of ageing. The reasoning is based on generalisations. Market-liberal thinking emphasises individual responsibility, which includes the obligation to stay involved in change, self-responsibility and self-direction, self-service and self-care.

Older people, comprising a population segment typically seen as being more vulnerable to social isolation during the later stages of life, are often more likely to be excluded from the focus of ICT research (Ihm and Hsieh 2015). Statistics Estonia, commissioned by the Ministry of Economy, carries out a household internet usage survey, in the framework of which only people up to 74 years of age are questioned. The survey's objective is to gather data about information technology devices and internet usage among residents of Estonia. Thus, older people, who make up 10% of Estonia's population, are excluded from the survey on internet use. The data from internet usage surveys are used to develop and implement the development plan for Estonia's information society. Moreover, collected data are used to develop and design digital services. Considering such needs, the Chancellor of Justice advises the Statistical Office to also collect internet usage data from people older than 74 years of age (Chancellor of Justice 2019). By disregarding one-tenth of the population, the bias in such data collection may lead policy makers and commercial organisations to over-estimate the number of people who can access online services, and to under-estimate the need for alternative delivery channels and support (Olphert and Damodaran 2013).

One of the reasons why older people are prone to digital exclusion is that their needs and experiences are ignored. In this context, relatively little is known about how older people are embracing constantly evolving digital innovations and how they adapt to rapid change. Against this background, several questions arise. For instance, what does it mean when services are provided by mobile apps? Are websites providing e-services user-friendly, including for older adults? How easy is it to navigate websites to find the services or other information that people need?

Our view is that the needs of older users are often ignored in the shift towards digital services. This happens not only in Estonia and Finland, but also elsewhere because digital service users are not involved and not engaged in the co-creation of the service. The situation is aggravated by the fact that technology applications are being developed separately from the user experience, whereby technology is driven by technology instead of user control. This gives rise to technology determinism, in which digitalisation seems to become a self-governing actor, a goal or a value in itself, rather than a tool for society to achieve its goals. Services are largely developed on the basis of digital solutions, with an instrumental and organisational focus, whereby customers' everyday needs are neglected. Older people will have to adapt to a constantly changing technological environment, rather than adapting technology to the needs and capabilities of older people (Pohjola 2017).

Typically, digital service providers, designers and developers represent younger age-groups who find it difficult to understand the needs of older people [see Poli et al. this volume for a discussion of the exclusion of older people from design processes]. The perceptions of different age cohorts are based on their own experiences. Service designers belonging to the youngest age groups may find it challenging to understand the needs of the older user and their customer journey.

32.1.4 Discussion

Digital forms of exclusion are part of a wider pattern of exclusion that affects people in later life. The challenge for policy makers wishing to reduce social exclusion in general is to place a stronger focus on reducing exclusion from digital technologies. Given the progressive ageing of Europe's populations and the associated shrinking populations of working-age, societies are increasingly cautious when using public funds. As a consequence, the European Economic and Social Committee argues that civil society representatives, including potential beneficiaries of innovations to maintain health and independence, should be included in dialogue arrangements (Batut 2016).

The issue of digital exclusion raises a fundamentally new social policy challenge if a significant and growing part of the population is not to be displaced by the increasing complexity and rapid social structural change. Matters of social responsibility need to be considered in relation to the situation of different population groups and in terms of digital accessibility. A socially sustainable digital society requires not only individual responsibility but also social solidarity in order to bridge the gap between population groups with differing degrees of access to and understanding of digital technologies.

The requirement of social responsibility is built on the fact that digital solutions are in any case social because they arise from human action. Technologies are merely platforms and tools for social action. The role of technologies is to bend the development of services to meet people's needs in order to support their well-being (Niemi 2017; Pohjola 2017). Key elements in the design of digital solutions for older people, as well as for other citizens, are shown in Fig. 32.1.

The starting point for designing a digital environment is to start with everyday practicalities (Koskiaho and Saarinen 2019). The goal is a human, workable everyday life and finding coping strategies. Everyday perspectives highlight the diversity of human social activity, its resources, networks and social capital. Digital solutions can, at best, support human social empowerment, deliver social support and inclusion, and reduce loneliness (Blazun et al. 2012), which in turn promote technology utilisation.

It is necessary to move from traditional technology- and organisation-oriented design to human-centred development (Leikas 2014) if we are to build solutions that are functional both for older people and for service providers. However, this often requires "interpreters", "translators" who are knowledgeable and informed about people's situations, such as social workers, who can help clarify needs and usability requirements. User-driven design is demand-driven and recognises the

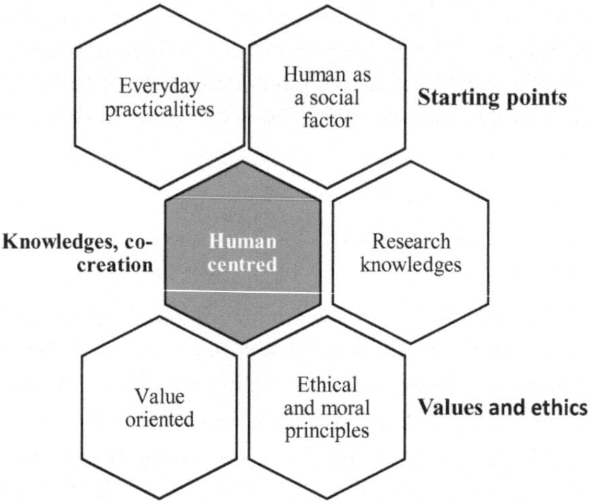

Fig. 32.1 Key elements of design for digital solutions

various factors that influence human-technology interaction, as well as people's different capabilities and conditions (Niemi 2017). At its best, user-driven digitalisation provides accessible solutions for older people. The human-centred (user-driven) concept implies a co-creation process where the user should be seen as an expert on the context (that is problem, need for service, implication of the result) while the service provider is the expert on the solution created during the service (Pohjola 1993).

Planning would also require a much better research knowledge base. The use of ageing-related scientific knowledge in technology development is still limited. Research is needed on the fundamental issues of how digitalisation affects people's daily lives, and what benefits or disadvantages it brings to different groups of people in different contexts and the unintended consequences (Niemi 2017; Koskiaho and Saarinen 2019). In a similar vein, value orientation is also key to designing digital solutions. It includes the basic question of what kind of social actors older people are perceived to be. A dignified old-age is a human right (Leikas 2014). The perspective on ageing differs depending on whether older people are seen as active and functioning citizens, consumers, clients or as recipients of care and services. According to the European Economic and Social Committee (Batut 2016), digitalisation for older people should not be limited just to "technical/medical aid". That is, user inclusive policy refers to taking into account both the provider's perspective and needs regarding value co-creation and the user's view and expectations (Kukk et al. 2014). The focus on value orientation is to avoid producing stigma. Understanding the different ethical and moral issues in the use of technology in society is also essential. For example, awareness of the self-determination of older people and insight into their resources is needed. Ethics are at the heart of digital services design (Niemi 2017; Koskiaho and Saarinen 2019).

32.1.5 Conclusion

Both in Estonia and Finland more effort and investment in digital solutions development is needed to ensure equal access to digital services. Policies can be shaped either to support the needs and values of older citizens as a target group or oriented mainly towards the needs and values of service providers. When it comes to reducing digital exclusion, we suggest that policy makers consider how best to find a balance between service-centred thinking and user (human)-centred understanding and implementation.

Editors' Postscript

Please note, like other contributions to this book, this chapter was written before the COVID-19 pandemic of 2020. The book's introductory chapter (Chap. 1) and conclusion (Chap. 34) consider some of the key ways in which the pandemic relates to issues concerning social exclusion and ageing.

References

Batut, L. (2016). *Opinion of the European Economic and Social Committee on the digital pillar of growth: E-seniors, a potential 25 per cent of the European population.* https://www.eesc.europa.eu/en/our-work/opinions-information-reports/opinions/digital-pillar-growth-e-seniors-potential-25-european-population. Accessed 8 Aug 2019.

Blazun, H., Saranto, K., & Rissanen, S. (2012). Impact of computer training courses on reduction of loneliness of older people in Finland and Slovenia. *Computers in Human Behavior, 28*(4), 1202–1212.

Cahill, M. (1994). *The new social policy*. Oxford: Blackwell.

Castilla, D., Botella, C., Miralles, I., Bretón-López, J., Dragomir-Davis, A. M., Zaragoza, I., & Garcia-Palacios, A. (2018). Teaching digital literacy skills to the elderly using a social network with linear navigation: A case study in a rural area. *Journal of Human Computer Studies, 118*, 24–37.

Chancellor of Justice. (2019) *Statistics Estonia should collect data on Internet usage by the elderly*. https://www.oiguskantsler.ee/en/statistics-estonia-should-collect-data-internet-usage-elderly. Accessed 16 Sept 2019.

Chen, K., & Chan, A. H. (2014). Predictors of Gerontechnology acceptance by older Hong Kong Chinese. *Technovation, 34*(2), 126–135.

Czaja, S. J. (2017). The role of Technology in Supporting Social Engagement among Older Adults. *Public Policy & Aging Report, 27*(4), 145–148.

Freese, J., Rivas, S., & Hargittai, E. (2006). Cognitive ability and internet use among older adults. *Poetics, 34*(4–5), 236–249.

Friemel, T. N. (2016). The digital divide has grown old: Determinants of a digital divide among seniors. *New Media & Society, 18*(2), 313–331.

Grundy, E. (2006). Ageing and vulnerable elderly people: European perspectives. *Ageing & Society., 26*(1), 105–134.

Helsper, E. J. (2012). A corresponding fields model for the links between social and digital exclusion. *Communication Theory, 22*(4), 403–426.
Ihm, J., & Hsieh, Y. P. (2015). The implications of information and communication technology use for the social well-being of older adults. *Information, Communication & Society, 18*(10), 1123–1138.
Kestilä, L., & Karvonen, S. (2019). *Suomalaisten hyvinvointi 2018* [The welfare of Finns 2018]. Terveyden ja hyvinvoinnin laitos Helsinki: THL [Finnish Institute for Health and Welfare].
Koskiaho, B. & Saarinen, E. (Eds.) (2019). *Ihan pihalla? Vanhat ihmiset digitaalisen maailman myllerryksessä: neuvonnan, ohjauksen ja asioiden ajamisen järjestäminen* [Old people in the turmoil of the digital world]. Helsinki: Soste, Suomen sosiaali ja terveys ry. [Finnish Federation for Social Affairs and Health].
Kukk, J., & Leppiman, A. (2019). The significance of value-in experience in the age of digitalisation. In S. Miettinen & M. Sarantou (Eds.), *Managing complexity and creating innovation through design* (pp. 132–140). London: Routledge.
Kukk, J., Leppiman, A., & Pohjola, A. (2014). Designing a business service experience: customer's perspective on value co-creation. *Journal of Research in Economics and Business: Central and Eastern Europe, 6*(1), 51–64.
Leikas, J. (Ed.). (2014) Ikäteknologia [Aging and Technology]. Tutkimuksia 2/2014. Helsinki: Vanhustyön keskusliitto [The Finnish Association for the Welfare of Older People].
Leppiman, A. & Tulva, T. (2005). Entwicklung und Probleme der Sozialarbeit in Estland nach der Wiedererlangung der Unabhängigkeit [Development and Problems of Social Work in Estonia after Regaining Independence]. – *Soziale Arbeit im öffentlichen Raum, Soziale Gerechtigkeit in der Gestaltung des Sozialen.* Berlin: VS Verlag für Sozialwissenschaften, 19. [CD-ROM].
Leppiman, A. (2010). Arjen Elämyksiä – Leiri-ja elämyspohjainen Arkipäivät Perhepalvelu Sosiaalisen Kokemuksen Tuottajana [*Everyday Experiences: Camp-and Experience Based Weekdays Family Service as a Producer of Social Experience*]. Rovaniemi: Lapland University Press.
Martin, C., Hope, S., & Zubairi, S. (2016). *The role of digital exclusion in social exclusion.* Scotland: Ipsos MORI.
Niemi, M. (2017). Ikääntyminen ja teknologia – Gerontologisen sosiaalityön näkökulmia [Aging and technology - perspectives on Gerontological social work]. In Kivistö, M. & Päykkönen, K. (Eds.), *Sosiaalityö digitalisaatiossa.* [Social work in digitalization. Social science publications]. Yhteiskuntatieteellisiä julkaisuja C 58. (pp. 97–111). Rovaniemi: Lapin yliopisto [University of Lapland].
Nordic Institute for Interoperability Solutions. (2019). https://www.niis.org/. Accessed 29 Sept 2019.
Olphert, W., & Damodaran, L. (2013). Older people and digital disengagement: A fourth digital divide? *Gerontology, 59*, 564–570.
Päykkönen, K. (2017). Sosiaalinen media ikääntyneiden kotona asumisen tukemisessa [Social media in supporting older people living at home]. In: Kivistö, M. & Päykkönen, K. (Eds.), *Sosiaalityö digitalisaatiossa.* Yhteiskuntatieteellisiä julkaisuja C 58 [Social work in digitalization. Social science publications]. (pp. 125–135). Rovaniemi: Lapin yliopisto [University of Lapland]. https://lauda.ulapland.fi/handle/10024/63035
Peral-Peral, B., Arenas-Gaitán, J., & Villarejo-Ramos, A. F. (2015). From digital divide to psycho-digital divide: Elders and online social networks. *Comunicar, Media Education Research Journal, 45*, 57–64.
Pohjola, A. (1993). Asiakas sosiaalityön määrittäjänä [Client Defining the Social Work]. In Granfelt, R., Jokiranta, H., Karvinen, S., Matthies, A.-L., & Pohjola, A. (Eds.), *Monisärmäinen sosiaalityö* [Multifaceted Social Work]. (pp. 55–91). Helsinki: Sosiaaliturvan Keskusliitto [Finnish Federation for Social Welfare].
Pohjola, A. (2017). Sosiaalityöohjautuva digitalisaation kehittäminen [Social work-driven development of digitalisation]. In Kivistö, M. & Päykkönen, K. (Eds.), *Sosiaalityö digitalisaatiossa.*

Yhteiskuntatieteellisiä julkaisuja C 58 [Social work in digitalization. Social science publications]. (pp. 181–190). Rovaniemi: Lapin yliopisto [University of Lapland].
Siegel, C., & Dorner, T. E. (2017). Information technologies for active and assisted living – Influences to the quality of life of an ageing society. *International Journal of Medical Informatics, 100*, 32–45.
Sourbati, M. (2007). 'It could be useful, but not for me at the moment': Older people, internet access and e-public service provision. *New Media and Society, 11*(7), 1083–1100.
Statista. (2018). Forecast of the internet user penetration rate in Finland from 2018 to 2024. https://www.statista.com/studies-and-reports/. Accessed 16 Sept 2019.
Statistics Estonia. (2019) Statistical Database. Population figure and composition. Modified 09.05.2019. https://www.stat.ee/population. Accessed 16 Sept 2019.
Statistics Finland. (2016). Official Statistics of Finland (OSF): Use of information and communications technology by individuals, 2016 [e-publication]. http://www.stat.fi/til/sutivi/2016/sutivi_2016_2016-12-09_tie_001_en.html. Accessed 16 Sept 2019.
Statistics Finland. (2019). Official Statistics of Finland (OSF): Population structure, 2019 [e-publication]. http://www.stat.fi/til/vaerak/index_en.html. Accessed 16 Sept 2019.
Turu-uuringute AS. (2019). Nationwide representative survey in Estonia, May.
Vehko, T., Ruotsalainen, S., & Hyppönen, H. (Eds.). (2019). *E-health and e-welfare of Finland* (Check point 2018. Report 7/2019). National Institute for Health and Welfare: Helsinki.
VM. (2017). Digituen toimintamalliehdotus [Digital support policy proposal]. AUTA-hankkeen projektiryhmän loppuraportti. Valtiovarainministeriö VM [Final Report of the AUTA Project. Ministry of Finance].
Walsh, K., Scharf, T., & Keating, N. (2017). Social exclusion of older persons, a scoping review and conceptual framework. *European Journal of Ageing, 14*(1), 81–98.
Yu, R. P., Ellison, N. B., McCammon, R. J., & Lange, K. M. (2016). Mapping the two levels of digital divide: Internet access and social network site adoption among older adults in the USA. *Information, Communication & Society, 19*(10), 1445–1464.

Chapter 33
Social Exclusion in Older-Age and the European Pillar of Social Rights

Maciej Kucharczyk

33.1 Introduction

Framed by an understanding of the role of the European Union in member states' social policy making, this chapter has a focus on analysing the potential of the European Pillar of Social Rights to address social exclusion of older people, the challenges that might impede its efforts, and the measures necessary to overcome such challenges.

To understand the place of European Pillar of Social Rights (the Pillar) in the EU policy context and its most likely impact on policy making, it is helpful to consider the evolution of the EU's evolving role in shaping national social policies since the beginning of European integration in the period that followed the Second World War. Already the Treaty of Rome (1957), which established the original European Economic Community (EEC), today's European Union (EU), contained first social policy measures, such as the free movement of labour and the provision of equal pay for men and women (Scharf 2010). These measures emphasised solidarity as one of the founding principles of European integration. EEC member states considered solidarity to be an intrinsic element of their common vision for development in the post-war period, combining economic growth with high living standards and good working conditions. However, in the 1960s and 1970s progress on harmonising EEC member states' social policies was limited to reaching agreement on broad policy goals (Scharf 2010). This already modest approach was challenged even further by the growing influence of neo-liberal economic and social policy thinking at the beginning of the 1980s. Eventually, "the resulting policy blockage was overcome by the Single European Act (1986), which confirmed the need to 'improve the Community's economic and social situation by extending common policies and pursuing new objectives'."

M. Kucharczyk (✉)
AGE Platform Europe, Brussles, Belgium
e-mail: maciej.kucharczyk@age-platform.eu

K. Walsh et al. (eds.), *Social Exclusion in Later Life*, International Perspectives on Aging 28, https://doi.org/10.1007/978-3-030-51406-8_33

With the Treaty of Maastricht (1992), the name of the European Economic Community was changed to the European Community. Omitting the term "economic" was all but semantic – it indicated member states' willingness to pursue integration beyond its purely economic objectives. Article 2 of the Treaty of Maastricht emphasised a high level of employment and of social protection, economic and social cohesion and solidarity. In 2000, the supra-national coordination received a new impetus, including in the social field, with the introduction of the Open Method of Coordination (OMC). The OMC was intended as a method of soft governance, aiming to spread best practice and achieve convergence towards EU goals in those policy areas which fall under shared or supporting competences of member states, such as social inclusion, health, education, youth or vocational training. Applied to the areas of social inclusion, health care and long-term care and pensions (Social OMC), the new framework provided further opportunity at European level to address social exclusion in older-age. Member states had the opportunity to exchange policy ideas and mutually learn from one another in relation to social policies. The aim was to strengthen well-being and cohesion in ageing societies, specifically in terms of the affordability, availability and quality of health and long-term care services underpinning older people's capacity to participate fully in society; and adequate and sustainable pension systems determining older people's income and de facto their social inclusion.

In 2009, the Treaty of Lisbon introduced additional measures with a social policy focus, including the social market, human dignity, justice and social integration, and gender equality. The EU was charged with a mission to contribute to overall sustainable development in the world, based on solidarity and reciprocal respect, where trade is simultaneously both free and just (Stjernø 2011). Article 151 of the Treaty on the Functioning of the European Union (TFEU) details the EU's key social policy objectives: promoting employment, improving working and living conditions, equal treatment of workers, adequate social protection according to need, social dialogue, developing human resources aimed at achieving a high and sustainable level of employment, as well as combating exclusion. In addition, Article 6 of the Treaty on European Union (TEU) gives binding force to the social rights in the EU Charter of Fundamental Rights. Consequently, the Charter consolidates all the fundamental rights applicable at the EU level. Finally, Art. 9 of the Lisbon Treaty, the so-called "horizontal social clause" proclaims that the Union has to take into account […] the guarantee of adequate social protection […] when implementing new policies.

Notwithstanding these attempts, over the decades, the EU action in the social field has remained limited to supporting member states in the organisation and implementation of national policies. It was only in the aftermath of the global financial and economic crisis of 2008 that a new approach emerged. Under public pressure to recognise the EU's responsibility to address the social consequences of the crisis, national governments and European institutions recognised the need to rebalance EU action. The objective of further economic integration was linked closer to progress towards greater social cohesion and equality. A new comprehensive vision for Europe to achieve "smart, sustainable and inclusive growth" was proposed in the form of the Europe 2020 Strategy. Launched in 2010, the Strategy set five "headline" targets to achieve within the next decade, including ones to lift 20 million people out of poverty, reduce rates of early school leaving to below 10%, and ensure participation of 75% of 20–64 year-olds in the labour market. Yet, once again, the attempt to add a strong social dimension to EU policy making failed. The Europe 2020 Strategy has largely failed in achieving its social goals, most evidently in terms of eradicating poverty. The Strategy's fate was sealed before even reaching 2020 and de facto paved the way to the proclamation of the European Pillar of Social Rights.

33.2 European Pillar of Social Rights

The European Pillar of Social Rights was proclaimed jointly by the European Parliament, the European Council and the European Commission at the Social Summit for Fair Jobs and Growth on 17th November 2017 in Gothenburg. The proclamation was more than symbolic. After years of loose and patchy initiatives in the social field, the EU institutions and member states agreed on a common set of social rights and principles to improve the lives of Europeans through greater equality, inclusion and well-being. This is emphasised in the Pillar's Preamble, which states that "The Union shall combat social exclusion and discrimination, promote social justice and protection, equality between women and men, solidarity between generations and protection of the rights of the child." Built upon 20 principles and rights clustered in three categories of "equal opportunities and access to the labour market", "fair working conditions" and "social protection and inclusion", the Pillar offers a broad policy agenda addressing various social needs.

The proposed rights-based approach makes the Pillar "potentially more powerful than harmonisation of overly divergent policy instruments or attempts at convergence on overly vague objectives" (Cantillon 2019). To be implemented properly, the Pillar could follow the examples of the European Charter of Social Rights or the United Nations' system of human-rights treaty bodies. The two frameworks are articulated around rights, promoting them through indicators and monitoring, establishing action plans and checking if progress is being made towards agreed benchmarks.

However, there remain uncertainties around how national governments and European institutions will fulfil their joint commitment. The Pillar's preamble explicitly states that dedicated measures or legislation must be adopted at the appropriate level for the 20 rights and principles to be legally enforceable. This means that while the EU institutions can propose initiatives and actions, either through legislation or soft policy measures, the responsibility to deliver on the Pillar lies principally in the hands of member states. However, member states can refuse to implement the proposed initiative evoking the lack of dedicated measures or legislation at the national level. Moreover, the implementation of the Pillar is supposed to take account of member states' different socio-economic environments and respect the fundamental principles of national social security systems.

At the same time, expectations of the Pillar are high. Stakeholders, including civil society, hope that the political engagement made by member states in Gothenburg will have a positive impact on improving people's daily realities. This should happen through rebalancing social versus economic considerations in national and EU policy making. According to Garben (2019), the Pillar:

> '...has put a surprising social spin on the Better Regulation Agenda that was threatening to erode the social acquis, it has rekindled the EU's relationship with the International Labour Organization and Council of Europe, and it helps rebalance the EU's output by reviving the use of the Treaty's Social Title'.

While it is too early to draw definitive conclusions, one can at least welcome the Pillar's first concrete achievement – the proposal for an EU directive on carers' leave to support informal carers. However, even this very first attempt to put the Pillar's principles into practice to strengthen EU social acquis is challenged by some member states. An open question remains as to what extent future initiatives of the Pillar will effectively combat social exclusion and discrimination, or consider the intersection of inequalities and multiple discriminations, such as, for example, of older women or older persons with disabilities. Moreover, the Pillar's reference to non-discrimination made under Chapter I, referring to "Equal opportunities and access to the labour market", may impede its efforts to addresses the causes of social exclusion beyond the employment-related perspective and working-age population. Such a limited approach to ageing policy may distract attention from various forms of exclusion in later life that reach beyond work and employment [see also Walsh et al. this volume]. This would include, for example, attention focused on disadvantages arising from age discrimination, limited material resources, lack of access to services, or one's place of residence (Scharf et al. 2004).

In terms of governance, there is no clear vision of how the Pillar will be implemented or of how it will be embedded in the EU's overall economic agenda. The absence of a post-Europe 2020 strategy with a social component puts additional risk on the policy impact of the Pillar. Neither legally binding, nor underpinned by sanctions for no-action, the Pillar's long-term implementation is thus unclear. Notwithstanding several references to the Pillar in the political guidelines of the new Commission President, Ursula von der Leyen, who included an explicit call for an implementation plan, no-one can predict the scope of future initiatives that the Commission will propose to fulfil the engagements of the Pillar. The ultimate impact of the Gothenburg 2017 social summit to make the EU agenda more socially oriented remains to be demonstrated.

33.3 The Pillar's Relevance to Addressing Social Exclusion of Older People

Several of the Pillar's rights and principles are relevant to older people on a general level, in relation to social protection and inclusion. They also apply in more specific ways, in terms of the adequacy of old-age income and pensions, facilitating the transition from work into retirement, or guaranteeing quality and affordable long-term care. However, the Pillar's ability to address social exclusion in older-age and its ultimate impact on policies depends on the level of understanding of the multidimensional nature of exclusion (*e.g.* Scharf and Keating 2012). This in turn undermines the capacity of policy makers to develop and implement policies which will reduce adequately social exclusion in later life (Walsh et al. 2017).

33.3.1 Principles Relating to Specific Forms of Old-Age Exclusion

A combination of factors such as low income, poor health, age and/or gender-based discrimination, reduced physical or mental capacity, unemployment, isolation, abuse, and limited access to services can all play a part in increasing the risk of poverty and social exclusion as people age (Walsh et al. 2017). The following principles of the Pillar are particularly relevant to address the multidimensionality of exclusion in later life (*i.e.* economic, social relations, services, community/spatial, civic and symbolic exclusion):

- Principle 1: The right to education, training and lifelong learning when applied to persons of all ages – when it is understood that this is a precondition for maintaining employability, social inclusion and health across the whole life span.
- Principle 3: The right to equal opportunities regardless of gender, racial or ethnic origin, religion or belief, disability, age or sexual orientation in respect to employment, social protection, education and goods and services – to foster cohesion in society where all population and age groups participate on an equal basis.
- Principle 4: The right to active support to employment – key to older jobseekers, who are often left out of active labour market policies that should support their (re)integration within the labour market.
- Principle 5: The right to secure and adaptable employment – indispensable to adapt labour markets and working conditions to provide for the socio-economic needs of an ageing population, including those workers who either need or want to continue working at an older-age (*e.g.* due to inadequate retirement savings, because of job satisfaction or the need for social interaction).
- Principle 9: The right to work-life balance which took the most concrete form of the European Directive including a paid leave (equivalent to sick leave) to care for dependent relatives – when adequately transposed and implemented at national level, the Directive will enable a more equitable sharing of child care and introduce remunerated carers' leave; this will be a major achievement for many women who must withdraw from the labour market to take on informal care responsibilities.
- Principle 12: The right to social protection for both workers and self-employed people regardless of the type and duration of their employment relationship – key to extending the benefits of social protection to everyone in a constantly changing labour market context (*e.g.* digital platform workers).

- Principle 14: The right to minimum income "at all stages of life" recognises the challenge of adequacy of minimum income schemes beyond the working-age population. An additional reference made to "effective access to enabling goods and services" indicates that non-monetary aspects, which are vital for many older persons to live in dignity, should be taken into consideration.
- Principle 15: The right to old-age income and pensions with the stated aims of "living in dignity" and "equal opportunities of women and men to acquire pension rights" – echoes the challenge of eroding older people's incomes due to declining replacement rates, the shift from pay-as-you-go to funded pension schemes or the persisting gender pension gap.
- Principle 16: The right to health care, referring both to preventive and curative health as well as affordability and quality – the features are indispensable for enabling not only longer, but also healthier lives and equity in health outcomes.
- Principle 17: The right to inclusion of persons with disabilities including adequate income and access to services with an objective to enable them "participate in society" – this broad approach recognises the need to extend social inclusion and participation beyond merely the labour market.
- Principle 18: The right to "affordable long-term care services of good quality, in particular home care and community-based services" – this is a first such implicit reference made at EU level to the challenge of adequate support and assistance to older persons; this also reflects the provisions of Article 25 of the Charter of Fundamental Rights of the European Union, recognising "the rights of the elderly to lead a life of dignity and independence and to participate in social and cultural life".
- Principle 20: The right "to access essential services of good quality, including water, sanitation, energy, transport, financial services and digital communications including support for access to such services" – provides a comprehensive approach to social inclusion beyond solely income-related aspects.

33.3.2 Example of the Pillar's Challenges to Address the Economic Risk of Exclusion in Later Life

In relation to economic exclusion, the right to "Minimum Income" (Principle 14) provides space for new EU policy action. However, first, it requires further clarification of what income adequacy should entail. One can hope that the reference made to "effective access to enabling goods and services" translates into a willingness to address and cover by minimum income schemes access to goods and services that reach beyond individuals' basic and monetary-related needs. For example, promoting and encouraging member states through the Pillar to develop and use national baskets of goods and services, based on a common reference budget methodology, would be helpful. Reference budgets are priced baskets of goods and services that represent a given living standard (Bradshaw 1993). While such budgets are widespread and increasingly applied across European countries, there are considerable differences in their methodologies and the ways in which they are implemented. The EU and member states use the at-risk-of-poverty-threshold (ARPT) – calculated as a percentage (60%) of median equivalent household income – as a benchmark against which an adequate minimum income can be assessed. However, the method ignores that the opportunities to participate fully in society are also determined by other structural and individual factors, such as the availability and accessibility of public goods and services and the extent to which human needs of health and autonomy are fulfilled (Storms et al. 2014). Therefore, the Pillar provides the EU with further responsibility to promote an adequate income across the life span and should focus more on the respective needs of different age and population groups. In regard to older persons, reference budgets should be broken down by gender and by age groups (65–75, 75–85 and over 85 years) in order to reflect older people's evolving needs as they age, including, for example, the higher cost of long-term care for the oldest old. Reference budgets could be part of the EU's further reflection and action on adequacy of minimum income schemes. Although not meant to be used in a prescriptive way, such as determining what people should or should not do, reference budgets provide information about the financial conditions necessary to ensure a person's full social participation. Therefore, reference budgets could be useful when evaluating the adequacy of national minimum income benefits and for guiding EU and national policy choices in social protection and social inclusion policies (Storms et al. 2014).

The right to "old-age income and pensions" (Principle 15) suggests that "workers and the self-employed in retirement have the right to a pension commensurate to their contributions and ensuring an adequate income". This formulation broadens the scope and goes beyond existing acquis by recognising the right of self-employed people to access social protection, even though the reference to individual contributions reflects the general tendency in pension reforms across EU countries to introduce an ever-closer link between earnings/contributions and benefits [see Ogg this section]. On a more positive note, the mention of equal opportunities for women and men to acquire pension rights echoes the evidence concerning the persisting gender pension gap and the European Commission's efforts to address this phenomenon in recent years. Equally important, the notion that "everyone in old-age has the right to resources that ensure living in dignity" represents another step forward in debates about the adequacy of pensions and old-age income for all. It encompasses not only people who can accrue pension rights through employment, but also all those who are permanently or temporarily unable to work due to disability and people who for justifiable reasons are no longer available to work, or have shorter or interrupted working carriers and therefore are unable to build adequate pension rights.

33.4 The Pillar to Socialise the European Semester

The key EU policy instrument to guide national macroeconomic and structural reforms, the European Semester (Semester), remains largely disconnected from the reflection on social aspects and their place in the overall economic growth paradigm. Actors at the national and EU levels, such as trade unions, civil society and academia, argue that the Pillar, if meant to underpin the EU's social agenda, should steer member states' policies through the Semester, to ensure a closer connection between the two processes (*e.g.* Vanhercke et al. 2017). Arrangements for implementing the Pillar through the Semester were already specified by the European Commission in the Annual Growth Survey 2018 and the Draft Joint Employment Report 2018. However, an open question remains as to what extent the Pillar's principles and rights will be considered through the implementation of the Semester at national level (*i.e.* the National Reform Programmes). The main challenge faced by the EU and member states is the ability to ensure consistency between economic, employment and financial policies with a view to strengthening the social dimension. Two years after the proclamation of the Pillar, it seems that the Semester has been paying more attention to social issues, including those relevant for older people, such as life-long learning, employment of older workers or quality long-term care systems. In its annual assessment of the Semester in 2018, AGE Platform Europe (AGE) considered the impact of the Semester's implementation on the social realities of older persons (Age Platform 2018). According to AGE, the adequacy of pensions had been addressed by the European Commission in its recommendations to those member states where the level of pensions is dramatically low. However, AGE members regret the lack of further focus on the most vulnerable groups of pensioners, such as older women, the very old or older persons with health issues. Moreover, other barriers that prevent older people from exercising their social rights, including those listed in the Pillar, are not addressed in the Semester. This includes barriers such as the investment gap in long-term care, the lack of accessibility of physical and digital environments, or the difficult situation of older jobseekers. Instead of emphasising its potential opportunities, population ageing remains perceived by many policy makers more as a burden to the public purse, which needs to be contained, than as an achievement and opportunity.

33.5 Conclusion

Considering the multiple crises that Europe has been facing over the last decade and growing public scepticism towards the European project, the proclamation of the European Pillar of Social Rights was a first attempt by EU institutions and member states to create conditions for greater fairness and solidarity at both the macro level (among countries and regions) and at the grass-roots level (among age and population groups and individuals themselves). The Pillar recognised the key role played by social rights in empowering all population and age groups as equal holders of social and, broadly, human rights. Consequently, the Pillar has the potential to improve not only daily realities of Europeans, but, equally importantly, to improve their perception of the EU as such. Eventually, this could have a positive spill-over effect beyond the strictly socio-economic sphere by helping to (re)adhere European people back to the European values and the common integration project.

Since the Pillar does not confer new competences or tasks upon the European Union, the EU does not have an enlarged competence in relation to the design of pension systems. Nor are the 20 rights and principles directly enforceable without implementing measures. Therefore, the ultimate impact of the Pillar will depend on the political will of both EU institutions and member states to develop concrete policy actions to implement the Pillar. In the long run, the European Court of Justice could refer to the Pillar when interpreting EU law, and de facto exercise pressure on policy makers to implement measures addressing the social needs of European people, including of those in later life.

Political will, commitment and accountability are all and equally needed for the Pillar to succeed and to avoid mistakes of the past, such as the lack of progress on the Europe 2020 Strategy's social headline targets (*e.g.* on poverty reduction). There remains a question concerning how the Pillar's implementation will inform the post-Europe 2020 strategy and how the latter will articulate and align its policy objectives with the Agenda 2030 and the Sustainable Development Goals. Stakeholder involvement, including involvement of civil society, will be another key element to enable the EU to steer national policies using the Pillar's principles and rights. At a broader level, further reflection is needed on other political processes that can underpin the EU's social dimension provided by the Pillar. Other policy standards, such as the International Labour Organisation's core convention and the Council of Europe's Social Charter should be used as inspiration.

Europe is still suffering the consequences of the 2008 economic crisis. Older people have not been spared in this process: the gender pension gap is close to 40% and poverty persists among many older women, the oldest old, those who were not able to build an adequate pension, or older persons whose income has eroded over time, in particular due to the growing costs of health care. The individualisation of old-age dependency risks, with increased out-of-pocket payments for health care, is undermining the universal character of health care that is a part of the European social welfare model. Pension reforms that delay the age at which people become eligible to receive their pensions are hitting vulnerable groups, such as the 48% of people aged between 55 and 64 years who are not in employment, not yet of pensionable age and who have very low prospects of finding a job.

Most of the Pillar's 20 principles and rights are directly relevant to older people and, therefore, of key importance. The ultimate impact they will have on the improvement of older people's social realities will depend on how comprehensive and mutually reinforcing the future policy actions proposed under the Pillar will be. Their overarching objective should be to address the multidimensionality of exclusion in later life from a rights-based perspective, for example by enhancing the rights to quality and affordable health and long-term care, to adequate pensions to live in dignity, to age-friendly working conditions and an inclusive labour market, or to access goods and services. To do so, member states and EU institutions must align any forthcoming Pillar proposals with Article 25 of the European Charter of Fundamental Rights, thereby acknowledging the right of older persons to live independently and in dignity.

Author's Postscript

Beyond the immediate challenges of saving lives and keeping healthcare systems functioning, the COVID-19 crisis has triggered an unprecedented shift in national and European policies. In this context, the Pillar of Social Rights acquires new importance; the full implementation of all its principles is more indispensable than ever and should underpin the recovery strategies that Member States and the EU put in place. With regard to older people, the Pillar's various principles are particularly important during and after the pandemic. These include universal health and long-term care services, and ensuring adequate social protection for all, including minimum safety nets or inclusive employment policies. The Pillar, together with the EU's environmental objectives and the UN's Sustainable Development Goals, should guide recovery strategies based on human rights, social inclusion and solidarity between all age and population groups.

References

AGE Platform Europe. (2018). Assessment of the European Semester 2018, with country perspectives from France, Italy, Malta and Spain. Brussels: Age Platform Europe. Available at: https://www.age-platform.eu/sites/default/files/AGE_Position_on_EUSemester2018.pdf

Bradshaw, J. (Ed.). (1993). *Budget standards for the United Kingdom*. Aldershot: Avebury.

Cantillon, B. (2019). The European Pillar of Social Rights: ten arguments for prioritising principle 14 on minimum incomes, Working Paper 19.02. Antwerp: Herman Deleeck Centre for Social Policy. Available at: http://www.centrumvoorsociaalbeleid.be/sites/default/files/CSBWorkingPaper1902.pdf

Garben, S. (2019). The European pillar of social rights: An assessment of its meaning and significance. *Cambridge Yearbook of European Legal Studies, 21*, 101–127.

Scharf, T. (2010). Social policies for ageing societies: Perspectives from Europe. In D. Dannefer & C. Phillipson (Eds.), *The SAGE handbook of social gerontology* (pp. 497–512). London/New York: Sage.

Scharf, T., & Keating, N. (2012). Social exclusion in later life: A global challenge. In T. Scharf & N. Keating (Eds.), *From exclusion to inclusion in old age: A global challenge* (pp. 1–16). Bristol: Policy Press.

Scharf, T., Phillipson, C., & Smith, A. E. (2004). Poverty and social exclusion: Growing older in deprived urban neighbourhoods. In A. Walker & C. H. Hennessy (Eds.), *Growing older: Quality of life in old age* (pp. 81–106). Maidenhead: Open University Press.

Stjernø, S. (2011). The idea of solidarity in Europe. *European Journal of Social Law, 3*, 170–173.

Storms, B., Kurcharczyk, M., Leydet, L., McKinney, C., & Perek-Bialas, J. (2014). *What should an adequate old-age income entail to live in dignity? Learnings from France, Ireland and Poland*. Brussels: Age Platform Europe. Available at: https://www.age-platform.eu/sites/default/files/AGE_EMIN_publication_Dec2014_EN.pdf.

Vanhercke, B., Natali, D., & Bouget, D. (2017). *Social policy in the European Union: State of play 2016*. Brussels: European Trade Union Institute. Available at: https://www.etui.org/fr/content/download/33096/306832/file/17+Social+policy+in+EU+2017+OSE+Web+version.pdf

Walsh, K., Scharf, T., & Keating, N. (2017). Social exclusion of older persons: A scoping review and conceptual framework. *European Journal of Ageing, 14*(1), 81–98.

Section IX
Conclusion

Chapter 34
Advancing Research and Policy on Social Exclusion of Older People: Towards a Coherent and Critical Discourse

Thomas Scharf, Kieran Walsh, Sofie Van Regenmortel, and Anna Wanka

34.1 Introduction

A key starting point for the contributions to this book has been the pressing need to address stagnation in research and policy debates on social exclusion in later life. As noted in recent reviews of the relevant academic literature (Van Regenmortel et al. 2016; Walsh et al. 2017), research relating to social exclusion of older people has been characterised by limitations in conceptual and theoretical development. While there is broad agreement on the different forms of exclusion that serve to reduce well-being in later life, the absence of a body of research that provides a comprehensive account of forms of social exclusion and considers the connections between them has limited the scope of policy makers to develop well-evidenced responses to the multifaceted challenges faced by ageing societies. Drawing on insights generated from the pathbreaking work of the interdisciplinary and international ROSEnet COST Action (CA15122), the chapters of this book reflect different disciplinary perspectives, contrasting methodological approaches, and a wide range of national and international contexts. With its five working groups addressing different domains of exclusion (economic; social; service; community and spatial; and civic) and a focus on the interrelationships between the domains, ROSEnet has been well

T. Scharf (✉)
Population Health Sciences Institute, Newcastle University, Newcastle upon Tyne, UK
e-mail: thomas.scharf@ncl.ac.uk

K. Walsh
Irish Centre for Social Gerontology, Institute for Lifecourse and Society, National University of Ireland Galway, Galway, Ireland

S. Van Regenmortel
Department of Adult Educational Sciences, Vrije Universiteit Brussel, Brussels, Belgium

A. Wanka
Research Training Group 'Doing Transitions' Goethe University Frankfurt am Main, Frankfurt am Main, Germany

K. Walsh et al. (eds.), *Social Exclusion in Later Life*, International Perspectives on Aging 28, https://doi.org/10.1007/978-3-030-51406-8_34

positioned to advance scientific knowledge and methodological rigour in the field of social exclusion. Moreover, ROSEnet's direct engagement with policy and practice stakeholders, including some who have contributed chapters to this book, ensures that the book offers valuable insights aimed at supporting policy development focused on reducing social exclusion in later life. Taken together, the chapters therefore provide the much-needed ideas and empirical evidence that are essential in defining a new agenda for future research on ageing and social exclusion.

In this concluding chapter, we return to the four key objectives that underpinned our choice of topics for the book. These were, in abbreviated form, to: (1) produce a comprehensive analysis of social exclusion of older people; (2) develop cross-national and interdisciplinary perspectives on social exclusion of older adults; (3) institute a dialogue between conceptual and empirical perspectives; and (4) nurture crucial research capacity in the field of social exclusion and ageing. Reflecting these objectives, we use this chapter to draw together some of the major themes emerging from the book's different sections and demonstrate interconnections between the contributing chapters. In this respect, we seek to deepen our understanding of the conceptual framing of social exclusion of older people, noting where gaps in knowledge still remain. Moreover, within the context of the far-reaching impacts of COVID-19 on older people and on the framing of later life, as noted in Chap. 1, we conclude by suggesting ways in which the insights developed in this book can be used as a basis for shaping a new research agenda relating not only to future empirical and conceptual research, but also to policy development in the field of social exclusion in later life.

In the introduction to this book, we identified features of the policy context around ageing and demographic change as playing a role in the lack of progress in debates on social exclusion in later life. This involves the widespread absence of age in equalities debates, the prevailing view of ageing as being a burden on welfare states, the systemic ageism that marks our societies, and a lack of attention to the risks of social exclusion in later life. Equally, research debates have failed to progress in meaningful ways owing to a lack of conceptual clarity about social exclusion and the resulting challenges of operationalising exclusion in empirical studies.

The various contributions to this book emphasise the importance of viewing social exclusion as a relative, dynamic and multidimensional construct. These characteristics are a longstanding feature of work on social exclusion relating to older people, picking up on ideas developed initially in research conducted in the UK (Scharf et al. 2002, 2005; Barnes et al. 2006; Kneale 2012) but subsequently acknowledged more widely (*e.g.* Moffatt and Glasgow 2009; Burns et al. 2012; Scharf and Keating 2012). The evidence presented in the various parts of the book, and aligning to the book's four objectives, emphasises the value of deepening knowledge about specific domains of social exclusion and the interrelationships between them, rather than focusing attention on the broader concept of exclusion. There is a general acceptance in the gerontology literature that the domains of exclusion that have the greatest impact on older people's lives and their well-being relate to individuals' material resources, social relations, access to services, civic and cultural participation, and socio-spatial context (Jehoel-Gijsbers and Vrooman

2008; Van Regenmortel et al. 2016; Walsh et al. 2017). Equally important is the need to improve our knowledge about the most appropriate policy and practice responses to different forms of social exclusion in older-age in order to build inclusive societies and consequently fight negative consequences of old-age social exclusion such as lower quality of life (Bayram et al. 2010), higher rates of depressive symptoms (Tong et al. 2011) and higher suicide rates (Yur'yev et al. 2010). We begin by reviewing the contributions across the different domains of social exclusion before considering the interrelationships between them and the role of policy in tackling risks of exclusion in later life.

34.2 Domains of Social Exclusion

The chapters in this book have addressed five domains of exclusion: economic, social, service, civic, and community and spatial exclusion. In relation to the economic domain, Jim Ogg and Michal Myck's introduction in section II (Chap. 2) emphasises the need to move beyond a narrow focus on poverty and pension entitlements in addressing economic and material forms of exclusion in later life. Reflecting a life-course approach, they argue that there is a need to take account of the ways in which circumstances earlier in life strongly influence risks of economic exclusion in older age. These risks are experienced differently according to individuals' social locations and political context, a point developed by Merle Sumil-Laanemaa and colleagues in their analysis of material deprivation of people aged 50 and above in different welfare regimes (Chap. 3). The authors make the key point that risks of economic exclusion vary considerably according to socio-demographic characteristics. While some demographic characteristics increase the risk of exclusion in all welfare regimes, particular subgroups of older people encounter disproportionately high risks of material deprivation in some of the clusters. Sumil-Laanemaa and colleagues suggest that, as ageing populations continue to become more diverse as demographic change continues apace, policy makers will increasingly need to consider how best to respond to the material needs of particular groups of older adults. In Chap. 4, Elke Murdock and colleagues focus on one specific group who experience a heightened risk of economic exclusion in later life. They highlight the impacts of unemployment in the later stages of working life, identifying it as an under-explored feature of debates in exclusion from material and economic resources. Given the potentially severe consequences of late-career unemployment within the context of policy measures aimed at extending working lives and the increasing numbers of older workers in many societies, Murdock and colleagues suggest the need for a stronger focus in research on older unemployed people. Another group whose material circumstances merit closer attention in research and policy are older women who are widowed, divorced or separated. Reflecting on the experiences of this group in Turkey and Serbia, and life-course determinants of low incomes in older-age, Hande Barlin and colleagues place value on social policy measures aimed at reducing risks of poverty (Chap. 5). In the absence of acquired pension rights, there is an obvious role for the state in providing survivor pensions and other types of income support to older women who experience widowhood, separation or divorce.

Noting the growing focus in gerontological research on issues relating to social relationships in later life, Vanessa Burholt and Marja Aartsen address the domain of exclusion from social relations with reference to older adults' social resources, social connections and social networks (Chap. 6). Drawing on a new conceptual model of exclusion from social relations (Burholt et al. 2019), they identify a range of personal attributes and life experiences associated with this form of exclusion and highlight its impacts on older people's health, well-being and sense of belonging. The conceptual model is grounded in a dynamic, life-course perspective that recognises the ways in which exclusion from social relations varies according to time and place, social norms, cultural values and policies and, hence, across societies. These ideas are developed in the three chapters that follow, illustrating the value of deepening understanding of the eco-bio-psychosocial factors associated with exclusion from social relations in later life. Sofie Van Regenmortel and colleagues (Chap. 7) draw on data from Belgium and rural Britain to demonstrate the presence of exclusion of social relations and at the same time analyse features of exclusion from social relations, showing how this form of exclusion connects to other features of disadvantage. In making a strong case for further cross-national and methodologically comparable research on the subject, the authors point to the need for social policy responses that acknowledge the impact of life-course factors on experiences of exclusion from social relations in older-age, while at the same time building and investing in age-friendly and prosperous environments to cultivate social inclusion. In Chap. 8, Deborah Morgan and colleagues explore micro- and macro-level drivers of loneliness, regarded as a key form of exclusion from social relations, and seek to measure changes over time in loneliness rates in a number of European countries. An important feature of the analysis developed in this chapter is the evidence provided to indicate how macro-level drivers, including perceived neighbourhood safety and normative levels of social connectedness, influence loneliness across nations. Although the two-year time frame of the analysis served to limit how much could be said about change over time, the authors hold out hope that future studies can draw on additional waves of data arising from longitudinal studies to provide more robust evidence of the dynamic nature of loneliness in later life. A similar case for longitudinal analysis emerges from Chap. 9, in which Charles Waldegrave and colleagues consider the complex nature of the conflicted, abusive and discriminative relations of older people and their differential exclusionary impacts in five contrasting countries (Norway, Israel, Italy, Finland and New Zealand). The authors expose the influence of discriminatory attitudes in excluding groups of ageing adults or individual older people from opportunities to develop or maintain supportive social relations. Their analysis highlights the need for qualitative studies that can improve understanding of the interconnections between vulnerability, dependency and abuse. The chapter notes the value of an exclusion perspective in terms of understanding non-normative social relations in later life, not least its potential to inform professional practice.

In considering the domain of service exclusion in later life, Veerle Draulans and Giovanni Lamura use their introduction in section IV to develop a new definition of this form of exclusion (Chap. 10). They define exclusion from services as the "condition (and the processes leading to it) that involves the lack or denial of services in later life, to a larger extent than what might be considered as 'normal' for the majority of people, with a negative impact both at individual and societal levels". This conceptualisation is helpful in contextualising the three substantive chapters that follow, each of which relates to a different type of service that plays a central role in older adults' opportunities for social integration. In Chap. 11, Florent Cholat and Luca Daconto describe the risks of spatial- and mobility-related exclusion from services that have the potential to affect older people who live in the unique environmental context of mountain areas. A key argument concerns the idea of "reversed" mobilities – the idea that people whose mobility is limited by their residential environment become more reliant on receiving products and services provided by relatives, caregivers or mobile shops in order to overcome the lack or denial of services. The chapter suggests that, by identifying areas potentially exposed to service exclusion as a result of interlinkages between individual and contextual vulnerabilities, research has a major role to play in informing policy innovation. In Chap. 12, Zsuzsa Széman and colleagues also consider factors that shape service exclusion, drawing on examples from the relatively under-researched context of countries in Central and Eastern Europe and the Russian Federation. The particular focus is onhome care services, underpinned by a combination of a strong tradition of familisation and a general lack of institutional care facilities. The authors suggest that while home-based care can potentially support more person-centred forms of care in the countries under investigation, some people may experience heightened risks of exclusion from social relations as a result of receiving care in their homes. Consequently, the chapter highlights the need for research that focuses on the cultural contexts in which services are provided to, and accessed by, older people. This is also an argument picked up in Chap. 13. Faced by increasing digitalisation of societies, accessing services online has become a key feature of many countries' health and care systems. Arianna Poli and colleagues analyse the role of digital technologies in supporting health care provision of older adults. Their work explores key drivers of exclusion from digital health services, demonstrating the interconnections between macro-, meso- and micro- decisions in shaping people's access to essential services in later life. The authors emphasise the importance of deepening understanding of barriers to the inclusive and equal implementation of digital health services in ageing societies. Responding to the challenges of digitalisation implies creating opportunities to improve health services in ways that can better meet the needs of a diverse older population.

Turning to community and spatial aspects of social exclusion, a consistent feature of chapters in section V is the perspective that national contexts appear to be less central than regional and place-specific contexts in framing experiences of exclusion in later life. Isabelle Tournier and Lucie Vidovićová's part introduction connects conceptual debates on exclusion with recent developments in the field of environmental gerontology (Chap. 14). In presenting an adapted framework model of life-space locations, ranging from clearly defined indoor spaces to more abstract global and digital spaces, they argue that risks of exclusion require responses from policy and practice at all spatial scales. These ideas frame the three chapters that follow. In Chap. 15, Matthias Drilling and colleagues introduce a new conceptual model of "Age, Space and Exclusion" that accounts for the triangular relationship between materialisations, conceptions and experiences of space in older-age. The "ASE-Triangle" is tested with reference to empirical evidence drawn from studies conducted in Ireland and Cyprus, illustrating the ways in which age, space and exclusion interact in different national and regional contexts. The authors highlight the considerable potential of their model in deepening understandings of spatial and community forms of exclusion, suggesting the potential to refine the model based on evidence collected from contrasting environmental contexts in other countries. The benefits of cross-national comparative frameworks that are attuned to regional variations within nations are also raised by the chapter that follows. In their comparative study, based on analysis of cases from Germany, Ireland and Poland, Anna Urbaniak and colleagues identify a need for researchers to deepen their understanding of the multifaceted connections between place, normative life-course transitions and social exclusion in order to contribute to more appropriate policy responses aimed at reducing exclusion in later life (Chap. 16). In particular, future research should examine more systematically the intersections between major life transitions and features of older people's neighbourhoods and communities. This would assist in casting light on the role of place in influencing how experiences of social exclusion change over time. Reflecting a longstanding concern in social gerontology with urban and rural places as contexts for ageing, Lucie Vidovićová and colleagues make the point that older people who live in rural areas are often ignored in research and policy (Chap. 17). With examples drawn from different types of rural location in the Czech Republic, Germany and Poland, the authors argue that lack of care provision amounts to a form of place-based social exclusion that is disproportionately experienced by older people in rural communities. Recognising the need for more evidence from other rural contexts, the chapter emphasises the value of developing better coordinated policy responses to place-based exclusion that reflect the diversity of both older adults and rural places. More inclusive policy responses require mutual learning between the different actors that belong to the older adult care sector, including non-governmental organisations, civil society groups and private actors.

Acknowledging that the domain of civic exclusion has historically been the least well-developed component of research on social exclusion in later life, Sandra Torres in section IV contextualises the three chapters that examine this domain by introducing key conceptual features of civic and cultural forms of exclusion (Chap. 18). She addresses the ongoing attention that has been paid to the idea of civic exclusion, noting the many evidence gaps that still remain in terms of its social and political aspects, before focusing attention on the under-developed socio-cultural dimensions of exclusion. She describes these as "the ways in which societal discourses lead not only to the exclusion of older people, but also to neglecting the complex identities they have, and the variety of circumstances, experiences and needs with which these are associated". Different features of civic and socio-cultural forms of exclusion are considered in the chapters that follow. In Chap. 19, Rodrigo Serrat and colleagues' scoping review of civic engagement in later life deepens our understanding of the construct of civic exclusion and identifies the knowledge gaps that will need to be addressed in future research. Aligning closely with themes raised in other parts of the book, four key dimensions of older people's exclusion from civic engagement merit particular attention: the multidimensionality of civic engagement; the diversity of older populations; the dynamics and experiences of engagement across the life course; and the culturally embedded processes that characterise civic engagement. The focus in Chap. 20 turns to socio-cultural aspects of exclusion from civic activities in older-age. Using evidence from Austria, Vera Gallistl's analysis of changing patterns of cultural consumption as people age emphasises the central influence of socio-economic status on non-participation in forms of culture that many people take for granted. She argues that future research in gerontology should consider older adults' exclusion from cultural practice as a question of both spatial and (cultural) taste marginalisation. According to Gallistl, given how particular groups of older adults experience structural and symbolic forms of marginalisation in late-modern societies, participation and non-participation in culture and the arts should become core themes in social gerontology, and especially in the study of social exclusion in later life. In Chap. 21, Ada Lui Gallassi and Lars Harrysson address a different dimension of civic exclusion. Their chapter connects socio-economic status and the conditions of ageing migrants to civic and broader forms of social exclusion emphasising how these processes influence older migrants' sense of status in a host society. Taking an intersectional approach, and using evidence from Sweden, the authors signal the importance of a future research agenda that takes account of the ways in which features of migrants' working life trajectories interact, leading to forms of symbolic exclusion in a post-work phase of life. The chapter makes a case for policy responses that emphasise individuals' right to work and the access social security entitlements, with equality and anti-discrimination approaches being identified as mechanisms for tackling social exclusion of ageing migrants.

34.3 Interrelationships Between Domains of Social Exclusion

As noted above, many of the chapters in sections II to VI of this book have already considered ways in which the various domains of social exclusion connect with one other. This demonstrates the value of adopting a dynamic, multidimensional exclusion lens when seeking to understand forms of disadvantage that characterise later life. In section VII, Lena Dahlberg therefore introduces four chapters that consider different types of interrelationship between specific domains of exclusion (Chap. 22). Her contribution is especially valuable in summarising previous research on multidimensionality of exclusion of older people, observing the various associations that have been identified between most of the domain combinations addressed in different chapters of this book. Drawing on studies across a range of countries, Dahlberg makes the key point that "being excluded on one domain increases the risk of exclusion from another domain". She identifies particular gaps in relation to longitudinal research that can capture dynamic features of multidimensional exclusion as well as research that considers different country settings. In Chap. 23, Feliciano Villar and colleagues address the experiences of older people who live in long-term care institutions, framing this in terms of their potential risks of exclusion from social relationships, civic participation and socio-cultural life. In Chap. 24, Michal Myck and colleagues analyse the relationship between people's material circumstances in later life and their risk of exclusion from social relations, operationalised with reference to loneliness. A notable finding from this longitudinal analysis is the strong and significant association between material deprivation and loneliness over time, with material conditions shaping both the degree to which people experience loneliness as well as the likelihood that loneliness will increase over time. Anu Siren's focus in Chap. 25 is on the role played by transport in older adults' risks of social exclusion. Her argument is that transport mobility, typically viewed in relation to exclusion from services, affects all domains of social exclusion. As a result, policy responses that fail to tackle the structural dimensions of age-related mobility will fail to achieve the social inclusion of older adults. In Chap. 26, Nilufer Korkmaz-Yaylagul and Ahmet Melik Bas consider homelessness of older adults in relation to multidimensional forms of social exclusion. Drawing on their analysis of current research, they highlight the ways in which homelessness in later life is related in one way or another to all forms of social exclusion. A particular concern of research on this topic has been on exclusion from services, amenities and mobility, presenting key challenges for policy makers tasked with reducing social exclusion of this especially marginalised population of older adults.

34.4 Policy Responses to Social Exclusion in Later Life

A common feature of many of the chapters in sections II to VII of this book is their direct engagement with policy responses directed towards reducing risks of social exclusion experienced by older people. The contributions to section VIII deal explicitly with policy challenges, laying the foundation for a series of actions that, taken together, provide opportunities to promote the social inclusion of ageing adults. The chapters in section VIII provide a more considered analysis of the range of policy issues impacted by and influencing social exclusion in later life than is typical for political and public debates on social inclusion in later life. In Chap. 27, Norah Keating and Maria Cheshire-Allen introduce social exclusion as a values-based policy framework for population ageing and older persons. They identify social exclusion as a "timely and relevant approach to the development of meaningful policy and practice", necessitating an examination of policy drivers and policy actions. Whilst accepting the importance of a sound evidence base to underpin policy, they caution that key policy actors may need to be won over to embrace the values that underpin a reinvigorated focus on social exclusion. These ideas are picked up in the chapters that follow. Taking a global perspective, Patricia Conboy analyses the potential of the United Nations' Sustainable Development Goals and the 2030 Agenda for Sustainable Development to serve as a global framework for addressing multidimensional old-age exclusion (Chap. 28). She identifies a range of processes and barriers associated with national governments' engagement with this global framework, highlighting actions that might reduce older people's risks of social exclusion across the world. In his review of pension policies, Jim Ogg shows how Europe's pension systems are responding to new social risks arising from a rapidly changing political, technological and economic context (Chap. 29). While pension systems act as the principal mechanism for preventing economic exclusion in later life, Ogg emphasises the risk that policy measures, such as those aimed at extending working lives, will typically increase the likelihood that future cohorts of older people will experience economic exclusion. Pension policies, alongside social care policies, are also a core focus of Irina Grigoryeva and colleagues (Chap. 30). Taking the examples of recent policy developments in Russia and Ukraine, they argue that reform measures run the risk of exposing greater numbers of older people to forms of economic and service exclusion. In both countries, low retirement incomes, poor health, and lack of access to services are associated with heightened risks of intense forms of social exclusion in later life. In Chap. 31, John Andersen and colleagues consider policy responses to risks of exclusion faced by residents of nursing homes. Their focus is on older adults' important connections to neighbourhood social relationships, showing how innovation in the design of nursing homes has the potential to improve opportunities for neighbourhood and social engagement of a heterogeneous population of older nursing home residents, including people living with cognitive impairment. In Chap. 32, within the context of policies aimed at digitalising access to public services in Estonia and Finland, Anu Leppiman and colleagues examine some of the contradictions associated with digitalisation for ageing adults. On the one hand, digitalisation has the potential to reduce exclusion of older people by providing access to information and services. On the other hand, given lower levels of digital literacy amongst older people, the shift to digital forms of service provision has the potential to exclude current cohorts of ageing adults. In Chap. 33, Maciej Kucharczyk analyses the potential of the European Pillar of Social Rights to address social exclusion of older people in Europe. The Pillar encompasses a set of social rights and principles aimed at improving the lives of people in Europe by focusing on promoting equality, inclusion and well-being. In line with its rights-based approach, the Pillar has the potential to overcome social policy blockages in many European countries to promote social inclusion of ageing adults.

34.5 Reducing Social Exclusion in Later Life: New Directions for Research and Policy

Taken together, the contributions to this book decisively push forward the current state of knowledge on social exclusion in later life. In response to the book's objectives, presented in Chap. 1, the multinational team of authors provide an insightful and comprehensive account of social exclusion in later life, exploring the multidimensionality of exclusion across different life domains, the interrelationship between these domains, and the involvement of individual and societal/policy levels (objective 1). The wide range of spatial and place-based contexts that underpin the chapters, representing different spatial scales ranging from local to global, as well as the contributions of a variety of scientific disciplines and methodological approaches, represent one of the book's core strengths. Drawing on the work of Walsh et al. (2017) in conceptualising social exclusion in later life, the chapters display a shared understanding of the exclusion construct, its meanings and its various domains (objective 2). In a number of chapters, contributing authors develop new theoretical perspectives that will help to shape future work on domains of exclusion and the relationships between domains. All chapters succeed in linking conceptual and empirical perspectives in a mutually supportive dialogue, deepening awareness of the methodological approaches needed to build the empirical evidence base as well as the conceptual tools that are required to inform future empirical studies (objective 3). The fact that many of the book's chapters have been written jointly by early-stage researchers and mid-career as well as well-established researchers, and by researchers drawn from multiple disciplines and a range of countries, has contributed to building the capacity of the research community to support future work that will extend even further knowledge about social exclusion and ageing (objective 4). Meeting these objectives is vital in moving forward research and policy agendas on the dynamic and multidimensional forms of social exclusion that characterise later life.

Against this background, and reflecting many of the arguments developed by contributors to this book, we conclude by outlining a future agenda for research on old-age social exclusion and for policy aimed at reducing social exclusion in later life. This is a collective task that will require collaboration between all sectors of society – a task made all the more necessary by the wide-ranging impacts of the COVID-19 pandemic on older people. To succeed, it will need to engage actors involved in policy making, civil society, service providers and scientific research. There is also a key role to be played by older people, including people with experience of exclusion, and their representative organisations in developing appropriate policy and practice responses. Working across sectors, the different actors will need to demonstrate their shared commitment to tackling social exclusion in later life and to addressing the multiple forms of disadvantage that reduce the well-being of far too many older adults across the world. Where policies are being developed that may impact on older people, they should be evaluated on the basis of their potential intended and unintended consequences in terms of social exclusion risks in later life. This applies, for example, to the ongoing pension policy and health and social care reforms being introduced in many countries in response to demographic ageing. Reflecting the pervasive nature of ageism and age discrimination in many societies, there is a fundamental need for coordinated responses that address symbolic, culturally embedded forms of social exclusion and engage in challenging negative representations of ageing and later life. These ideas are picked up in the next sections in terms of responses to the multidimensional nature of exclusion in later life, and responses to accumulated disadvantage and risk groups, and to multilevel shocks that are associated with risks of exclusion of older adults.

34.5.1 Responding to Multidimensionality of Social Exclusion in Later Life

From a research perspective, the contributions to this book emphasise the value of further deepening our knowledge of the ways in which different forms of exclusion combine in older people's lives, and of the implications of social exclusion for older adults' health and well-being. Future research should also focus on identifying key causes and drivers of multidimensional exclusion, and how these factors interact with the ageing process to impact on older people's lives. While considerable progress has been made by the research community in developing conceptual frameworks that explain the connections between different forms of exclusion, including by contributors to this book, there is scope to revisit these frameworks in order to identify the type of interventions that might best respond to different forms of exclusion. In relation to the multidimensionality of exclusion in later life, a key task will be to improve the quality of data that can be used to provide evidence across the domains of exclusion and to improve understanding of the connections between different domains. For example, while some domains, such as economic exclusion or exclusion from social relations, can draw on high quality quantitative data collected in longitudinal and cohort studies, other domains are not as well operationalised in major surveys. Equally, numerous qualitative studies have focused on older adults' material or social well-being but have not connected these domains to other forms of exclusion such as socio-cultural or socio-spatial exclusion. There is also a further empirical challenge to be addressed in research on social exclusion in later life. Measures of exclusion need to assess exclusion across multiple areas of older people's lives, such as economic, social relations, services, civic, and community/spatial domains. It is common for empirical studies to measure only one or two of these domains sufficiently well, whilst ignoring others entirely or using single indicators that fail to capture the breadth of the domain in question. Where feasible, in order to assess the links between different forms of exclusion, empirical work should consider the ways in which different exclusion outcomes can combine to generate further disadvantage.

Turning to policy responses, integrating a multidimensional understanding of social exclusion in later life into policy making, at different levels of the political system, would represent a major achievement. This would imply moving away from a narrow focus on ageing in ageing policies (*e.g.* as a health and care concern) and from an equally narrow focus on specific domains of exclusion in poverty policies (*e.g.* economic exclusion). Most notably, there has been a longstanding policy concern with forms of economic disadvantage. Contributions to this book, especially those in section VIII, have demonstrated the need for a more active engagement by policy makers with the full range of issues relevant to social exclusion in later life. In the case of economic exclusion, connecting features of low incomes, limited assets and poor material conditions to other forms of exclusion, whilst also extending the focus to all life stages, has the potential to create coordinated policies that are better suited to the needs of a diverse older population. This aligns with the point made by Norah Keating and Maria Cheshire-Allen in Chap. 27 that there is a strong case to be made for using social exclusion as an integrative policy framework for understanding the interconnections between different policy challenges and the interdependency of a range of policy solutions.

In addition, including in policy making older adults who are themselves experiencing or are at risk of exclusion is key to addressing challenges of social exclusion in later life. Engaging disadvantaged people in policy making not only improves understanding of such individuals' experiences, but it can also strengthen their position and inclusion (Lister 2002, 2007) and, as a result, overcome power imbalances. Despite research that emphasises the impact of political decision making and programmes in the field of poverty and social exclusion (*e.g.* Phillipson and Scharf 2004), too often older adults on low incomes are ignored in poverty programmes (Rissanen and Ylinen 2014). In reforming welfare states, it is important to give voice to people who will be or are affected by these reforms (Henderson and Tickamyer 2008). As Lister (2007, 2008) argues, giving financially excluded older people a voice has the potential to reduce their risk of exclusion.

34.5.2 Responding to Accumulated Disadvantage and Risk Groups

Reflecting the need to adopt a life-course approach to understand the dynamic nature of social exclusion in later life, as suggested in many contributions to this book, implies a need for future research not only to focus on specific groups at risk of social exclusion but also to consider the ways in which individuals and groups are prone to experiencing the accumulation of disadvantage over time. Social exclusion is best understood as a process that evolves over the course of individuals' lives and the experiences of different birth cohorts. Longitudinal quantitative and qualitative research approaches hold out the promise that researchers can deepen our knowledge of the dynamic relationship between individual life experiences and group-level factors in generating exclusion in older-age. These approaches can assist in identifying critical points in people's lives where policy and practice responses might be most effective in reducing risks of exclusion later in life. They also engage with challenges arising from increasing digitalisation of societies and changing labour markets that can be associated with the increasingly precarious working lives of key social groups. Where possible, research should focus on the diversity of and intersectionality with old-age, assessing how such factors as age, gender, race and ethnicity, socio-economic status, sexual orientation, health status, geographic location and their combinations influence old-age social exclusion. This also implies ensuring that key subgroups of ageing adults are sufficiently well represented in empirical studies. Given the importance of spatial dimensions of exclusion in older age, future research will benefit from a stronger focus on the different meanings associated with ageing in place, and the barriers and enablers that apply to diverse groups of older people who live in different place contexts.

For policy, responding to the later life consequences arising from the accumulation of risks across the life course suggests a need to build on awareness of the impact of critical life events and precarious living and working lives on individuals' vulnerability to exclusion in later life to inform the timing and nature of policy and practice interventions. Such interventions should be attuned to the diversity of older populations, individuals' evolving needs, and the nature of the subgroups that they belong to. A strong case exists for targeting policy measures and practice interventions at groups recognised as being at greatest risk of accumulated social exclusion across the life course.

34.5.3 Responding to Multilevel Shocks

As suggested by the authors of numerous chapters in this book, older people can be susceptible to the multifaceted impacts of unanticipated events that alter the broad societal contexts that shape their lives and local environments. Before the COVID-19 pandemic, the most obvious example of such a multilevel shock was the period of austerity that affected a number of countries in the aftermath of the Global Financial Crisis of 2008 (Ginn 2013; Walsh et al. 2015; Phillipson 2020). Other shocks that demonstrated the interlinkage between macro-, meso- and micro-level consequences for risks of social exclusion in later life were associated with economic downturns, environmental disasters, climate-related events, and conflict situations. However, the experience of COVID-19 provides a textbook example of how an unanticipated crisis cuts across the dimensions of social exclusion to reduce older adults' well-being. While the impact varies across countries and between regions of different nations, the global pandemic has been associated with heightened risks of exclusion from social relations arising from enforced restrictions on older people's social connections (*e.g.* Berg-Weger and Morley 2020), the increasing potential of economic exclusion as a result of unemployment amongst older workers (*e.g.* Morrow-Howell et al. 2020), and well-publicised risks of civic and cultural forms of exclusion linked to overt expressions of ageism and age discrimination (*e.g.* Ayalon et al. 2020). In the absence of a critical gerontological lens that develops a critique of such forms of exclusion, there is a danger that already marginalised groups of older people are at risk of being left behind as policy makers focus on meeting the needs of younger age groups and people of working age.

34.6 Concluding Remarks

The ideas presented here, and those noted in the individual chapters within this book, are essential as part of a response to the multifaceted challenge of exclusion in later life, but not exhaustive. Demographic ageing is rightly regarded as one of the key achievements of the modern age. Improving understanding of the ways in which ageing interacts with other far-reaching social and economic trends to increase the risks of exclusion faced by older adults around the world continues to be a key task for research on ageing. This is a task that will benefit from the insights of researchers at all career stages. A notable feature of the ROSEnet COST Action was its focus on nurturing research capacity and cross-national collaboration in the field of social exclusion and ageing. This is reflected in the contributions of early-stage researchers to many chapters in this book. Continuing to invest in the development of meaningful partnerships between early-stage researchers and more senior scholars across nations is fundamental to the further development of research on social exclusion in older-age. Responding to the challenge of exclusion also requires concerted action by policymakers and practitioners in all world regions. Our hope is that the different contributions to this book can become part of a necessary response, assisting in developing understanding of multidimensional social exclusion in later life and helping to shape debates around appropriate interventions that might contribute to overcoming the types of disadvantage faced by many people in later life.

References

Ayalon, L., Chasteen, A., Diehl, M., Levy, B., Neupert, S. D., Rothermund, K., Tesch-Römer, C., & Wahl, H. W. (2020). Aging in times of the COVID-19 pandemic: Avoiding ageism and fostering intergenerational solidarity. *The Journals of Gerontology: Series B.*https://doi.org/10.1093/geronb/gbaa051.

Barnes, M., Blom, A. G., Cox, K., Lessof, C., & Walker, A. (2006). *The social exclusion of older people: Evidence from the first wave of the English longitudinal study of ageing (ELSA), final report*. London: Institute for Fiscal Studies.

Bayram, N., Bilgel, F., & Bilgel, N. G. (2010). Social exclusion and quality of life: An empirical study from Turkey. *Social Indicators Research, 105*(1), 109–120.

Berg-Weger, M., & Morley, J. E. (2020). Loneliness and social isolation in older adults during the Covid-19 pandemic: Implications for gerontological social work. *Journal of Nutrition Health and Aging, 24*(3), 456.

Burholt, V., Winter, B., Aartsen, M., Constantinou, C., Dahlberg, L., Villar, F., et al. (2019). A critical review and development of a conceptual model of exclusion from social relations for older people. *European Journal of Ageing*. https://doi.org/10.1007/s10433-019-00506-0.

Burns, V. F., Lavoie, J. P., & Rose, D. (2012). Revisiting the role of neighbourhood change in social exclusion and inclusion of older people. *Journal of Aging Research, 2012*. https://doi.org/10.1155/2012/148287.

Ginn, J. (2013). Austerity and inequality. Exploring the impact of cuts in the UK by gender and age. *Research on Ageing and Social Policy, 1*(1), 28–53.

Henderson, D. A., & Tickamyer, A. R. (2008). Lost in Appalachia: The unexpected impact of welfare reform on older women in rural communities. *Journal of Sociology & Social Welfare, 35*(3), 153–171.

Jehoel-Gijsbers, G., & Vrooman, C. (2008). *Social exclusion of the elderly: A comparative study of EU member states* (ENEPRI Research Report No. 57), Ceps. https://doi.org/10.2139/ssrn.2027886.

Kneale, D. (2012). *Is social exclusion still important for older people?* London: International Longevity Centre UK (ILC-UK).

Lister, R. (2002). A politics of recognition and respect: Involving people with experience of poverty in decision making that affects their lives. *Social Policy and Society, 1*(1), 37–46.

Lister, R. (2007). From object to subject: Including marginalised citizens in policy-making. *Policy & Politics, 35*, 3.

Lister, R. (2008). Inclusive citizenship, gender and poverty: Some implications for education for citizenship. *Citizenship Teaching and Learning, 4*(1), 3–19.

Moffatt, S., & Glasgow, N. (2009). How useful is the concept of social exclusion when applied to rural older people in the United Kingdom and the United States? *Regional Studies, 43*(10), 1291–1303.

Morrow-Howell, N., Galucia, N., & Swinford, E. (2020). Recovering from the COVID-19 pandemic: A focus on older adults. *Journal of Aging & Social Policy, 32*(4–5), 526–535.

Phillipson, C. (2020). Austerity and precarity: Individual and collective agency in later life. In A. Grenier, C. Phillipson, R. Settersten Jr (eds) *Precarity and ageing: Understanding insecurity and risk in later life*, (pp. 215–236). Bristol: Policy Press.

Phillipson, C., & Scharf, T. (2004). *The impact of government policy on social exclusion among older people*. London: Social Exclusion Unit, Office of the Deputy Prime Minister.

Rissanen, S., & Ylinen, S. (2014). Elderly poverty: Risks and experiences – A literature review. *Nordic Social Work Research, 4*(2), 144–157.

Scharf, T., Phillipson, C., Smith, A. E., & Kingston, P. (2002). *Growing older in socially deprived areas: Social exclusion in later life*. London: Help the Aged.

Scharf, T., Phillipson, C., & Smith, A. E. (2005). Social exclusion of older people in deprived urban communities of England. *European Journal of Ageing, 2*(2), 76–87.

Scharf, T., & Keating, N. (Eds.). (2012). *From exclusion to inclusion in old age: A global challenge*. Bristol: The Policy Press.

Tong, H. M., Lai, D. W. L., Zeng, Q., & Xu, W. Y. (2011). Effects of social exclusion on depressive symptoms: Elderly Chinese living alone in Shanghai, China. *Journal of Cross-Cultural Gerontology, 26*(4), 349–364.

Van Regenmortel, S., De Donder, L., Dury, S., Smetcoren, A. S., de Witte, N., & Verté, D. (2016). Social exclusion in later life: A systematic review of the literature. *Journal of Population Aging, 9*(4), 315–344.

Walsh, K., Carney, G., & Ní Léime, Á. (Eds.). (2015). *Ageing through austerity: Critical perspectives from Ireland*. Bristol: Policy Press.

Walsh, K., Scharf, T., & Keating, N. (2017). Social exclusion of older persons: A scoping review and conceptual framework. *European Journal of Ageing, 14*(1), 81–98.

Yur'yev, A., Leppik, L., Tooding, L. M., Sisask, M., Värnik, P., Wu, J., et al. (2010). Social inclusion affects elderly suicide mortality. *International Psychogeriatrics, 22*(8), 1337–1343.

The manufacturer's authorised representative in the EU is Springer Nature Customer Service Centre GmbH, Europaplatz 3, 69115 Heidelberg, Germany. If you have any concerns regarding our products, please contact ProductSafety@springernature.com

Printed and bound by CPI Group (UK) Ltd, Croydon, CR0 4YY
30/09/2026
02225690-0015